HEALTH INEQUALITIES IN EUROPEAN COUNTRIES

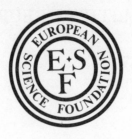

EUROPEAN SCIENCE FOUNDATION

The European Science Foundation is an association of its 49 member research councils and academies in 18 countries. The ESF brings European scientists together to work on topics of common concern, to co-ordinate the use of expensive facilities, and to discover and define new endeavours that will benefit from a co-operative approach.

The scientific work sponsored by ESF includes basic research in the natural sciences, the medical and biosciences, the humanities and the social sciences.

The ESF links scholarship and research supported by its members and adds value by co-operation across national frontiers. Through its function as a co-ordinator, and also by holding workshops and conferences and by enabling researchers to visit and study in laboratories throughout Europe, the ESF works for the advancement of European science.

Further information on ESF activities can be obtained from:

European Science Foundation
1 quai Lezay-Marnesia
67000 Strasbourg
France

Health Inequalities in European Countries

Edited by
JOHN FOX
Social Statistics Research Unit, City University

Gower

Aldershot, Brookfield USA, Hong Kong, Singapore, Sydney

Published by
Gower Publishing Company Limited
Gower House
Croft Road
Aldershot
Hants GU11 3HR

Gower Publishing Company
Old Post Road
Brookfield
Vermont 05036
USA

British Library Cataloguing in Publication Data
Health inequalities in European countries.
   1. Western Europe. Man. Health. Social
aspects
   I. Fox, John, *1935–*
362.1'042'094

Library of Congress Cataloging-in-Publication Data
Health inequalities in European countries / edited by John Fox.
   p. cm.
Bibliography: p.
Includes index.
   1. Health status indicators—Europe. 2. Mortality—Social
aspects—Europe. 3. Diseases—Social aspects—Europe. 4. Social
medicine—Europe. I. Fox, John, 1946, April 25–
RA407.5.E85H45 1988
362.1'094—dc19

88–11133
CIP

ISBN 0566 05497 3

Printed and bound in Great Britain at
The Camelot Press plc, Southampton

Contents

Figures

vii

Tables

Acknowledgements

The chapters presented here are revised papers presented at a series of three workshops held at City University in 1984, 1985 and 1986. These workshops were organised by Professor John Fox, Professor Raymond Illsley and Dr Julian Le Grand, under the auspices of The European Science Foundation and the Economic and Social Research Council.

Mrs Maureen Brierley was responsible for the arrangements for the three workshops and for organising the preparation of the material for publication with support from Miss Sharon Clarke. Illustrations were drawn by Mrs Anne Church.

Chapters 5, 7, 9 and 13 contain information from the Office of Population Censuses and Survey's Longitudinal Study which is subject to Crown Copyright.

I hope the scientific content of these chapters reflects the valuable exchange which took place at the workshops and encourages further attempts to undertake comparative research in this area.

My appreciation goes to those mentioned above, to the ESRC and ESF for their support and to participants for having made the task of coordinator a simpler one.

John Fox
January 1988

Contributors

Pierre Aiach is a Sociologist, working in the French 'Institut National de la Sante et de la Recherche Medicale'. His main interest in social inequalities is in symptomatology, in the context of general medicine and specific conditions such as mental disorders and cancer.

Aaron Antonovsky is Kunin-Lunenfeld Professor of Medical Sociology and Chair of the Department of the Sociology of Health, Faculty of Health Sciences, Ben-Gurion University of the Negev, Beersheba, Israel. His most recent book is *Unravelling the Mystery of Health*. He is engaged in research on the health consequences of retirement.

Sara Arber is Senior Lecturer in the Department of Sociology, University of Surrey. Her current research is on inequalities in health, stratification and early retirement, and the circumstances of the elderly disabled. She is co-author of *Doing Secondary Analysis* and *Exploring British Society*.

Mildred Blaxter is currently working on the National Health and Lifestyle Survey at the University of Cambridge Clinical School. Publications include *The Meaning of Disability; Mothers and Daughters; A Three-generational Study of Health Attitudes and Behaviour;* and *The Health of the Children*.

Roy Carr-Hill is Senior Research Fellow in Medical Statistics at the Centre for Health Economics, York. He has written widely in criminology and educational planning as well as in the epidemiology of birth outcomes and the more general area of inequalities in health.

Roderick Floud is Professor of Modern History at Birkbeck College, London. He is currently writing a book (with K. W. Wachter and A. Gregory) on *The Heights of the British 1700–1980* to be published by Cambridge University Press.

Ken Fogelman is a Deputy Director of the Social Statistics Research Unit at City University. Through his long association with the 1958 British Cohort (The National Child Development Study), he has wide research interests in education, health and social welfare. His publications include *Growing Up in Great Britain* and *Britain's Sixteen-Year-Olds*.

John Fox is Professor of Social Statistics and Director of Social Statistics Research Unit at City University. His main research has been on occupational and socio-economic differences in mortality. He was the author of the 1970–72 *Decennial Supplement on Occupational Mortality* and with Peter Goldblatt wrote *Socio-demographic Mortality Differentials*, the first report on the OPCS Longitudinal Study.

Nicky Hart is a Lecturer in Sociology at the University of Essex. She served as Research Fellow to the DHSS Working Group on Inequalities in Health 1978–80 (The 'Black' Report). Publications include *Sociology of Health and Medicine.*

Jeddi Hasan is Professor of Occupational Health at the University of Tampere in Finland. He has for several years conducted research on the determinants of health of occupational classes in an industrial population.

Lars-Gunnar Horte is Chief of Section at Statistics Sweden. He is currently working with the Swedish occupation-death registers.

Peter Jozan is Chief of Population Statistics Section at the Central Statistics Office in Budapest, Hungary. His current research is on the epidemiology of the transition of mortality differentials in Eastern Europe, especially in Hungary.

Annette Leclerc is a researcher at INSERM (National Institute for Health and Medical Research), Paris; she is an epidemiologist, specializing in the study of occupational and social risk factors.

David Leon is a Lecturer in the Department of Epidemiology at the London School of Hygiene and Tropical Medicine. He is author of *The Social Distribution of Cancer* and has conducted research on occupational cancer.

Julian LeGrand is Professor of Public Policy at Bristol University. He co-directs the Welfare State Programme at the London School of Economics with Professor A. B. Atkinson. His publications include *The Economics of Social Problems* (with R. Robinson), *The Strategy of Equality* and *Not Only the Poor: the Middle Classes and the Welfare State.*

Elsebeth Lynge is head of research section at the Danish Cancer Registry. She was the author of the first Danish study on occupational mortality to use a record linkage approach and of a Council of Europe review of socio-economic differences in mortality.

Sally Macintyre is Director of the MRC Medical Sociology Unit, Glasgow. Her main research interest is in the social patterning of health, and she is currently working on a prospective study of everyday life and health among young people.

Oriol Ramis-Juan is a community doctor working at the Planning

Office of the Department of Health and Social Security of the Government of Catalonia (Spain). His research has been on health inequalities in south Europe.

Julia Szalai is a senior researcher at the Institute of Sociology of the Hungarian Academy of Sciences. Her main interest is in social policy and social problems for the health care system under state socialism. She lectures on the social history of social policy at the University of Budapest.

Alex Scott-Samuel is a Specialist in Community Medicine with Liverpool Health Authority and Honorary Lecturer in Community Health, University of Liverpool. He was founding editor of Radical Community Medicine, 1979–85, and is convenor of the Unemployment and Health Study Group. He writes and researches in materialist epidemiology and health policy.

Johannes Siegrist is Professor of Medical Sociology at the Medical School, University of Marburg, West Germany. He and his group are involved in extensive studies on the role of social factors in the development of cardiovascular disease.

Katherina Sokou is Senior Health Research Scientist at the Institute of Child Health, Athens, Greece. She has conducted research in social inequalities with special emphasis on the child, focusing on sociological aspects of infant mortality and morbidity, school achievement, health services and health policy. At present she is engaged in research on youth unemployment and the effects of unemployment on the family unit.

Tapani Valkonen is Professor of Sociology and Demography at the University of Helsinki. His current research is on the development of socio-demographic mortality differentials in Finland.

Richard Wilkinson is a Research Fellow at the Centre for Medical Research, University of Sussex, where he is working on the relationship between income and mortality. He edited *Class and Health: Research and Longitudinal Data*.

PART I
BACKGROUND

1 Introduction
John Fox and Roy Carr-Hill

> To crystallise tendencies into epigrams is always to overstate the antithesis, but we shall perhaps help the reader to grasp the distinction if we say our grandfathers believed that in the case of consumption what was the matter with the poor was poverty and that consumption would not be eliminated without the eradication of poverty; since they did not believe that poverty could be eradicated they did not expect to 'stamp out' consumption. The latter day view is less pessimistic (or, if we look at it from another point of view, more pessimistic) and suggests that consumption might be eliminated without any obliteration of the distinction between class and class (Collis and Greenwood, 1921).

Inequalities in health – and commentary about them – have obviously been around for a long time. But Collis and Greenwood were writing at the time of the First World War. Surely, given the massive changes in living standards since then, not only consumption but many other infectious diseases have been eliminated, so even if our societies remain class-bound in other respects (education, housing, income and wealth) at the very least gross inequalities in risk of serious disease or death between social groups would have been eradicated. So why this book?

The principal reason is simple: these inequalities have not been eliminated.

This is particularly poignant when we recall that Collis and Greenwood were commenting before the misery of the 1930s and of the Second World War had encouraged the creation of welfare states. The institutional form varied between countries but the overall aim was similar: to guarantee all citizens minimum standards in terms of health as well as education and housing. Just as nearly all of our populations now go to school for a minimum number of years and most have a roof over their heads with basic amenities, one would expect a basic minimum life expectancy to be available to all. What happened?

First, it is clear that average income has risen substantially. In the period following the Second World War, up until the end of the 1970s, most countries experienced very high rates of economic growth. Table 1.1 presents data showing the growth in the Gross Domestic Product (GDP) at constant prices between 1960 and 1983. Clearly, the growth has been very large. Moreover, despite starting

Table 1.1   Gross Domestic Product (in millions of national currency units) in selected European countries, 1960–83

Country	1960	1965	1970	1975	1980	1983
Austria	162,870	246,320	375,880	656,130	994,700	1,206,000
Belgium	557,018	829,955	1,262,110	2,271,144	3,419,567	4,095,006
Denmark	41,149	70,320	118,627	216,257	373,786	515,399
Finland	16,199	26,634	45,743	104,291	192,556	275,084
France	296,506	483,488	782,560	1,452,319	2,769,317	3,957,043
Germany	302,710	459,170	675,300	1,026,510	1,481,360	1,667,480
Greece	105,167	179,765	298,917	672,158	1,710,934	3,040,730
Iceland	85	214	437	1,977	13,841	56,070
Ireland	631	959	1,620	3,789	9,178	14,452
Italy (billions)	23,207	39,124	62,883	125,378	338,740	535,900
Luxembourg	26,029	35,142	54,043	86,631	135,200	163,200
The Netherlands	44,003	71,308	120,499	220,252	336,740	376,720
Norway	33,058	50,563	79,877	148,701	285,046	401,769
Portugal	71,441	107,484	177,792	377,203	1,231,501	2,289,000
Spain	685,500	1,398,900	2,576,200	6,019,300	15,185,100	22,682,900
Sweden	72,160	112,112	172,226	300,785	525,099	704,474
Switzerland	37,370	60,860	90,665	140,155	170,330	203,860
Turkey	46,977	76,440	145,491	519,300	4,332,400	11,210,000
United Kingdom	25,733	35,801	51,313	105,960	229,560	300,228
Czechoslovakia			311,100	404,000	482,500	
Poland			749,200	1,349,700	1,986,600	

Source: OECD, 1986, Table H3, p. 156.

from very low levels, the rates of growth have been quite similar. Thus Gillon and Hemmings (1985) present comparative data for OECD countries to show that in 1963–67 the average rate of growth in these countries was about 5 per cent with even the low-growth nations – Britain, Ireland, Germany and Finland – experiencing, in that period, growth rates that are enviable from the vantage point of the 1980s. In more recent years, nearly every nation – except Ireland and Finland – have experienced sharp reductions in economic growth, with the overall average down to around 2 per cent. But, with occasional and rare exceptions, GDP per capita has continued to grow albeit slowly.

Whilst it was realised that 'economic growth is not an end in itself, but rather an instrument for creating better conditions of life' (Interministerial Declaration at OECD Conference, 1970), it was assumed that living conditions had improved. Indeed, in the middle of the post-war period, rises in GDP per capita were associated with

Table 1.2 *Infant and perinatal mortality in selected European countries, 1950–83*

	Infant mortality (% of live births)					Perinatal mortality (% of live and stillbirths)				
	1950	1960	1970	1980	1983	1950	1960	1970	1980	1983
Austria	5.56	2.64	2.37	1.43	1.19	4.80	3.50	2.70	1.42	1.13
Belgium	5.40	3.12	2.11	1.10	1.12	—	3.20	2.30	1.40	—
Denmark	3.10	2.15	1.42	0.84	0.77	3.40	2.60	1.80	0.90	0.90
Finland	4.35	2.10	1.32	0.76	0.62	3.45	2.75	1.70	0.84	0.74
France	5.19	2.74	1.82	1.01	0.89	3.60	3.10	2.30	1.29	—
Federal Republic of Germany	5.53	3.38	2.34	1.27	1.03	4.99	3.58	2.64	1.16	—
Greece	4.09	4.01	2.96	1.79	1.46	3.10	3.05	2.79	2.12	—
Iceland	2.17	1.30	1.33	0.77	0.61	2.60	2.00	1.90	0.90	0.73
Ireland	4.60	2.93	1.95	1.11	0.98	—	3.80	2.40	1.50	—
Italy	6.38	4.39	2.96	1.43	1.24	5.10	4.20	3.10	1.75	1.52
Luxembourg	—	3.15	2.49	1.15	1.12	—	3.23	2.47	0.98	—
Netherlands	2.67	1.79	1.27	0.86	0.84	3.40	2.70	1.86	1.10	0.98
Norway	2.42	1.89	1.10	0.81	0.79	2.80	2.40	1.90	1.11	0.96
Portugal	9.40	7.75	5.51	2.60	1.90	4.80	4.11	3.70	2.55	—
Spain	—	4.37	2.81	1.11	—	—	—	—	1.57	—
Sweden	2.00	1.29	0.96	0.69	0.70	3.40	2.70	1.60	0.90	0.73
Switzerland	2.95	2.11	1.28	0.86	0.80	—	—	1.81	0.95	0.91
Turkey	—	—	12.30	11.00	—	—	—	—	—	—
United Kingdom	3.12	2.25	1.85	1.21	1.02	3.90	3.40	2.40	1.34	1.05
Czechoslovakia	—	—	—	(1.77 (1979))	1.57	—	—	—	—	—
German Democratic Republic	—	—	—	1.21	1.07	—	—	—	1.36	—
Poland	—	—	—	2.13	1.92	—	—	—	(1.72 1979))	—
Russia (1974, Infant Mortality 2.77)	—	—	—	—	—	—	—	—	—	—

Source: OECD, 1986, Table F2, p. 131.

progressive improvements in a whole range of living conditions, and specifically in gains in the expectation of life as mortality levels fell at all ages. However, in the late 1960s, health indicators started to suggest that expectations built upon a continuing fall in death rates may be over-optimistic. Tables 1.2 and 1.3 provide a crude overall picture for European countries. Infant mortality and perinatal mortality have declined throughout, but the rate of decline between 1960 and 1970 was less than that between 1950 and 1960, and there were only marginal improvements in life expectancies at age 40 between 1960 and 1970. The trend in the 1970s is more differentiated: infant

Table 1.3   Life expectancy at age 40 in selected European countries, 1950–80

	Females				Males			
	1950	1960	1970	1980	1950	1960	1970	1980
Austria	34.5	36.2	36.5	38.3	30.9	31.2	31.1	32.5
Belgium	34.8	36.1	36.9	37.5	31.1	31.4	31.7	32.0
Denmark	35.3	36.7	38.2	39.2	34.1	34.2	34.0	33.9
Finland	34.0	35.3	36.5	39.0	28.9	29.8	29.8	31.8
France	35.4	37.2	39.1	40.2	30.8	31.7	32.7	33.2
Germany	34.6	35.8	36.6	38.6	32.3	31.8	31.7	32.9
Greece	37.5	38.3	39.3	40.1	35.0	35.7	35.9	36.4
Iceland	37.4	37.8	39.1	41.6	34.2	36.0	34.5	36.5
Ireland	33.5	35.4	35.8	36.2	31.6	32.8	31.8	32.0
Italy	35.8	36.7	37.9	39.5	33.1	32.8	32.9	33.7
Luxembourg	33.4	35.8	36.4	37.1	30.3	31.7	30.8	31.3
Netherlands	36.2	37.8	38.7	40.7	34.9	34.8	33.7	34.7
Norway	37.1	38.3	39.3	40.4	35.1	35.1	34.1	34.7
Portugal	34.9	36.2	36.6	38.0	30.7	31.9	32.0	32.0
Spain	33.9	36.6	38.2	39.6	30.4	33.1	33.9	34.5
Sweden	35.6	37.3	39.3	40.4	34.1	34.6	35.1	34.9
Switzerland	35.5	36.9	38.4	40.7	32.3	32.9	33.6	35.1
Turkey	—	—	—	—	—	—	—	—
United Kingdom	35.4	36.9	37.5	38.2	31.3	31.9	31.8	32.7

Source: OECD, 1986, Table F1, p. 130.

and perinatal mortality fell at almost the same ratio as in the 1950s but not much thereafter, whilst life expectancy at age 40 showed improvements for women but not for men. In most developed countries therefore it looks as if the 'diseases of affluence' were starting to take their toll at older ages, even if improvements could still be expected in childhood. The argument was that improvements in basic diet, antibiotics and new medicines and higher standards of health care were being offset by vehicle accidents, tobacco and alcohol consumption and a diet too rich in animal fats.

Those kinds of figures and arguments have been tossed back and forth in many a conference and publication. But, regardless of the extent to which lifestyle and/or medical innovation affect the overall levels of health, the changes in living standards have been so great and medical standards have improved so much that one might expect that inequalities in serious illness or death would have disappeared, simply because many of the diseases that affected the poor have disappeared. The purpose of this book is to explore that simple proposition: what is the current situation in Europe in terms of inequalities in mortality? inequalities in morbidity? and how should they be explained?

Table 1.4   *Estimates of poverty in selected European countries in the early 1970s (per cent of population below relative poverty line)*

	National Definition	Standardized Definitions[a] ILO	Standardized Definitions[a] OECD
France	15–20	—	16
Germany	—	—	3
United Kingdom	13	10[b]	7½
Belgium	14	6	—
Ireland	24	—	—
Norway	—	7½	5
Sweden	—	—	3½

Notes:
[a]For definitions, see original sources.
[b]Great Britain. Sources: W. Beckerman, *Poverty and the Impact of Income Maintenance Programmes in Four Developed Countries*, ILO, Geneva 1979; OECD, Public Expenditure on Income Maintenance Programmes Paris 1976.

Source: Sawyer, 1982, Table 7.11, p. 210.

Of course, the question of inequality, or of whether some people are 'left behind' in welfare status, is not limited to health issues alone. In the aftermath of the Second World War, one of the major expressed objectives in overhauling health and welfare institutions was to create fairer societies. For some time, it was widely assumed that the problems of poverty had been overcome and that the 'pockets' that remained would soon be eradicated. However, the 1970s saw a revival of the 'poverty lobby' for a number of reasons: the growth in the elderly, often living on low incomes, as a fraction of developed countries' populations; increasing numbers of unemployed on low levels of benefit as a result of the recession; and the financial consequences of the increasing rates of marital break-up and single parenthood.

It is, however, almost impossible to provide coherent comparative data about levels of poverty, and this is not the place to rehearse arguments about absolute and relative definitions of poverty (see Townsend, 1979). It is complicated enough to resolve that issue in one country, let alone compare across countries. Nevertheless, the few data available for the early 1970s (see Table 1.4) suggest that, even at the end of the long boom, there were 'pockets of poverty' – in some cases quite large – in every country.

The impact and meaning of the numbers or proportions in 'poverty', however defined, is not the same as the impact and meaning

Table 1.5   Shares of post-tax income between bottom and top deciles in selected European countries around 1970

	Year	Bottom 10%	Bottom 20%	Top 20%	Top 10%
Finland	1971	2.5	6.6	38.5	23.5
France	1970	1.4	4.3	46.9	30.4
Germany	1973	2.8	6.5	49.1	30.3
Italy	1967	2.3	6.2	43.9	28.1
Netherlands	1967	2.6	6.5	42.3	27.1
Norway	1970	2.3	6.3	37.3	22.2
Spain	1973–4	2.1	6.0	42.3	26.7
Sweden	1976	2.2	6.6	37.0	21.3
United Kingdom	1973	3.2	6.6	39.1	23.6
Average		2.4	6.3	41.5	25.9

Source: Sawyer, 1982, Table 7.10, p. 207 and Table 7.12, p. 211.

of inequalities in material standards. Table 1.5 presents comparative data on the distribution of post-tax income around 1970 for nine countries. It is clear that, along with poverty, there was extensive inequality in all countries, with the top decile receiving between nine and 22 times as much as the bottom decile and more than 40 per cent of income in every case accrues to 20 per cent of the households.

Of course, most of the data antedates the present recession. Table 1.6 presents data for the few countries where over time data are available since 1970. Whilst Italy and Sweden became progressively more equal during this period and Finland registered little change, a widening gap between the top and bottom deciles is evident for Austria and the UK.

The apparently conflicting picture of ever greater increases in average wealth coupled with sharp rises in the numbers of poor in some countries highlights the inadequacy of statistics which focus only on one aspect of the wealth or health distribution in countries. The average as depicted by the GNP or by life expectancy may conceal quite different patterns of change experienced by different sections of the community and, whilst income distribution data was presented only for a few countries in Tables 1.5 and 1.6, the pattern of inequality can clearly be very different between countries. This volume focuses on the statistics of inequalities in health – on the differences in health status between sections of the community within countries. Our interest is in whether changes implemented after the Second World War have indeed led to fairer societies in terms of

Table 1.6 Recent changes in distributions of income in selected European countries

Austria – Growth of earnings by decile

	1974–78 (1974=100)	1978–82 (1978=100)
Top Decile	138.9	134.6
Bottom Decile	139.8	129.9

Finland – Share of disposable income: household

	1977	1980
Top Decile	21.2	21.4
Bottom Decile	2.5	2.5

Italy – Distribution of post-tax income

	1972	1977
Top Decile	30.2	28.1
Bottom Decile	1.8	2.3

Sweden – Growth of real income: all households

	1975–80
Top Decile	−0.5%
Bottom Decile	+15.5%

United Kingdom – Shares in total income (after tax)

	1975–76	1978–9	1981–2
Top 10%	23.1	23.4	25.6
Bottom 10%	3.0	2.9	2.4

Source: Sawyer, 1982, Table 7.14, p. 214 for Italy, and
    Sawyer, 1985, Tables 1, 3, 5 and 6 in Appendix 1 for all other countries.

health as was their explicit objective, and in which countries has most progress been made.

In 1979 the United Nations and the World Health Organisation co-sponsored a meeting in Mexico City on the socio-economic determinants and consequences of differential mortality. A number of points became apparent. Participants were concerned with differences in mortality between different sub-groups of their populations, defined in terms of their socio-economic background and circumstances. The evidence presented, which included reviews of a substantial body of literature, pointed to differences in almost all countries studied (UN/WHO, 1981). These differences were based on comparisons of disparate groups such as educational groups, income groups, housing groups or occupational groups such as social classes. Nonetheless, in each case 'better-off' sections of the community had longer life expectancies than 'less well-off', sections. Clear differences were noted for infant mortality, child mortality, and mortality during early adulthood, middle and older ages.

The diverse nature of the evidence allowed one to draw the above conclusions but offered little in the way of a common basis for comparisons between countries. As a result several important questions were left unanswered. In particular, differences in life expectancy between different countries could not be related to the state of economic development or to their health and welfare systems. Were differences in life expectancy between socio-economic groups in, for example, Scandinavia, where life expectancy is greatest, smaller than those in Latin America or Africa, where life expectancy is particularly low? How did countries like the United Kingdom and the United States of America, with their different systems in provisions of health and welfare, compare in terms of differences in life expectancy between the poorest and richest deciles of their populations? The questions raised by this meeting have received wide attention in national and international meetings around that time and since. For example, in the United Kingdom a government Working Group considered the evidence but its findings (Black, 1980), coming at a time when a new administration was intent on increasing economic incentives, fell on deaf ears. Nevertheless as momentum has built up behind the World Health Organisation's programme 'Health for all by the year 2000', so more countries are developing statistical systems which allow progress towards a target of reducing inequalities by at least 25 per cent to be evaluated. One might therefore expect that the data available by the mid-1980s would provide a firmer basis for contrasting inequalities in health in different countries.

European Science Foundation workshops

With encouragement from the World Health Organisation and the United Nations a number of groups from different countries have been meeting regularly since 1979 to try to address these comparative issues (CICRED, 1981, 1982, 1984 and 1986). The first step was a major exchange in expertise between countries, allowing statistical sources and methods of measurement to be tested in different national contexts. By 1982, when the European Science Foundation organised a meeting in London to consider suggestions for topics to be covered by its future programme, a number of people felt that a series of workshops on 'inequalities in health in European countries' could benefit from and add to these recent advances. A draft programme for three workshops was then considered by the European Science Foundation Council and endorsed by national social science research councils who agreed to fund participants from their own countries. Three workshops were planned in order to maximise the collaboration between people from different countries and to emphasise the comparative dimension.

These workshops brought together 35 researchers from 13 European countries on 5–7 September 1984, 4–6 September 1985 and 25–27 June 1986. Experts were drawn from medical sociology, health economics, demography, economic history, social statistics, epidemiology, child health and community health. The first workshop was devoted to researchers introducing themselves and their research interests to each other and to planning their contributions to the next two workshops. We wished to create a climate in which people from different countries did not talk at each other from a national standpoint, as frequently occurs when people from different countries and different disciplines are brought together in international meetings, but one which would enable participants at the series of meetings to consider together the product they were aiming at. We felt this was essential if researchers were to identify a common basis for exchange. The theme was pursued both in the preparation of papers for meetings and in discussions at the meetings.

The second and third workshops heard a series of papers under three main headings:

1. between-country comparisons of mortality differentials;
2. between-country comparisons of differences in health, illness and health care, and
3. explanations of differentials.

In an ideal world, in which historic data were available for each country of interest, we would also have wished to ask 'how do inequalities in health vary between countries?' and 'how have these patterns changed over time?'

Even though suitable statistical sources have been made available in most of the European countries this is only a recent development. It means that we were left to construct many a picture with only a small fraction of the pieces of the puzzle. We were able to describe the patterns for only those countries represented at the workshop and those for which data were readily available. Nevertheless the picture presented here should encourage and provoke policymakers, researchers and health professionals both in these countries and in those not represented to put some effort into seeing how the picture unfolds as more pieces of the puzzle become available in the future.

This book presents papers originally prepared for the second or third workshops and revised in the light of discussions. Five themes cut across the discussions at the workshops: these were

1. the value and contribution of comparative research;
2. the care needed in choosing measures and methods of comparison;

3. the persistence across time and similarity between countries of the inequalities themselves;
4. the continuing debates over aetiology; and
5. the poverty of policies.

Purpose and value of comparative research

It is always difficult to study phenomena such as inequalities in health which involve complex data on all persons in a society. The use of comparative techniques to help interpret complex social issues has a long history. Durkheim, in his celebrated study of suicide, employed the techniques of cross-cultural and international comparisons; and both Marx and Weber, in their analyses of the rise of capitalism, made frequent use of international comparisons and cultural paradigms. Whilst the topic of inequalities in health may not have as broad a sweep as these, some of the problems of explanation recur.

First, some factors or features believed to be associated with inequalities in health are stable or very nearly stable within one country over time. This may be because changes in those features are slow and unremarkable, making the differences and similarities difficult to identify and isolate in one country. It is, for example, almost impossible to study the impact of the health care system as a whole on reducing or sustaining inequalities in isolation from the wider economic trends in the country. Within the confines of this series of workshops it was not possible to attempt a thorough comparative systems study of this type. Moreover, the paper by Macintyre (Chapter 15) shows how little comparative data is available on health care systems. However, the country sketches presented in the annex to Chapter 2 tend to support the conclusion of other authors (Maxwell, 1981; OECD, 1986; and WHO, 1986) that wide variations in the mode of provision of health care are associated with very similar patterns of mortality.

Secondly, the importance of differences and similarities can only be properly evaluated with reference to an international comparison such as is presented here. Several papers in this volume illustrate this rather well. Lynge *et al.* (Chaper 8) show how the overall similarities between the Nordic countries in fact conceal quite wide differences among them in terms of patterns of mortality. At the other end of the continent, Ramis-Juan and Sokou (Chapter 14) show how apparently large overall differences conceal basic similarities between Greece, Portugal and Spain. Finally, Valkonen (Chapter 7) shows how 'years of education', a variable which has been under-used in Europe, in fact betrays an astonishing constancy of effect across several countries.

Third, the assessment of the comparative weight of different factors in accounting for a given configuration may, in fact, depend upon a feature specific to that country which cannot be understood from studies of that country alone. Several of the papers illustrate this theme. Aiach and Carr-Hill (Chapter 2) compare the debates on inequalities in health among countries and find that the existence and nature of any debate, and therefore the kinds of explanations advanced, often depend on a specific configuration of history, ideology and policies in each country. Leclerc (Chapter 5) shows how variations in the cause of death patterns of mortality among groups in a country are more a reflection of mortality patterns specific to that country than of social variations *per se*.

Measurement and methodology

It is sufficient to say that this workshop, at least in part, follows on from an earlier series on health indicators in appreciating the importance of measurement issues. This series was also financed by the European Science Foundation (Culyer, 1983). Partly because of this, there was less emphasis in these workshops on the problem of measuring health than might have been expected. For example, those participants who concentrated on variations in mortality quickly agreed on a common set of age groups for comparison.

There was, however, some discussion of the measurement of morbidity. Antonovsky (Chapter 19) provided a salutory reminder that the issue for the workshop was inequalities in health not inequalities in illness; and Floud (Chapter 11) argued strongly for the use of height as a measure of health status. Blaxter (Chapter 10) also discussed measures of health as well as illness in a thorough overview of which measures of morbidity are used and how comparative they are.

Much more attention was devoted to the choice of criteria for measuring inequality and of methodologies appropriate to the investigation of inequality. One debate concerned the need to identify the dimension, or structure, of inequality. Le Grand (Chapter 4), for example, considers the variation about the average age of death (using a modified Gini coefficient) to describe the differences in life chances between individuals in a country. This summarisation of the traditional survival curve has its parallel in statistics describing national income distributions, but does not point to the structure of the variation observed.

Other participants argued that, while socio-economic and income inequalities were indistinguishable, health and socio-economic inequalities were interrelated in a variety of different ways, and that it was essential that various dimensions be separated for policy purposes. Farr, in his early analyses of mortality patterns in England

(1864), had compared the life expectancy in different parts of the country with that in 'healthy districts' in an attempt to gauge the improvements in health which might be gained by 'environmental' changes. In the present context, participants were interested in disaggregations of the population in terms of occupational and socio-economic group; geographic groups such as regions, counties and urban or rural aggregates; or groups defined in terms of their migration histories, their ethnic origins, their family or household circumstances, their educational background, their housing, their income or their employment (between those with jobs and those without).

Although these various dimensions were discussed, it must be appreciated that data are rarely available for all of these in any one country, let alone for a group of countries or over an extended period. This volume therefore contains but a few examples – remembering that participants at these workshops had access to their own national data and a determined effort was made to exchange data thereby allowing participants to focus on one particular dimension of inequality.

None of the papers considers the fate of immigrants in different European countries, nor of internal migrants. We also do not use marital status, housing or income to define socio-economic groups. With the exception of income for which there is relatively little data linking individuals' incomes to health or mortality, these exclusions principally reflect the interests of participants. The potential for building on this foundation should not however be overlooked.

One further division is being recognised to have socio–economic implications, that is the comparison between men and women. Hart (Chapter 6) was able to compare most countries over a long period of time.

Finally, there was some purely technical debate about research design. There appears to be a growing consensus, particularly among demographers, statisticians and epidemiologists responsible for the production of national mortality statistics, that the most reliable results on socio-economic differences are to be derived from longitudinal rather than cross-sectional studies. New sources of this type are being developed in Scandinavia, France, England and Wales, Austria, Hungary and the USA and these will substantially increase the scope of national mortality statistics.

Inequalities in death and illness

Several of the papers document inequalities in death. The various participants were asked to write about inequalities among groups defined by socio-economic characteristics considered in the previous section. Leclerc compared the pattern of mortality by cause of death (Chapter 5), Hart compared sex differences (Chapter 6), Valkonen differences by level of education (Chapter 7), Lynge *et al.* occupational differences (Chapter 8), and Jozan geographic differences (Chapter 9).

The methodological advantages of making intercountry comparisons have already been commented upon; but each of the papers also makes a substantive contribution to the received wisdom about inequalities. In some cases, the findings depend upon the methodological advantages of making the particular comparisons. Thus Leclerc concludes that 'excess mortality' in any country from a specific cause is specific to that country rather than a consequence of (social) class membership; in a more (relatively) homogeneous group of countries, Lynge *et al.* are able to conclude that the occupational differences indicate effects over and above those of social structure; and Valkonen can turn an apparently weak argument about a relationship between the level of education and mortality into a strong thesis because he obtains consistent results across a number of countries.

In other cases, whilst the descriptive findings might be obvious, the intercountry comparison adds another dimension to the interpretation. This can be seen in comparisons of mortality differences between men and women, between urban and rural areas and between those in employment and those without jobs.

The evolution of wide differences in mortality between the sexes, common to most European countries this century, tells us something about the inherent differences between men and women. The recent trends in some countries for men to start to catch up with women in terms of life expectancy reflect the extent to which women following men into the labour market adopt male harmful behaviours such as cigarette smoking. Similarly we find that comparisons of urban and rural areas depend upon the general direction of migration at the time. For those countries where there is a development of new urban industrial areas, movement to these areas might be associated with good health, and the mortality of the rural areas might reflect the relative depression which affects agricultural communities at the time. Equally, when the general tendency is for people to move away from historically important inner cities to suburbs and rural commuting areas, the reverse picture might be expected. International studies of unemployment and mortality help us understand the influences of socio–economic circumstances and health selection on the adverse effects of unemployment on people's health and help us anticipate the effects of the higher levels of unemployment observed throughout Europe in the early 1980s.

The analysis of inequalities in morbidity presented here is more wide ranging, and did not focus on distinct breakdowns in the same way. It was, perhaps inevitably, also more tentative. Thus Blaxter's (Chapter 10) first conclusion is 'that there is little possibility of comparing morbidity data across Europe in detail'. Yet she does feel able to make some very important generalisations: economically poor groups and populations in poorer regions suffer worse health as well as die younger, and this is especially true for chronic rather than acute illnesses.

These 'broad-brush' conclusions are amplified in two other chapters in Part III. First, Arber (Chapter 12) digs deeper into the class-gender interaction. She shows how the typical analysis of (social) class inequalities in health confronts major problems when considering women; and using a 'dominance' measure of household status, she shows how the gradients are as large for women as for men and that women suffer from their low economic activity status in British society. Ramis-Juan and Sokou (Chapter 14) advance an altogether much wider hypothesis about the relation between poverty and inequalities in health. They compare levels of death and health across countries and over time, concluding that as Mediterranean countries 'develop' economically, the gap between rich and poor in those countries is likely to widen.

A rather different perspective on relative health is presented by Leon and Wilkinson (Chapter 13) who demonstrate that lower status groups may not only have a higher risk of contracting certain diseases but also worse prognoses. It should be recognised that this may be of major importance for conditions such as breast cancer with potentially good survival but not for fatal conditions like lung cancer.

Explanations
Nearly every paper presented to the workshop addressed the problem of explanation in one form or another; any other situation would have been surprising. For example, the chapters in Part II on differences in mortality which have displayed inequalities according to different characteristics also provide interpretations of the observed differences. In every case, whilst none of the authors is claiming that the characteristic on which they have concentrated provides the explanation for inequalities, they would each argue that the process by which these inequalities are generated and maintained can be better understood by an examination of that particular empirical breakdown. Again, although they focus on very different issues, the papers by Arber, Leon and Wilkinson and Ramis-Juan and Sokou each confront the problem of explanation.

In general, they have argued that an understanding of the impact of structural/materialist features is essential. Thus Leclerc (Chapter 5) and Hart (Chapter 6) suggest that there are some features specific to each country which lead to the observed differentials (whether by cause or by gender); educational attainment, employment status, occupation and area of residence are shown to be powerful discriminators even if the interpretation of these differences is by no means clear. That message is reinforced by the papers on inequalities in morbidity. Thus Floud (Chapter 12) argues that height inequalities have been maintained over 150 years or more and Ramis-Juan and Sokou refer to national economic development as major determinants of their population's health. On a more detailed level, Arber concentrates on the joint effect of class and gender (Chapter 12) upon self-reported morbidity and Leon and Wilkinson (Chapter 13) on the pervasive effects of class at all stages in the development of illness.

It is important to remember this context in considering the papers in Section 4, which have addressed the problems of explanations on a more micro level. Thus, whilst Antonovsky (Chapter 19), Hasan (Chapter 18) and Siegrist (Chapter 17) all focus on the psychosocial level of explanation (whether in terms of coherence or stress), each would insist that these processes can only be understood against a powerful backdrop of structural social determinants. Equally a similar conclusion would be drawn from Fogelman *et al.* (Chapter 16), who considered evidence for the selection hypothesis, the oft-favoured explanation in some circles in Britain.

Policy implications

It is only fair to ask – so what? Which kinds of policy reforms, costing how much, and implemented by whom will work the miracle of decreasing inequalities in health? What are the obstacles to such reforms? And who cares?

Because the largest number of participants came from Britain there was a tendency for the discussion to be driven by the British debate. However, it was appreciated that each country not only has its own problems, but also its own health policy. It was wrong to think that any one priority could be established across all countries. In the Nordic countries, for example, it was thought that current concerns of health policy revolved around a rapidly ageing population. This possibly reflects a belief which has existed until very recently that post-war policies had dramatically reduced inequalities so that the problem no longer existed. In contrast, a country such as Spain needed to be most concerned about inequalities in service provision at this stage in its development.

Despite these complexities of pronouncing upon comparative

public policy, the group saw it as important to draw out some tentative implications of their findings. Three approaches were tried. Two surveys, one by Aiach and Carr-Hill (Chapter 2) before the second workshop and one by Scott-Samuel and Szalai (Chapter 3) before the third workshop, solicited views both of participants and others who might shed insights. Neither survey was designed to provide a representative sample but both were intended to identify the main parameters influencing the policy debate in European countries.

The third approach was to use one of the participants, in this case Alan Williams, as a 'sympathetic but sceptical' politician seeking evidence:

(a)   that there is a significant problem;

(b)   that it would not prove self-corrective or self-limiting if ignored;

(c)   that the underlying causal mechanisms were clearly enough established, so that one could be confident that the recommended action would have the desired effect (without undue side-effects);

(d)   that recommended policy actions would have a clear favourable effect within two or three years (or perhaps if dramatic effects cannot be expected, that clear trends in the right direction could be established);

(e)   that recommended policies would not mean unacceptable sacrifices of other policy objectives, such as raising the general living standards or improving the general level of health.

We must emphasise that the group recognised its limited qualifications for discussing policy issues. The way the group was selected meant that it was equipped to document the nature and extent of inequalities in health in each of the countries and to talk about explanations. To discuss policy authoritatively we would have needed to invite a number of policy experts from each of the countries represented and this would have meant quite a different kind of meeting. We all felt, nevertheless, that it should be appreciated that we were dealing with a topic which had policy relevence and implications. We hoped that this volume might persuade countries throughout Europe to continue to fill the gap in their statistics on this important issue and to develop the policy debate we have started here. As indicated by Aiach and Carr-Hill (Chapter 2), the existence and nature of a debate is affected 'more by political and socio-cultural considerations than by the "objective" state of inequality, or even whether or not adequate statistical data exist'. It matters whether or not some powerful group is prepared to fight for placing the issue of health inequality on the national agenda.

Assuming there is a concerned caucus, what can the concerned politician do or endorse? Macintyre's paper (Chapter 15) shows how the two opposing views about the efficacy of health services are hardly sensible as general statements but that the current approach is to investigate the circumstances in which particular components of health care can do harm or good to specific conditions or social groups. She goes on to show how the problem of assessing the effect of health services on inequalities in health is compounded by the lack of appropriate data and the multiplicity of causes and of effects.

Moreover, given that many 'explanatory variables' are probably not there for themselves but as proxies for something else (e.g. class, tenure) they are not really credible as policy instruments. Thus we are left with those things which are credible and manipulative as causes of inequality – Williams' list included (a) disposable real income (and access to other tangible resources); (b) physical environment (including occupational hazards); (c) social environment (household, family, neighbourhood etc); (d) education; and (e) access to treatment and support.

The discussion brought out three main priority areas. First, and of greatest importance, was the need to redistribute real disposable income to those groups who have the poorest health. It was argued that there would be several multiplier effects of such a policy and that whereas increments, or decrements, in wealth at the top end of the scale would have little health impact, those at the bottom end would be most important, particularly with regard to child health and development.

The second priority area concerned the use of knowledge about particular substances and the development of coherent well understood national programmes of prevention. The areas which currently receive wide publicity are drug addiction and AIDS. However, despite extensive knowledge of the problems for some time, only a few countries have developed adequate population programmes to tackle cigarettes and alcohol.

The third priority area was the design of preventive health programmes. A variety of examples exist which should be used to reduce differences in antenatal care, in child health and development, in dental health as well as in adult conditions such as breast and cervix cancer and heart disease. In these areas it is important that providers of services draw on what is known about socio-economic factors affecting take-up of services and treatment in the design of those services.

It is clearly difficult to give a simple answer to our concerned politician. Perhaps one of the main impacts of all this research is simply to remind the politician and bureaucrat that nearly every policy omission or proposal may well cost lives.

References

Beckerman, W. (1976), *Poverty and the Impact of Income Maintenance Programmes in Four Developed Countries*, Geneva: ILO, 1979; OECD, Public expenditure on income maintenance programmes, Paris.

Black, D. (1980), *Inequalities in Health*, Report of a research working group, London: Department of Health and Social Security.

Collis, E.L. and Greenwood, M. (1921), *The Health of the Industrial Worker*, London: Churchill, p. 127.

CICRED (1981), *Socio-economic Differential Mortality in Industrialised Societies 1*, Committee for International Cooperation in National Research in Demography, Paris.

CICRED (1982), *Socio-economic Differential Mortality in Industrialised Societies 2*, Committee for International Cooperation in National Research in Demography, Paris.

CICRED (1984), *Socio-economic Differential Mortality in Industrialised Societies 3*, Committee for International Cooperation in National Research in Demography, Paris.

CICRED (1986), *Socio-economic Differential Mortality in Industrialised Societies 4*, Committee for International Cooperation in National Research in Demography, Paris.

Culyer, A.J. (1983), *Health Indicators. An International Study for the European Science Foundation*, Oxford: Martin Robinson.

Farr, W. (1864), 'Letter to the Registrar General' in *Supplement to the 25th Annual Report of the Register General of Births, Deaths and Marriages in England*, London.

Gillon, C. and Hemmings, R. (1985), 'Social expenditure in the United Kingdom in a comparative context: trends, explanations and projections' Chapter 2, pp. 22–36 in Klein, R, and O'Higgins, M. (eds) *The Future of Welfare*, Oxford: Blackwell.

Maxwell, R.J. (1981), *Health and Wealth: An International Study of Health Care Spending*, Massachusetts and Toronto: Lexington Books.

Organisation for Economic Cooperation and Development (OECD) (1970), *Economic Growth: Quantitative and Qualitative Objectives for the 1970s*, Interministerial Declaration, 20–22 May 1970, Paris.

OECD (1986), *Measuring Health Care 1960–1983*, Paris.

Sawyer, M. (1982), 'Income distribution and the welfare state'. in A. Botho (ed.), *The European Economy: Growth and Crisis*, Oxford University Press.

Sawyer, M. (1985), *Trends in Income Distribution, Equality and Wealth*, Report on a meeting of trades union experts under the OECD Labour/Management Programme, June 1985.

Townsend, P. (1979), *Poverty in the United Kingdom*, Harmondsworth: Penguin.

UN/WHO (1981), *Proceedings of the Meeting on Socio-Economic Determinants and Consequences of Mortality, Mexico City, June 1979*, New York and Geneva.

WHO (1986), *The Health Burden of Social Inequities*, Copenhagen: WHO Regional Office for Europe, (ICP/HSR 801/MO4).

2 Inequalities in health: the country debate
Pierre Aiach and Roy Carr-Hill

Introduction

This workshop is concerned with the analysis of, and eventually recommendations about, inequalities in health in the various countries. It should, however, be evident that such analyses do not take place in a vacuum. To assess them in a comparative context, it is therefore essential to locate the analyses in their cultural, economic, political and social contexts.

The point can be illustrated from our respective studies of the British and French cases (summarised in Annex 2B). These make it clear that there are structural (whether economic, ideological or political) and conjectural factors which interact to influence the nature of the debate.

For example, there is the fact that the British NHS has no equivalent in France: instead the French instituted a Social Security system founded on the insurance principle. This was due, at least in part, to the weight of tradition and thus Laroque (1981) comments: 'We wanted to remain faithful to the French tradition of syndicalism and mutality' (*Le Monde* 30 September 1981). But this has resulted in an almost permanent preoccupation with financing the reimbursements. In contrast, in the UK, the emphasis is on the efficient and 'proper' management of the NHS: issues such as accessibility and administrative fairness – see for example, the deliberations of the Resources Allocation Working Party (DHSS, 1976). These concerns were, of course, highlighted by the Black Report (DHSS, 1980) and, in turn, reiterated by those interested in an eventual privatisation of health care.

Another example in scientific terms is the origin of the longitudinal studies. The longitudinal study in the UK fuelled an already existing debate. In France, differential mortality had also been studied for a long time but the Institut Nationale des Statistiques et des Etudes Economiques (INSEE) staff argued that the evidential basis for the debate was not sufficiently rigorous. Whilst the results have been published (since 1965) and provide irrefutable evidence of social differentials, there has been no discernible political debate or policy impact.

This probably reflects an even more fundamental issue: these inequalities in death are a reflection of social structure and to question them implies questioning the social structure itself. Hence the ideological utility – at least for the élite – of a notion that the Great Reaper is egalitarian; and similar notions such as 'riches don't make you happy . . . nor ensure your health' and 'everyone dies sometime'.

The purpose of this paper is therefore to examine the variety of debates about inequalities in health which have flourished over the last decade in the countries of the European Region: to ask whether there actually has been any debate in the different national contexts, how it has arisen, what form it has taken, who supports it, and so on. This kind of understanding provides an essential backdrop to any empirical comparison that might be made.

Material available
A thorough study of questions such as these would require prolonged study visits in each of the 25 countries of the European Region. As a poor substitute, a very primitive questionnaire was distributed to the participants both of the European Science Foundation Workshop on Inequalities in Health and of the WHO–Europe meeting in Copenhagen in 1984 and we received some 30 replies from colleagues in 19 different countries.[1]

These responses, together with other material available to us – principally the papers from the Copenhagen meeting[2] – have been used in two ways. First, as a means of constructing thumbnail sketches of the nature of the debate in each country (presented in Annex 2A). These are very sketchy indeed, but we hope to have picked out the features of interest in each case, with slightly longer 'summaries' for France and Great Britain with which we are more familiar (in Annex 2B). Secondly, we have used the material as a way of testing some of our own ideas about the differences and similarities between countries and the factors influencing the development of the debate in a particular country. This does not claim to be the conclusion of an exhaustive study, which would require extensive and intensive study but impressions gained from the various papers that were available to us and a more detailed analysis of the British and French situations.

Discussing the debate
It should be evident that we cannot presume that the nature and tenor of argument and debate about inequalities in health in a country can be deduced simply from an analysis of the actual extent of inequalities in health over that period, for the specific approach to the discussion of issues of social inequality and the way in which such issues are

eventually resolved reflect the economic, political and social situation in each country. This does not mean, of course, that we can simply ignore the level of inequalities in health.

For example, the 'issues' are not at all the same in developing and developed countries. Thus, in most African, Asian and Latin American nations, there are huge differences in living standards between the majority of the population and the situation of the privileged élite. These 'inequalities' are far greater than those observed in Europe now but correspond to what might have been observed at the beginning of the nineteenth century. There is, of course, the added spice of colonial exploitation and an international context of very large disparities in consumable wealth between countries (see, for example, Hayter, 1981; World Bank, 1986) in comparing the nature and tenor of the debate between these countries. One would therefore expect to base much of the analysis on the comparative extent of actual inequality.

In contrast, whilst the experiences of the countries represented at the ESF Workshop are diverse (as reflected, for example, in the documents prepared for the Copenhagen meeting, WHO Europe, 1986), they are much more homogenous than when comparing on a world scale. Yet Annexes 2A and 2B which are drawn both from the replies to our questionnaire and documents submitted to the Copenhagen meeting, suggest that there are considerable differences between the countries in the way in which these inequalities enter into political and scientific debate. Our problem is therefore to find a way of understanding those different views about the issue of inequalities in health in order to assess them in their cultural, economic, political and social contexts.

One approach which tempted at least the pragmatic half of this coalition, was to classify the replies in terms of a broad structuring of the implicit ideologies of health and of health care in each of the countries. Thus one could contrast the Scandinavian countries (and Germany and Israel) which have extensive health and social welfare systems with other countries having a relatively longstanding welfare state with yet other countries which have recently instituted a health service (Greece, Italy, Spain). Thus the Scandinavians worry about the particular impact of specific cuts and the new 'NHS' countries are relatively enthusiastic about what will be a rosy future when the recession goes away. The difficulty arises with the middle category which includes countries like Belgium and France who are concerned with academic research into differential medical consumption and Hungary and the UK where the debates are, for different reasons, *sui generis*.

Another possible division is between those who are concerned to situate the distribution of health care services within a general debate about the *distribution of resources* and those who concentrate on differential *medical consumption*. The former issue is usually only opaquely expressed, whilst the form of the latter varies according to the reimbursement system adopted. A similar division is that between authors who raise the issue of inequalities in *health* compared to those who concentrate uniquely upon *health care*. Indeed, it is striking how few papers or responses dealt with *health as such* even though many talked of 'health resources'. In principle this makes it very difficult to compare the approaches across countries at all.

A third emerging or possible division might be between those who see (ill-)health as something that happens to people and those who see the individual as largely responsible for his own health (although, in fact, very few actually said that). Within the first category, we could distinguish between those who appear to concentrate on inequalities between individuals so that the question of access to curative services is crucial and those who emphasise the group membership of individuals so that the question becomes one of the relative poverty of that group and so on.

Yet another line of attack is to look at the categories by which inequality is defined and, subsidiarily, the dimensions of health over which inequality is measured. For example, although several kinds of disadvantaged groups are cited, there is very little consideration of ethnic minorities or of immigrants. Again, given that the crucial inequalities probably occur in childhood, the relative prominence given to the elderly in several countries is interesting.

The difficulty with all or any of these intercountry comparisons is twofold:

1. The material available to us is very partial. Thus the apparent coherence of a country paper or questionnaire reply dissolves when we realise that another source from the same country is equally coherent but contradicts the first on crucial points. The apparently correct classification of a country according to one reply might therefore be due more to our (mis)interpretation or (mis)understanding of a given reply rather than a reflection of any 'objective' feature of that country.

2. The comparisons would neglect essential historical dimensions of how the debate has arisen and is articulated in a particular economic, political and social context. It is not therefore a question of comprehending a series of one-dimensional comparisons but of how those factors combine and have combined in a specific context.

Therefore, instead of attempting to classify the country replies according to their expressed position on a number of dimensions of comparison, we have attempted to provide a 'theory' of how the debate about inequalities in health might be constructed and to illustrate that theory with examples from the papers and the questionnaire replies.

Theses and antitheses
The argument is that, in order to discuss and eventually propose action about particular forms of inequalities in health, there are a series of factors which need to be taken into account in each country: the overall *ideology* towards the existence of inequality and the collection of relevant data; the prevailing views about *what affects health* and the efficacy of health care in general; the moves between *prosperity and restrictions* and how these are perceived; and finally, the *relative power* of different interest groups in society.

Ideologies of inequality
First, the ideological/political climate has to permit discussion of inequality. Thus, in some countries, it is difficult to discuss publicly the existence of inequalities because the political regime sees such discussion as a direct attack upon its legitimacy. Indeed, the WHO Regional Conference took as its theme 'Social Equity and Health' precisely because of this difficulty. This might seem a very liberal, very obvious position but it has important consequences in other situations. For even if the political regime permits discussion of inequalities, not much can be said or talked about if no data exists. Thus, it is not only in Hungary and Poland where people complain about the lack of good data but also in Belgium.

The lack of data, or at least the inappropriate nature of the data, can also be linked to the administrative/political structure of the country. Thus in the FDR, there are no data at the national level sufficient to generate epidemiological research because of the decentralised federal structure of the country: for example, there is no national cancer registry. In other countries, such as in ex-Franco's Spain and ex-Salazar's Portugal, the administrative structures are rigid for historical reasons.

Another type of problem arises from the socio-professional classifications which are used: for example, in Belgium there are different categorisations for white-collar workers and for blue-collar workers; again in FDR, there is no agreement on the appropriate classification so that researchers use their own which makes it difficult to accumulate research results.

Second, there has to be a view that the inequalities do exist: whether or not there are any differences; whether such differences are large or small. For example, in Sweden the consensus for some time has been that the welfare state had eradicated the important inequalities so they were rarely discussed; in Switzerland the view is that the inequalities which remain are so small that they are not worth discussing. In both these countries, therefore, any discussion of inequalities tends to be restricted to specific forms of morbidity where state intervention might make a difference.

In contrast, there are countries where the inequalities are so flagrant that they are also 'forgotten' or at least normally accepted as part of a daily existence. Whilst this is more obviously the case in Third World developing countries than in Europe, the fact that the subject seems not to be discussed with great fervour in Greece, Italy or Spain is perhaps indicative of this. In these cases, inequalities in health are apparently less important or less urgent to tackle. What matters first is to establish the country economically, to introduce more social justice in respect of incomes, housing, and schooling and, of course, to give care to those who need it . . . the rest will follow. At the same time, there does appear to be a demand for more research in these countries. But this seems to come up against powerful opposition groups who are ideologically very close to their former positions in socio-political structures. In Spain for example, the medical profession and university researchers seem to hold back. Clearly in these countries the development of an adequate research base will take some time.

Lastly we should not forget the East European countries where researchers have an extremely difficult task, both because the administrative structures make it difficult to obtain adequate data and because, ideologically and politically, it is often not appropriate. Where it does prove possible to conduct research, as in Poland, it is usually very descriptive.

The whole question of the extent to which a debate or issue is determined by (the knowledge of) existing data or, of itself, generates the data necessary for a 'response' is a very difficult one. It includes a view about the neutrality of scientific (statistical) information; a theory as to how knowledge is generated, maintained and reproduced; and comparisons not only between countries but over time. Whilst we believe therefore that the precise role played by information in a particular economic, political and social context is very important, we do not know how to incorporate it other than under this rubric.

Views about health and health care
The third factor is the prevailing ideology of health. Thus in nearly every country there has been an emphasis on the individual's responsibility for their own (ill-)health – and eventually death – because of their behaviour or the lifestyle they adopt. Once these kinds of factors are thought to be at the origin of the inequalities (as,

for example, in FDR where some epidemiologists argue that cultural differences in individual behaviour are the principal cause of inequalities in health) the role of collective factors – which are, of course, always *expressed* individually – are forgotten. If this latter ideology were re-adopted *in toto* ('re-adopted' because, in a certain sense, that was the view in the first half of the nineteenth century) then the question of inequalities would not exist, or at least, not be publicly debated; and, of course, such an ideology is very useful for legitimising cuts in health care expenditures.

The fourth factor is the kind of health care system which has been designed or has evolved to deal with illnesses. In some systems access to primary health care in some form might be very easy, so that the important point is to understand the factors influencing the quality of care which one receives. For example, in Ireland, O'Hare (1986) sees it as curious, and to be explained, that women report less illness and make less use of hospital services than men in contrast to other countries. The Irish health care system does not of course provide equal and open access to all, and this might explain the differential use of hospital services, but not the differences in self-reported illness which are more likely to be related to what counts as illness for men and women in their society. In Poland, with free access for all, the concern is with social differentiation on the functioning of the health care system (waiting times, access to hospitals and availability of certain drugs). There are similar concerns in the UK within the National Health Service. The concentration is on the measurement of the quality (or outcome?) of care.

In other systems, whilst the quality of care might be more or less equivalent, the question is one of financial access to the care in the first place. The French obsession with differential consumption of medical services is an obvious example but so is Ireland where the difficulties faced by the travellers, the single homeless, single mothers, the elderly living alone and the unemployed are regularly raised by politicians. The issue is the extent to which different groups have access to the various forms of health care.

Material conditions

Fifth is a series of conjunctural factors. It has already been emphasised several times that the question of social inequalities has an historical past which will be unique to the particular country being considered. It is therefore of considerable interest to note that the problem of inequalities in health is being raised in more or less the same way in several countries at the same time. We think that the reason is relatively simple: many of the European countries have had a very similar history over the last 30 years.

Table 2.1:   Share of social expenditure in GDP, the (relative) share of health care expenditure and its growth rate, 1960 and 1981

(i) In Capitalist Countries

	Social Expenditure Share in GDP		Health Share in Social Expenditure		Annual Growth Rates in Health Expenditure			
					1960–75		1975–81	
	1960	1981	1960	1981	Real Exp.	Real Ben.	Real Exp.	Real Ben.
Austria	17.9	27.7	16.2	17.0	—	—	—	—
Belgium	17.4	37.6[a]	14.9	13.3[a]	—	—	—	—
Denmark	—	33.3[b]	—	—	—	—	—	—
Finland	15.4	25.9	14.8	19.9	11.9	11.5	3.9	3.6
France	13.4[c]	29.5	18.7	22.0	10.9	8.7	6.3	5.6
Germany	20.5	31.5	15.1	20.6	6.6	5.0	2.1	2.1
Greece	8.5	13.4[a]	20.0	26.1[a]	—	—	—	—
Ireland	11.7	28.4	25.6	29.6	7.7	−0.4	6.6	4.7
Italy	16.8	29.1	19.0	20.6	6.7	5.1	7.7	8.2
Netherlands	16.2	36.1	8.0	18.6	11.4	8.7	4.4	1.2
Norway	11.7	27.1	23.9	23.6	9.0	8.2	5.2	4.8
Sweden	15.4	33.4	22.1	26.6	11.3	10.6	3.4	3.1
Switzerland	7.7	14.9[b]	—	—	—	—	—	—
UK	13.9	23.7	24.5	22.8	3.4	3.0	2.0	2.0

(ii) COMECON Countries

	1960	1979	1960	1979	1960–70		1970–80	
Hungary	1.5	2.2	31.7	21.8	6.3	—	4.6	—
Poland	—	—	7.4[d]	7.7[d]	4.0[e]	—	11.9[e]	—

Notes
a 1980
b 1979
c Excluding education
d Share in total consumption
e Growth rate in current prices
f Allowing for changes in coverage and demographic structure
Source: OECD, *Growth in Social Expenditure*, Paris, 1985; UN National Accounts Yearbook, 1980.

Thus, from 1960–75 in all the capitalist countries of Europe there was a large proportionate increase in social expenditure (see columns 1 and 2 in Table 2.1). From around 1975 the rate of increase started slowing down in nearly every country (with the exception of Greece) and was less than half the rate in Belgium, Germany, Italy, Netherlands, Sweden, Switzerland and the UK (OECD, 1985, Table 4, p. 28), but 'over the period 1975–81 the growth rate of average real benefits still managed to keep pace with the growth rate of real GDP per capita' (OECD, 1985, p. 32).

With every country trying to curb state expenditure, from 1980 the increasing pressures of expenditures on pensioners and the unemployed meant that expenditures on health care have been relatively squeezed in many countries. The rate of increase has dropped by more than half in Finland, Germany, Netherlands and Sweden but has *increased* in Ireland and Italy (right-hand half of Table 2.1).

Whilst expenditure has to be controlled, there are strong pressures to do something for those who risk suffering most from any cuts. At the same time there is a (growing?) questioning of the efficacy of medical care: for, without necessarily being convinced by Illich (1971) or McKeown, Record and Turner (1975) these ideas are being accepted on some levels both by the medical profession and by politicians – partly because it is in their interest.

Government and opposition
Sixth, the particular political situation and respective roles of government and opposition can make a very great difference. Thus in countries where a welfare state was instituted and maintained when left-wing or social democratic parties were in government, the opposition (the centre and right-wing parties) are more likely to have concentrated on the potential expense of such a system rather than on the necessity of tackling the outstanding inequalities. In situations where the centre or right-wing parties have been in power for some time, then the opposition (of left-wing and social democratic parties) will have used the existence of social inequalities as one of their arguments against the government, whilst when in government, will tend to appear to be interested in the inequalities without making any serious attempt to reduce them.

This is certainly the case in France for, when the Socialist party came to power, despite having attacked the previous government about inequalities, they did little about health care. Instead, they have controlled expenditure with a relatively draconian policy of restrictions: hospitalisation is no longer free and the reimbursements for dental care and for opticians have not been increased. The changes that have been made in the hospital sector and the introduction of Regional Health Observatories were both introduced by the previous government and they do not, in any case, have any significant effect on social inequalities in health; and the same is true of the reform of medical studies. The only substantial change has been the elimination of the private hospital sector which had been allowed to survive by the previous reform in 1958.

Seventh, the nature of the debate will be affected by the relative position, power and recognition of various groups in society. Thus, despite the fact that the inequalities in death are possibly most flagrant between immigrants and nationals in most of the European countries, hardly anyone mentioned that in their replies. In contrast, many of the more 'developed' countries are very concerned about the situation of the elderly *vis-à-vis* those who are younger, which surely reflects the former's increasing power in those societies.

Although it is difficult to point to particular examples, there is an emphasis on the plight of those in rural areas especially in Finland and Hungary.

More parochially, it must be remembered that those who know the evidence are not the principal victims; indeed, they tend to be those who have the best chance of a long life. Thus, in France, it has often been claimed during the last 20 years that schoolteachers have the longest life expectancy even though many other groups were equally favoured. This enabled the explanation of inequalities to concentrate on lifestyle (stability, temperance) rather than on variations in conditions between the different social classes.

Synthesis

The nature of any debate about inequalities will, of course, depend upon the kind of inequalities being discussed. Inequalities in death between adults can be seen as the ultimate injustice even when they can be 'explained' by factors which are supposed to be an entirely individual responsibility. For, on one level, inequalities in death summarise, and are the consequence of, all the other inequalities; they show how one person's life has been very different from another because they die differently. In contrast, inequalities in infant mortality, whilst viewed as equally serious, are not seen in the same light: we 'know' that the important factors are independent of the baby (the living conditions of the mother before and during pregnancy etc). Moreover, we are successful in reducing the overall rate, if not in reducing the gap between the 'top' and 'bottom' of the social scale.

From this point of view the extent to which one views other inequalities as fair or unfair will depend upon their importance in producing these inequalities in death. For some countries that might eventually be a question of geographical or regional differences; for others, the kind of housing policy may have led to a specific set of problems, and so on.

This entirely 'rational' view ignores a number of crucial factors which facilitate or impede the development of a debate. Indeed, given that one could argue that inequalities in death are *the* central issue, there is surprisingly relatively little debate. It is as if policymakers and researchers are reluctant to dwell publicly on inequalities which are of such supreme importance. Is it because of the *lack of information* that, in Western countries, neither left-wing parties nor trade unions raise the issue, or is it for other reasons? Instead, even for existing data demonstrating differences to be recognised, let alone acted upon, there has to be a 'scandal' (as when inequality was rediscovered in Sweden in the late 1960s) or at least a spectacular (non-)presentation (as with the Black Report in Britain).

More systemically, this paper has argued that in European countries or, more generally, in industrialised countries, the extent to which the question of inequalities in health is seen as important and is acted upon depends on:

1. The extent to which the political regime in power is *prepared to recognise the existence of inequalities*. This could either be because social inequalities cannot exist, according to the prevailing doctrine, or because the regime does not accept any collective responsibility.

2. The existence or at least the perceived *existence of inequalities* in health between groups of individuals. It must be emphasised that the lack of appropriate data can be one effective impediment to debate as in (1).

3. The prevailing views about *what affects health* and in particular the extent to which it is an individual rather than collective responsibility: *in extremis*, inequalities are irrelevant.

4. The particular form of the *health care system* which has evolved to deal with illnesses and to cure people and, in particular, the form of access. For inequalities to be perceived, comparisons have to be made and the specific administration of health care will determine the data available.

5. The *economic and historical context* will also affect the salience of the debate as is evidenced by the fact that so many European countries were prepared to sanction this series of workshops.

6. In a parliamentary democracy, the respective ideologies of the groups and/or tendencies *which are in government or opposition* will structure the form of the debate as can be seen from the comparison between France and the UK.

7. The relative *position and power of disadvantaged groups* will also be an important factor in determining whether or not inequalities in health become an important issue. A society concerned with the growth of the elderly population will tend to focus on age at death; inequalities in health between the poor and the rich when young will be ignored.

The question remains whether anything has been learnt from this broad-brush comparative overview of the debate about inequalities in health in the European countries. There are two answers:

1. As has already been mentioned, in most countries, a particular combination of economic and historical factors led to the creation

of a health system which was intended to provide health care more or less equally to most citizens. But that epoch has been followed by another combination of factors which has led each of those countries to attempt to reduce health and social service expenditures and, consequently perhaps, to re-introduce those inequalities. The problems faced by each country are therefore similar; and hence there is a common analysis.

2. As is demonstrated in Annex 2A, many of the important factors which structure the debate seem to be specific to the context in each country. From this point of view it is difficult to see what can be gained from the comparison except complexity and confusion.

In general, we (the authors) have convinced ourselves that much can be learnt from a study of this material. The question as to why there are so many international forums with so few national policy changes is important. The analysis above suggests that whether anything is done about inequalities in death (or in health) depends not only on an understanding of the complexity of the issues involved but also on whether or not it is acceptable, to those in power, to do something about it. The answer unfortunately is usually 'no'.

Notes

1. The material for four of these countries was too slender to make even a thumbnail sketch, so only 15 countries have been analysed.
2. Edited by Raymond Illsley and Per-Gunnar Svenssen and published by the WHO Regional Office for Europe as *The Health Burden of Social Inequalities*, Geneva H/B/S/I/1986 (ICP/HSR 807–m04).

References

Department of Health and Social Services (1976), *Resources Allocation Working Party*, London: HMSO, Cmnd.

Department of Health and Social Services (1980), *Inequalities on Health*, Report of a research working group chaired by Sir Douglas Black, London: HMSO.

Hayter, T. (1981), *Causes of World Poverty*, London: Pluto.

Illich, I. (1971), *Medical Nemesis*, London: Calder Boyar.

Laroque, G. (1981), Report in *Le Monde*, 30 September.

McKeown, T. Record, R.G. and Turner, R.D. (1975), 'An interpretation of the decline of mortality in England and Wales during the twentieth century', *Population Studies*, 29, (3), pp. 319–422.

O'Hare, A. (1986), 'Ireland', WHO (1986), op. cit., pp. 117–126.

Organisation of Economic Cooperation and Development (1985), *Growth in Social Expenditures*, Paris: OECD.

World Bank (1986), *World Development Report*, Washington.

World Health Organisation (1986), *The Health Burden of Social Inequalities*, Copenhagen: WHO, Regional Office for Europe.

United Nations (1982), *National Accounts Yearbook 1980*, New York: UN.

Annex 2A   Country reports

Belgium

The debate has been taken up in scientific associations and, recently, by the Flemish Socialist Party with some research projects funded by the government.

Their colloquium emphasised that social inequalities in health have existed for a long time and indeed are probably increasing even though one might have expected a diminution in inequalities from the post-war system of social security. However, the poorer group is now smaller and more diverse but although inequalities have changed in form they are evident whichever indicators are chosen. Moreover, those social groups which are at risk from a variety of factors (occupational, income, housing, education) also tend to be in poor health which in turn influences their social situation.

There is a wide difference in mortality between the Dutch – speaking and French – speaking parts of Belgium, especially for men. Indeed, these are probably perceived as the most important social differences. Wunsch argues that 'anomie', housing and the pattern of prosperity are the principal factors; on the other hand he is surprised at the lack of relation between the level of health and the structure of medical services. The authors conclude by underlining the importance of individual behaviour 'e.g. in eating and smoking habits, exercise, alcoholism, sugar intake, and stress' at the same time as regretting the lack of appropriate longitudinal data.

There have been some studies of dental health and of disabilities/invalidities by cause, broken down by two social classes. But there is no general policy interest in the problem even though Belgium has a relatively low life expectancy. Instead, there are specific interests in the health of the 'Fourth World' and especially in the health of their children; in the health of immigrants; and in the impact of handicaps on employment.

The authors conclude that the social class variable probably provides the most powerful discrimination but this seems to be mostly related to consumption of medical services. On the other hand they also say that income, level of education and insured status are important determinants of the demand for medical services. The majority of death data are presented by region which is not very surprising given the cultural and linguistic differences between the

Flemish and the Walloons.

Conclusion
- There is lack of basic data for research and especially the lack of longitudinal studies;
- The subject is complex and the multicollinearities make casual explanatory analysis difficult;
- The partial state of research means that we cannot determine the possibilities for policy remedies.

Future research
They emphasise the importance of research into the chronically ill as the most at-risk group. There has been some research at Louvain on the financial implications of chronic illness in terms of what the sufferers receive and spend.

They also speak of research into regional differences in the services provided so as to ensure a more equitable distribution of health care resources.

There seems to be no real analysis of the political aspects of the issue. They concentrate only on the potential of financial or organisational reforms for improving access to health care.

Denmark
There has been a tradition of studying inequalities in health since the middle of the nineteenth century and there has recently been renewed scientific interest in the question. Study concentrates on three kinds of issues:

1. the link between economic status and occupational diseases;
2. the wide disparities in rates of mortality, of illness and disability pensions but little disparity in the use of the health care system;
3. links between health and lifestyle.

There is extensive data on mortality, disability and morbidity. The main criteria of classification are by gender, marital status, occupational structure and region.

There has not recently been any political debate about inequalities in health except among the left-wing parties. The little debate there is, is not, in general, linked to any wider debate about social inequalities although this was, briefly, a concern in the early 1970s. Instead the accessibility of health services and the increase in cost to the state have always been at the forefront of any debate about the health care system. The Copenhagen paper shows that they take the view that inequalities in health are manipulable through political effort. It underlines the difficulties of interpretation because of changes over time, confusion between exposure and selection, and validity of indicators.

Finland
The question of health inequalities has been raised recently in a political context with the left-wing parties asking for more public services and the bourgeois parties asking for the same or less. But the academic debate has existed for some time with three national health surveys (in 1964, 1968 and 1976) animated by demographers, occupational sociologists and social policy theorists. Perhaps this reflects the importance attached to health policies in Finland. The debate is framed both in terms of living conditions and of personal health habits. But there are differences in the focus of the three groups of academics: demographers concentrate on morbidity and mortality differentials between the regions, the sexes and socio-economic groups; occupational sociologists on the impact of the labour process on the health of workers; and social policy theorists on the use of resources (health differences can cause or indicate inequality). The emphasis on health habits is quite recent but relatively strong.

The recent emphasis on budget restraint has held back the projected development of personnel in the health care sector. Meanwhile private services have expanded. The summary says that there are large discrepancies between the general debate, government policy and any scientific discussion.

West Germany (FRG)
Since 1978 there have been several attempts to curb the inflation of medical expenditure. This led to the creation of a consultative committee to advise upon anti-inflationary measures and the restriction of services.

The debate assumed renewed importance after the Right took power in 1982 when new levels of poverty were discovered. The argument was whether or not the changes in benefits and subsidies had led to decreased utilisation and, therefore, increase in morbidity and mortality. The Ministry of Labour accordingly financed 16 epidemiological studies which were, however, of doubtful worth.

The focus of the debate has been upon those sectors where treatment might work, prompted by questions about whether an improved infrastructure of medical services might save money in the medium to long term. At the same time, the debate is linked by some protagonists to a broader concern about the social fabric for, in the same way as unemployment is/was seen as one of the major factors in the rise of Nazism, every political perturbation of the social peace, such as that which may arise from the *perception* of pronounced inequalities in health care, implies a possible danger for FRG democracy.

The Copenhagen paper discusses the fragmentary nature of the information available, the potential possibility of using the data routinely collected by local health insurance systems, but there is no epidemiological data at the national level. Thus, each study uses its own classification, perhaps a sign of disagreement on the nature of social stratification in West Germany. Despite this lack of comparable data, they say there are clear differences in morbidity and mortality between the social classes (infarctions and psychoses) and in particular the underutilisation of services by the poorer classes. The authors claim that this leads to a higher perinatal mortality rate.

In contrast, the Stuttgart study explains the differences as due to variations in individual behaviour – for example, the length of time poorer classes wait before consulting. But some sociologists do have a different approach emphasising instead collective factors. They make the point that epidemiology does not permit a thorough study of the question of inequalities.

The public perception is of major change in 1982: previously the concern with social inequality was quasi-universally taken as a prime motive for constructing the welfare state (prior to 1973) and for maintaining, preserving and possibly extending it until 1982 when the Welfare State itself began to be questioned.

Greece

The whole debate is very much a live issue as a National Health Service has recently been introduced with the specific objective of redistributing health resources [sic] and extending health insurance over the whole population. Note that redistribution here is understood primarily in terms of the regional distribution of health service but also includes the reallocation of resources within the health service.

The installation of a decentralised health care service and the training of adequate and appropriate personnel at the same time as ensuring universal coverage of the social insurance system dominates discussion of policy so that the problems of particular at-risk groups are less considered. The hope is that in tackling the problems among the majority of the population, many of the social injustices suffered by minority groups will be solved.

The disparities between rural and urban areas are given special attention but there have also been laws, regulations and services introduced to protect specific groups (such as the disadvantaged, the elderly, students etc.). The whole orientation of the health service has also been changed with, for example, the introduction of Primary

Health Care Centres, reorganisation of the hospital services, the introduction of psychiatric services and, academically, the foundation of new departments of social medicine and the introduction of sociology into the medical degree course.

Previously there was much less debate although specific forms of inequality were commented upon.

Hungary

The debate is seen as constrained in different ways by our three respondents. On the other hand, the debate is seen as being hampered by the paucity of data – none on health and only some on mortality. In any case, the debate is mainly scientific as the explicit recognition of inequalities is difficult politically. At the same time, there is a widespread public debate about the health care system which touches upon inequalities because it focuses upon shortages.

The realisation that the rates of mortality are increasing has led to a programme of research involving, mostly, sociologists. Inasmuch as there is a political recognition, it is limited to the access to grades and forms of health care and is focused on the differential availability in urban/rural areas, especially on the role played by under-the-counter payments.

There has been no change in the recent past: it is interesting to note that whilst the prospect of a wide-ranging economic and social reform is debated, the responsibility for ill health is being shifted to individuals as in some West European countries.

Ireland

There is very little political debate in Ireland on the general effect of social inequalities on health status. This is perhaps due to the assumption that, as 38 per cent of the Irish population, or those least well off financially, have full eligibility to all health services free of charge, this entitlement negates the effect of social inequalities on health status. Individual politicians occasionally raise the issue of inequalities in relation to the health of specific marginal groups, such as the travellers (formerly tinkers), the single homeless, single mothers, the elderly living alone and the unemployed.

In the Copenhagen paper, O'Hare (1986) starts out by saying that inequalities in income, in access to education, and in access to social mobility, are greater in Eire than in France, Great Britain and Sweden. She also shows how women report *less* illness, and make less use of hospital services in contrast to other countries.

O'Hare presents data on mortality by region and sex, but not by socio-economic group; she also discusses a wider range of vulnerable groups than most others – not only the young unemployed but also the elderly alone and the travellers. She concludes 'if health policy is to be responsive to the health needs of the most vulnerable groups in Irish society, then more data on the correlations between social class and morbidity are required' (p. 46).

Questions of social inequalities emerge in scientific discourse from relevant research findings when published or when used by pressure groups. There is ongoing but intermittent concern about marginal groups and occasional general debate on the extent of poverty and social inequality in the country. This concern generally takes the form of an appeal to the government to do something about the inequality concerned, for example, to provide accommodation for the single homeless. The dimension of inequality most often referred to is that of poverty, but it can be specific to the problem in question. For instance, it has been suggested that prejudice towards the travelling people prevents them from using existing health services.

The aspects of health focused on is both problem- and group-related: high infant mortality and lowered life expectancy associated with the travellers; tuberculosis, mental illness and chest infections with the single homeless and conditions of anaemia and toxaemia with single mothers. The question of inequalities in health reflects a more general debate about social inequalities, but health is always a central issue in any such debate.

There is a change today in how questions of inequality are put and understood from the recent past. Evidence of the change comes from the government's tacit recognition of the need for an anti-poverty policy: previous governments believed that the poor could best be helped within the framework of economic and social development. Limited economic resources have also forced the present government to declare its intention to direct resources more specifically towards those in greatest need and to develop accessible 'reach out' services to low-income groups who have an exceptionally high level of illness but make inadequate use of existing services.

Israel
There has been a loud and vociferous public debate recently because of budget cuts in the health service and in the resources provided via the health insurance system. The debate focuses in particular on the chronically ill, the elderly and low-income groups which were affected by these recent shifts in government policy.

There had not previously been any debate apart from that raised by speculation about the impact of the physicians' strike in 1983. This is relatively curious as there have been quite extensive studies by Antonovsky of mortality differentials. Perhaps the political and social conflicts between communities make it a touchy subject?

Indeed, the report presented to the WHO by Shuval (1986) gives almost no data on mortality or morbidity differentials whether by social class, socio-economic group or level of instruction, although the authors do refer in general terms to the higher levels of both infant and overall mortality among the Arabic population.

Fundamentally, however, the issue is treated in terms of disparities in the quality and quantity of health care between the regions and sometimes by country of birth and level of instruction. Data on occupation is only available from special studies.

Italy

There has been a debate around the introduction of the new Health Reform Act (Law No. 833/1978) which aimed at unifying and generalising the health care services. However, it is difficult for any scientific discourse to develop as there is very little valid data. On the whole, the view is that the Reform could have worked (to what purpose?) but the financial crisis brought on by world recession has meant that implementation has been very, very slow. The Copenhagen report dwells also on the impact of the economic crisis on the implementation of the 1978 Reform and on the financial cuts in services. They argue that this has led to a highlighting of inequity and the promulgation of a notion of solidarity. Thus health (care) policies should at least not aggravate existing inequalities, and notions of social justice are increasingly appealed to in political debate (p. 3).

The financial cuts have particularly affected the weakest (p. 31) and this problem has attracted researchers from several disciplines under the banner of 'Health and Justice'. They talk in terms of 'new' health inequalities which have arisen through regional differences and social transformation. Despite the interest, there is still too little information to assess how the various factors interrelate and to design appropriate prevention policies (especially for the new marginal populations).

Economists have concentrated on searching for macro-relationships between economic phenomena and health and on analysing the efficiency of service delivery on the grounds that 'an increase in equity in distributions normally corresponds to an increase in efficiency as a whole' (Mooney 1983). They also underline the effects of unemployment.

Sociologists have also concentrated on equities in access to and use of health care services and have underlined the importance of considering individuals in their specific social context so as to develop a range of policies more appropriate to their specific context.

Netherlands

Inequality in health was recently the subject of a congress held by the

Dutch Society of Social Medicine on 'Inequalities in Health and Health Care'. But there was no continuity to that congress: 'One reason seemed to be the economic recession. Neither policy makers nor researchers judged the theme as most relevant to health and health care in the eighties' (Social and Cullinal Planning Office, 1984, p. 274).

As indicators for social inequality, they use sex, age, region and socio-economic group. But most studies on mortality are descriptive with only the occasional plea for the investigation of causes.

Norway

Extensive data are available in Norway. There were the two national health surveys in 1968 and 1975, the Level of Living Survey in 1980, and the Regional Mortality Survey 1976–80, all carried out by the Norwegian Central Bureau of Statistics (NOS).

The Copenhagen paper presents analysis for differential mortality, levels of morbidity and psychiatric conditions by income and social class. Whilst these are the main axes of stratification, they are also interested in breakdowns by region and, indeed, one of the more spectacular differences is in dental health; and there is a mention of immigrants.

Overall, their paper is concerned with the problems of classification. Thus:

Acts of classification and the classification systems and the categories of these systems, however, are not pre-theoretical (p. 3).

What kinds of social inequity are expalined when 'structural variables' are employed? (p. 28).

but:

The problem with structural determinants is that they, as social and cultural phenomena, are produced and reproduced by the kind of social acts and processes, that should be determined by these 'structures' (p. 29).

Nevertheless, they feel able to conclude that:

. . . inequalities in occupational structure may explain a variation in mortality of 20%. A natural and general interpretation is that variation in life style and life condition create variation in mortality (p. 13).

There has been a recent political debate about the consequences of the introduction of private health care services but not much research. The questions are: (1) Will vulnerable groups be worse off with the new health care payment system? and (2), What will be the impact of private health care services?

These questions are explicitly linked with the overall political debate about socio-democratic welfare ideology. The focus of the debate has shifted in recent years because of the perceptions that demographic pressures will change future needs.

Poland
Our actual questionnaire received a negative response in that we were referred to the competent authorities. At the same time, the documents presented to the Copenhagen meeting are quite detailed and:

1. There has been an increase in mortality rates between 1970 and 1980 both for adults and for infants. This is seen as a serious problem.
2. Whilst there is little data relevant to social class inequality there is data on regional differences and on infant mortality by level of instruction.
3. There is also evidence on social differentiation in the functioning of the health care system (waiting time, access to hospitals and availability of certain drugs).

Once again, the sociologists seem to play an important role. Thus, the Copenhagen paper argues that they have carried out research but overall the data is hardly appropriate to the problem of studying inequalities. The authors of the Copenhagen report appeal for more studies of causes and explanations.

Spain
The arguments and evidence in the Copenhagen report is a little confusing about inequalities: first they invoke the inverse care law yet, whilst they point to wide gaps between classes both economically and ideologically, there appears to be only a small difference in the health status of different groups; later, however, they say that the poorer groups in the population use medical services more and their health status is lower. The real problem is that whilst there are some studies relating access to hospital care to social factors, there is no systematic data on health status or even mortality broken down by social group. Any political debate is only marginal and is restricted to considerations of inequality in access to health care. If the argument is pushed any further it is in terms of the access to *appropriate* health care and the differential availability of fashionable hi-tech medicine or expensive drugs to different groups.

The whole debate has shifted from before Franco's death. At that time, inequalities in health care – along with other perceived inequalities of service provision – were on the political genda. The subsequent normalisation of Spanish politics has ended open debate although a law inaugurating a National Health Service is being passed this session by Parliament.

Sweden

The prevailing mood of the 1950s and early 1960s was that social problems had been overcome. Thus:

> . . . the prevailing Swedish dogma seemed to be that such differences did not exist or that they were relatively unimportant. This was reflected in the 1960 Parlimentary decision to abolish social class as a category for official statistical purposes (Vagero 1986, p. 231).

However, a survey of levels of living showed that inequalities still existed although health issues as such were not studied. Indeed, there appears to be: 'Some reluctance . . . on the part of authorities . . . to commit themselves to the study of the health consequences of social inequity' (Vagero, 1986, p. 231).

There has been a political debate within the Social Democratic Party and among trades unions and some academic debate in the Social Medicine section of the Swedish Medical Association centred on two fronts: the possibility that privatisation leads to unequal access to services; and the link between inequalities in health and distributional issues. Overall, health has never been a prominent issue.

Switzerland

There is very little data although there has been a National Health Survey and the Statistical Office will publish mortality by occupational groups in 1986. Some academics have also mobilised around the general theme of inequalities in health but the lack of debate is explained in terms of the high standard of living and low levels of poverty.

However, some specific issues have been raised. Thus, there has been some debate around the revision of the coverage of the health insurance scheme.

References

Mooney, O. (1982), *Equity in Health Care: Confronting the Confusion*, Aberdeen: Health Economic Research Unit (Discussion Paper no. 11–82).

Social and Cultural Planning Office (1984), *Social and Cultural Report*, Netherlands: The Hague Govt Printing Office.

Shuval, J.T. (1986), in Illsley, R. and Svensonn, P.G. (eds), *The Health Burden of Social Inequities*, Copenhagen: WHO Regional Office for Europe.

Vagero, D. (1986), *The Health Burden of Social Inequalities*, WHO Europe, pp. 227–32.

Wunsch, G. (1979), 'Differential mortality and cultural differences. A case study: Belgium' in *Proceedings of the Meeting on Socio-Economic Determinants and Consequences of Mortality*, Mexico City, pp. 339–50.

Annex 2B   Data on inequalities in health in France and the UK

Political and scientific debate on inequalities in health in France

Social policies and inequalities since the War

The debate on inequalities in health in the French context can only be understood in terms of the specific ideological and political context since the Second World War which appears to have determined the kinds of questions which can and have been asked and the interpretations placed upon the researches which have been carried out.

Between 1945 and 1981 the political forces dominant in government have been the centre and right-wing parties with the left in 'permanent' opposition. For the first 30 years (until 1975) a rapid economic growth permitted the growth of a network of institutions together constituting a welfare state apparatus. In this period the fundamental idea was that, as the national cake increased, each individual share would be increased even if a certain degree of inequality would remain.

The arrival in power of Giscard d'Estaing coincided with the slowdown in the rate of growth and the realisation that not much had changed in 30 years. It is therefore not surprising that official ideology shifted from promoting social justice to the elaboration of a notion of 'merited justice' wherein each should receive according to the *value* of her/his work. Distributive justice would interfere with the functioning of the economy. Instead state interventions should be limited, according to Stoleru (1978) – principal ideologist of the regime and political advisor to the president, Giscard D'Estaing – to fighting absolute poverty.

This refurbished ideology – one could hardly call it new – was supported by various social movements. The new social strategy is characterised by the reintroduction of capitalist logic into social policies. It is interesting that the existing evidence suggests that prior to this new approach, there has been some narrowing in social differences since the beginning of the 1970s.

The situation has, in principle, changed radically since the Socialist Party came to power in 1981. Until then, the inequality theme was used by the left in opposition as a big stick with which to beat the government especially as they could show that inequalities in France were possibly the worst in Europe. It is, of course, difficult to know what has happened in the last five years but a recent colloquium organised by groups close to the governing Socialist Party (Les Inégalités Sociales en France) (reported in *Le Monde* for 6 March 1985) concluded that '. . . far from being reduced, inequalities are widening in France since the beginning of the crisis' (rough translation).

Social inequalities in the area of health
In the specific case of inequalities in health, there have been shifts during the 1970s. Thus, the VIth Plan (1971–75) went further than the previous Plans in emphasising collective services, primary prevention and priority actions in favour of particularly vulnerable social groups. The VIIth Plan (1976–80) was very different from its predecessors in concentrating on individual prevention. The business representatives, indeed, had begun to propose cut-backs in expenditures on health services.

Around this time, the trade unions began to develop a more global analysis of the development and maintenance of inequalities. For a workshop organised by the Association Santé et Socialisme in 1975 the preparatory text presented inequalities as a fall-out from the process of profit accumulation. The report by one of the organisers, Dr. Robin, was more sophisticated claiming that inequalities are produced by the nature of social relations and the living conditions of individuals.

Since the mid-1970s whilst the left-wing opposition emphasised the way in which health questions are part and parcel of the social system, the government tended to dissociate health service policies from the totality of state interventions. Moreover, health policies were made subordinate to financial limitations so that, for example, out of an ambitious programme of health education directed towards disadvantaged groups, the actual activities were a series of advertising programmes.

With the arrival of the left in power one might have expected at least a series of important reforms. In fact, after a brief honeymoon period, the policies of the socialist government became more prudent and similar to preceding administrations: economic expansion, 'fighting' inflation, and modernisation of information technology. Hence, the perceived necessity among socialist militants to organise a colloquium in 1985.

This overall U-turn is reflected in the domain of health care policies. Promises about increasing the reimbursable part of dental and opticians fees were not kept, the list of non-reimbursed medicines was increased and a daily hospital fee was introduced.

Inequalities in health have, however, not been absent from official preoccupations. Reference is made to the WHO target of 'Health for All by the Year 2000' in both the Health Charter of March 1982 and the IXth Plan published in December 1983. The concern appears, however, to be more a question of protecting against criticism than effective policies. It is worth contrasting the statements of the new Minister when commenting upon the introduction of a daily hospital payment 'we have to take account of economic realities' with his earlier arguments that 'we have to do everything to make inequalities in health disappear. Along with the inequalities in educational opportunities, they are the most intolerable. I'm surprised that the unions haven't already gone on strike' (reported in Badiou, 1985, pp. 225–6). In fact, of course, the main concern of the Socialist Government has been to reduce health care expenditure.

The scientific approach
The nature of debate on a scientific level generally depends on the political regime. The French case is very interesting where, despite data existing on differential mortality by socio-professional category and on medical consumption, social policies have hardly been affected.

Thus, the data on medical consumption comes from the enquiries conducted by INSEE (Institut National de Statistiques et Etudes Economiques) and CREDOC (Centre de Recherche et de Documentation sur la Consommation). They were probably then motivated by worries about increasing expenditure on health care. The longitudinal study on differential mortality conducted by INSEE was launched in 1955 with a sample of 464,000 men aged 30 to 69 and 328,000 wives. It appears to have been motivated more for methodological reasons so that, when the first report appeared in 1965, two-thirds of the text was concerned with methodology (Calot, February 1965).

Nevertheless, the overall results showing that the gap between the extreme categories (teachers and unskilled manual workers) is very large and that this is because the most at-risk group are more affected by tuberculosis, alcoholism, accidents and suicides, rapidly became integrated into official discourse. It is as if everyone found it more comfortable to support a belief in equality before death.

The extent of social inequalities in mortality, which were progressively better understood as INSEE continued to produce analyses, became a sort of ritual reference point in any scientific discussion of the health of the French population without implying any political action to rectify them nor even any further scientific research into the causes.

The lack of research is probably due to:
— the strict division between INSEE (the data gatherer) and

INSERM (Institut Nationale de la Santé et Recherche Medicale (the analyser) with the latter reluctant to include 'social class' (categorie socio-professionelle) in the analysis;

— the state of French epidemiology which is dominated by the medical profession or by mathematical statisticians;

— the weak development of social sciences and of sociology in particular, and the lack of interdisciplinary research.

Whatever the reason, the lack of analyses on the cause and the process has led to a certain reification of the results.

Indeed, since the first results were published, the question of social inequality in death has sometimes been presented almost as a moral problem contrasting teachers with the longest life expectancy with unskilled manual workers with the shortest (Desplanques, 1976). The teacher is presented as a model of virtue, with a well ordered and sober life which should be imitated by others. Implicitly, therefore, death can be postponed by individual moderation more than by the possession of power and wealth.

It is surprising that these kinds of arguments are supported by authors such as Sauvy '. . . income is not the essential factor, when it can be separated from the cultural factor . . .' (preface to Surault, 1979) or Charlot '. . . to live better, people should become teachers . . .' (Charlot, 1976, p. 60).

At the same time, given the existence of the studies on medical consumption, there has been a paradoxical temptation to ascribe the social inequalities in death to the disparities in medical consumption. Many authors imply that the inequalities in death can be explained by an insufficient or poor utilisation of health services. Given the simultaneous concern with reducing the growth in health expenditure, this has led to the emphasis on better accessibility and health education for the disadvantaged groups. The research has been peculiarly subservient to the needs of the dominant class.

The political and scientific debate on inequalities in health in the UK
The National Health Service

The debate in Britain can only be understood in the context of the inception of the National Health Service in 1948. The creation of the NHS (National Health Service), following the *Beveridge Report* in 1942 (Cmd 6404), represented an important part of the post-war settlement between capital and labour, and 'Aneurin Bevan drew enormous strength from labour in his struggles to set up a truly accountable service. Yet the organisation of the class politically and ideologically was insufficient for it to force itself upon the way in which the NHS was created' (Corrigan, 1977). As a result the final structure of the NHS was determined by the outcome of negotiations between the state and various establishment groups – the voluntary hospitals, the former approved societies and, most importantly, the leaders of the medical profession. The consultants as a group were able to maximise their control over the practice of medicine.

The White Paper introducing the NHS declared that

> The Government . . . want to ensure that in future every man, woman and child can rely on getting all the advice and treatment which they may need in matters of personal health; that what they get shall be the best medical and other facilities available; that their getting these shall not depend on whether they can pay for them, or any other factor irrelevant to real need (Ministry of Health, 1944).

Thus, a major justification for state intervention in health care which has been repeated ever since that 1944 White Paper has been the attainment of some kind of equality – whether of treatment, of access or of health itself. Moreover, the lack of scientific discussion on the subject from the end of the Second World War until the middle of the 1970s suggests that many thought it was no longer a problem.

From administrative solutions to the Black Report

The political concern with inequalities in health has concentrated almost exclusively on the geographic maldistribution of health care resources. Thus, one of the main arguments of Bevan against a local government health service was the fear of 'perpetuating a better service in the rich areas, a worse service in the poorer'. Yet the system ended up by simply controlling inherited local budgets which of course 'favoured most the authorities who shared the least degree of financial responsibility in the early years of their service (Guillebaud, 1956). At the same time, the NHS did succeed in reducing disparities in medical manpower between regions (Honigsbaum, 1979).

The concern resurfaced with Crossman (1972) which eventually led to the introduction of a resource allocation formula to even up the distribution of funds between Hospital Boards (DHSS, 1976) and eventually to the RAWP formula introduced in 1977–78 – thirty years after the foundation of the NHS. Klein (1983) suggests that this delay can be accounted for by the 1950s being a period of consolidation of the infant NHS and the period from 1960 to 1975 as being one technocratic change. It seems equally likely to suggest that a bureaucratic service will never, *per se*, be interested in the reduction of inequality but that the development of their own management tools may, of itself, stimulate debate.

The RAWP report itself clearly addresses the problem of equity in access to health care and relates this to the objective of equality in

health. They '. . . sought criteria [which would be] responsive to need
not supply or demand' (DHSS, 1976: para. 3). Of course '. . . even if
geographical variations were "eliminated", it does not follow that
other variations would be' (RSHG, 1977, p. 5). They aimed to assess
need in terms of morbidity levels and variations and to *measure* those
by standardised mortality ratios.

In the mid-1970s, however, concern arose at '. . . Britain's failure
to match the improvements in health observed in some other countries
. . .' (Townsend and Davidson, 1982, p. 14), and some felt that the
relative worsening of Britain's position in the world league table of
infant mortality (from eighth in 1960 to fifteenth in 1978) was due to
the persistence of inequalities. Indeed, the Department of Health and
Social Security themselves emphasised in 1976 that international
comparisons suggested that '. . . there is ample scope for improvement . . .' (DHSS, 1976, Chapter IV, p. 45) and arguing that '. . .
socio-economic factors seem to be of great importance . . .' (ibid, p.
57).

Pressures such as these led to the establishment of a Working
Group on Inequalities in Health under the chairmanship of Sir
Douglas Black in 1977. But the lack of public discussion during its
period of deliberation (1977 to 1980) is curious and suggests that it
was never intended to become part of the policy formation process
even by the Labour Government who set it up.

The *Black Report* was published in August 1980 showing that,
despite more than 30 years of a National Health Service committed to
offering equal care for all, there remained a marked class gradient in
standards of health. Specifically, there are marked differences in
mortality rates, so that, for example, 'those in unskilled manual
workers' families are four times more likely to die in their first year of
life', and differences in self-reports of long-standing illness and
inequalities in the utilisation of health and preventive services.

They made a wide range of proposals, but Patrick Jenkins, the new
Secretary of State for Social Services, called the recommendations
'. . . quite unrealistic in any present or foreseeable economic circumstance . . .'. He attempted to 'hide' the findings by restricting
circulation of the report but this backfired, and instead the issue
received wide publicity. For example, summaries of the report were
published by the trade unions (e.g. TUC, 1981), in professional
journals (e.g. Deitch, 1981), and by public health workers (e.g.
Radical Community Medicine, 1980).

It is tempting to conclude that the political debate in the UK is not
due to any change in the material circumstances – the inequalities
themselves – but to the cavalier treatment of the *Black Report* allied to
the search for some stick with which to beat the Conservative Party.

Scientific fashions and ideologies

Of course, data on occupational differences in mortality have existed since the beginning of the century, based on the decennial censuses, showing considerable inequality. But, during the recent period, whilst there was a growing body of research in medical sociology, much of the work was qualitative, conducted within the interactionist paradigm and did not bear directly upon the comparative health status of different population groups. Nevertheless, it should also be noted that the researchers at the Office of Population Censuses and Surveys (OPCS) started a major longitudinal study in order to analyse mortality differentials based on a one per cent sample from the 1971 Census. Whilst the first report was not published until 1982 (Fox and Goldblatt, 1982), the existence of the study during the 1970s was itself a comment on the importance of the inequality debate.

Scientific investigation and research into inequalities has therefore been on the agenda for over 50 years. The sudden upsurge around 1980 is obviously associated with the political fervour around the *Black Report*. Thus, in the following year the Secretary of State was forced to elaborate on his very brief introduction to the *Black Report*. In a speech at Cardiff, he drew attention to what he considered to be the Black Report's three principal shortcomings: first it did not adequately explain the causes of inequalities in health and therefore its enormously expensive programme of recommendations could not be accepted; second, he denied that 'new evidence' disproved the thesis that the working class suffered poorer access to health services; and third, there was no evidence that more money would make any difference.

The Introduction to the Pelican edition of the *Black Report* discusses and refutes these arguments at some length (pp. 19–31, and much of the subsequent research has been within this framework (see Carr-Hill, 1987). For example, the Working Group had emphasised materialist or structuralist explanations of inequalities in health (Townsend and Davidson, 1982, pp. 21–2). This has led to a flourishing of studies of the deprived and particularly of the unemployed, relative to a previous focus on the developmental health of children. Moreover, the emphasis on an aetiology of 'multiple deprivation' also has an implicitly ideological baggage, emphasising the individual deprivation and denying the social nature of inequality (see Carr-Hill, 1985).

But the report also made two other important claims which influenced the nature of the debate in the UK. First, that there has been an *increase in inequality*. The evidence presented by the *Black Report* itself showed that the widest gap was at the beginning of the 1960s, and others have disputed that claim (e.g., Illsley, 1987; Le

Grand, 1985). But that belief has certainly been an object of research. Second, that Britain is *lagging behind*. This viewpoint has focused on infant mortality and perinatal mortality rates because of the acknowledged difficulty of allowing for different and changing age structures (e.g. CSO, 1985, p. 27). The Social Service Committee drew attention to this in 1980 but Macfarlane and Mugford (1984) remain unconvinced that 'The international position of England and Wales is so completely unsatisfactory' (p. 245).

It looks suspiciously as if scientific debate flourishes only when convenient to powerful interest groups, playing a uniquely ideological role. More subtly, the existence of the NHS since the Second World War has precluded the discussion of many important aspects of the economic and social forces determining inequalities in health.

References
France
Badou, G. (1985), *L'Etat de Santé*, Paris, Buchet – Chastel.
Calot, G. and Febvay, M. (1965), 'La mortalité differentielle suivant le milieu social: Presentation d'un methode experimentée en France sur la periode 1955–1960, Premiers resultats', *Etudes et Conjunctures*, 11 November, pp. 75–159.
Charlot, M. (1979), *Vivre avec la mort*, Paris: Moreau.
Desplanques, G. (1976), *La mortalité des adultes selon le milieu social, 1955–1971*, Collections INSEE, Serie D, n. 44.
Stoleru, L. (1978), *L'équilibre et la croissante economique*, Paris: Dunod.
Surault, P. (1979), *L'inéqalité devant la mort*, Paris: Economics.

UK
Beveridge, W. (1942), *Social Insurance and Allied Services* London: HMSO (Cmnd 6404).
Carr-Hill, R.A. (1985), 'Distribution of and inequalities in health', *Radical Community Medicine*.
Carr-Hill, R.A. (1987), 'The inequalities in health debate: a Critical Review of *Class and Health* and of the *Decennial Supplement*', in *Journal of Social Policy*, **16**, (4), pp. 509–42.
Central Statistical Office (1985), *Social Trends 15*, London: HMSO.
Corrigan, P. (1977), 'The welfare state as an arena of class struggle', *Marxism Today*, **21**, (3), March, p. 91.
Crossman, R. (1972), *A Politician's View of Health Service Planning*, University of Glasgow.
Deitch, R. (1981), 'The Debate on the Black Report', *The Lancet*, 18 July.
Department of Health and Social Services (1976), *Sharing Resources for Health in England*, Report of the Allocation Working Party, London: HMSO.
Fox, A.J. and Goldblatt, P.O. (1982), *Socio-Demographic Mortality Differentials: Longitudinal Study, 1971–75*, Series L.S. no. 1, London: HMSO.
Guillebaud, G.W. (1956), *Committee of Enquiry into the National Health Service*, London: HMSO, Cmnd. 9663.
Honigsbaum, F. (1979), *The Division in British Medicine*, London: Kogan Page.
Illsley, R. (1987), 'Rejoinder to Richard Wilkinson', *Quarterly Journal of Social Affairs* 3.
Klein, R. (1983), *The Politics of the National Health Service*, London: Longman.
Le Grand, J. (1985), *Inequalities in Health: The Human Capital Approach*, Welfare State Programme Pamphlet No. 1, London: LSE.

Macfarlane, A. and Mugford, M. (1984), *British Counts: Statistics of Pregnancy and Childbirth*, **I, II**, London: HMSO.
Ministry of Health (1944), *A National Health Service*, London: HMSO (Cmnd. 6502).
Radical Community Medicine (1980), *The Black Report* (4), Autumn.
Radical Statistics Health Group, *RAW (P) Deals*, London: Radical Statistics Group, c/o British Society for Social Responsibility in Science.
Townsend, P. and Davidson, N. (1982), *Inequalities in Health*, Harmondsworth: Penguin.
Trades Union Council (1981), *The Unequal Health of a Nation: a TUC Summary of the Black Report*, London: TUC.

3 Policy issues in health inequality
Alex Scott-Samuel and Julia Szalai

Introduction

This chapter discusses a survey on policy issues in health inequality carried out in the first few months of 1986. We do not claim to cover comprehensively the wide range of issues concerning inequalities in health and their bearing on policy. However, we feel that for a number of reasons a consideration of these issues is an essential part of any discussion of inequality.

Firstly, the choice of inequality itself as a subject for research implies a concern about its existence. The word is not chosen arbitrarily: it is equally possible to study 'variations' or 'differences' without the implication, carried by 'inequalities', of departures from a more desirable state (of equality). In other words, the concept of inequality is not value-free. While we would argue that all research takes place in a context of socially constructed values, it is especially clear that research in a 'value-laden' area such as inequality cannot be divorced from its implications for policy.

Despite this, our area of study is one that has hitherto received relatively little attention from researchers. It is only in the last two decades that the health of Europeans has reached the crucial level of development when attention begins to turn from overall advances in the public health to the examination of differential levels of attainment and of their social implications. As a public health physician and a medical sociologist respectively, we are both aware that many such issues which inhabit the 'grey area' of the interface between science and policy are only just beginning to be clarified.

The social context of research and policy is in part also responsible. The medical model of health as the absence of disease, which dominates the health systems and policies of most European countries, has created the tendency for health research to be seen primarily as medical research, and even for social research in health to be narrowly focused on the social distribution of individual diseases or the economic costs of health care systems. Research which addresses social models of health has in general been slow to develop, has remained poorly funded by comparision with medical research, and has largely been kept at a distance from the agencies (government departments, health authorities) and individuals (doctors, politicians) that influence policy.

A recent initiative which is helpful in focusing the common health policy objectives of European countries is the approach to 'Health For All by The Year 2000' taken by the World Health Organisation's (WHO) Regional Office for Europe. Having adopted in 1981 a regional strategy for health for all, its member countries in 1984 endorsed a set of 38 targets and a provisional list of 65 detailed indicators for monitoring progress towards their achievement (Targets for Health for All 1985). Thus there is now, for the first time, a mutually agreed set of objectives and a broad, common policy framework for acheiving them throughout the 33 countries comprising the WHO's European Region.

Of particular relevance to the present discussion is what the Director-General of WHO describes as the 'central preoccupation' with equity in health. The theme of reducing health inequalities is one which runs throughout the European strategy, and which forms the first of its 38 targets: 'By the year 2000, the actual differences in health status between countries and between groups within countries should be reduced by at least 25%, by improving the level of health of disadvantaged nations and groups'. The strategy makes it clear that health inequality is conceptualised broadly in dimensions ranging from mortality and morbidity through health services expenditure and distribution to health behaviour and education, and housing and working environments. Socio-economic, gender and geographical inequalities are among those explicitly addressed.

The policy context required if 'Health For All' is to be achieved is made very clear – it is one of an 'actively participating community' against a background of 'effective legislation and permanent machinery' to ensure 'multisectoral coordination' between all government and other agencies concerned with health-relevant areas. Examples of such areas include physical planning, housing, industry, agriculture, transport, energy production and environmental protection. International cooperation is also emphasised. In the specific context of equity, the strategy calls for:

> willingness in recognising the problem, for initiative in actively seeking information on the real extent of the phenomenon, and for political will in designing social policies that go to the roots of social group formation, in terms of guaranteed minimum income, assurance of the right to work, active outreach services to assist the groups in need etc.

The survey

The survey was designed against the backcloth we have described, coupled with our own awareness of relevant issues in our respective countries (Szalai, 1986; Scott-Samuel, 1986) and of issues discussed at

Table 3.1   Responses to the survey on policy and health inequality

Sample	Sample size (%)	Responded (%)	Declined to respond (%)	No reply received (%)
ESF Workshop participants	30 (100)	18 (60)	5 (17)	7 (23)
Extended sample	45 (100)	8 (18)	10 (22)	27 (60)

Table 3.2   Countries represented by respondents (where more than one response the number is shown in brackets)

Sample	Countries represented			
ESF Workshop participants	Denmark	Finland	France	Greece
	Hungary	Israel	Norway	Spain
	Sweden	United Kingdom (6)		
	West Germany		Yugoslavia	
	TOTAL = 17 (6 UK, 11 others)			
Extended Sample	Hungary	Italy	New Zealand	
	United Kingdom (5)			
	TOTAL = 8 (5 UK, 3 others)			

the previous European Science Foundation (ESF) Workshops on Health Inequalities. Our aims were twofold: to obtain factual information from respondents on the handling in their countries of the major policy issues relating to health inequality and to allow them to express their views on these issues and on the appropriate responses. The questionnaire is shown in the Appendix 3A. It was sent to all 30 participants in the ESF Workshops, and in addition to 45 others known to us to be involved in this field of study, in order to extend the sample and to provide more detailed information relating to the United Kingdom. Respondents were given one month to reply, after which a reminder was sent. In all 18 of the ESF participants (60 per cent) and 8 of the extended sample (18 per cent) replied to the questionnaire (Table 3.1.). Two of the ESF participants produced a joint response, so that there were 25 responses in all.

The countries represented among the replies are shown in Table 3.2. One of these (New Zealand) is not a member country of the ESF or of the WHO European Region.

The aim of the survey was to address the broad policy questions posed by the existence of health inequality – questions which are, on the whole, common to all developed countries. It did not attempt to bring out in detail the specific ways in which particular inequalities had arisen and been dealt with in particular countries. These will clearly show enormous variation, reflecting the varying social, economic and political histories of countries; the same will be true of the development of their health care systems. The survey was therefore designed to answer questions common to all, while allowing respondents also to refer to those issues and agencies which they felt were relevant in their country.

Survey responses

Predictably, there was substantial variation in both length and quality of individual responses. This variation doubtless reflects differences in the degree of knowledge of respondents and in their interpretation of particular questions, in addition to genuine between-country variation in the actual situations. We would not therefore claim that this limited survey of a small and possibly unrepresentative sample could yield an accurate and comprehensive picture of policy issues in health inequality in Europe. Rather, we present our impressions of issues, problems and opinions illustrated in the survey by respondents from specified countries. Where possible we have quantified particular responses to questions and shown the total numbers of clear answers to that question among the 25 responses. We then go on to look in greater detail at the policy setting in one country (England).

The numbers and titles of the paragraph headings below correspond with those in the questionnaire, but the appendix should be consulted for the full details of questions.

1. Concepts of health inequality in policy

1.1 Is the reduction of health inequality a policy objective?
This fundamental question was mostly interpreted in terms of current government policy in the country concerned. Clear answers were as follows:

> United Kingdom (UK) respondents : Yes 3 No 6
> Other respondents: Yes 9 No 5

Some of the issues raised by this question can be seen in the following responses:

> To answer this question, it is necessary to distinguish between political rhetoric and evidence of a real commitment to implement policies which could have an impact on reducing differentials in the quantity and quality of life. (UK)

It is assumed that the problem of equal health care has been resolved by providing general access to the health system by establishing an insurance system. (W. Germany)

The main target must be to increase equality between different population groups by creating equal opportunities for all for the prevention and treatment of disease. (Health Policy Report) (Finland)

1.2 Is it seen as the responsibility solely of health agencies?
The majority of respondents answering "yes" to question 1.1 answered "no" to this question.

UK: Yes 1 No 2
Others: Yes 1 No 8
The general improvement of health conditions is not regarded as the sole responsibility of the health agencies. Regulations in other fields, eg food and nutrition, work environment, traffic and road conditions, pollution and housing standards are examples where other agencies have the formal responsibility but clearly consider health effects. Indirectly I would say that much of this regulatory framework functions in an equalising way since the bulk of the regulations are universalistic (the compulsory safety belt) or have the objective of eradicating the worst conditions (work environment legislation).

I guess you can also find counter examples. Furthermore, recent deregulatory trends (for instance in the field of housing) combined with changing roles for central authorities towards more advisory and educational effort and a general decentralisation of the policy-making process may result in adverse effects on health inequalities. It points to the importance of singling out not only general health improvement, but also reduction of health inequalities as a manifest objective and not only a latent function of universalistic welfare policies. (Sweden)

It is both the responsibility of official health agencies (eg Government Health Department) as well as of other agencies ... Among the non-health agencies are voluntary organisations, trade unions, political parties, self-help groups, women's organisations, mass media programmes, educational and research institutions. (Greece)

1.3 How is health inequality conceptualised by these agencies?
Differences in health state measures between social groups or geographically : deaths (of various kinds), low birthweight, breast feeding, immunisation take-up. (UK)

The regional aspect has been emphasised, especially since the early 1970s and perhaps the main aim in this area has been to provide equal access to the health services all around the country. Differences in income have also been considered and, consequently, a free primary health care system has been created. . . . Occupational health differences have been the main reason for a rapid development of occupational health care, starting from the occupations carrying greatest risks. (Finland)

The basic concept is the principle of solidarity executed at the level of work organisations, communes, regions, republics, provinces and the Federation which is contributing to the reduction of health inequality. Through this form of mutual assistance are satisfied all joint needs which cannot be equally provided for . . . because of different work and earning possibilities, level of economic development and different conditions of life and work. (Yugoslavia)

As a right for all citizens to greater and more equal access to health care; as a right to more services for citizens in need (eg the chronically ill). It is the expression of a political ideology of greater equality. (Greece)

By and large we can say that health inequality is conceptualised in terms of redistribution of health-related resources. This means that the emphasis is input-oriented rather than output-oriented. (Italy)

1.4 What dimensions of health inequality are considered in policy debate?

Probably area inequalities are more important in the public discussion than any other form of inequality and it is probably the only one which is measured and where action is actively taken : class (or income) inequalities are always discussed at a very non-specific level. Sex inequalities have been put into the political arena by the women's movement (especially abortion-related issues) and by government agencies (legal entitlement issues). (Spain)

Non-governmental debate : race, gender, occupation, social class, housing tenure, region/locality, language. Governmental debate: locality (occasionally). (UK)

The policy goal is equity, not equality, in order to

- decrease social class gradients
- support policies for access to services irrespective of age, sex, race, geography, social class
- make available stated minimal levels of a wide range of basic requirements of life (New Zealand)

1.5 Do policies aimed at reducing health inequality explicitly consider the influences of non-health policies?

UK: Yes 3 No 4
Others: Yes 7 No 3

Health is seen as a result of multisectoral cooperation in a participating community. (Norway)

Relevance of non-health policy is only considered by private individuals and voluntary groups. (UK)

The reduction of all inequalities (not differences) is a welfare goal. Reduction of non-health inequalities is then beleieved to reduce health inequalities. Right now we have a debate on the health aspects of the agricultural policy. It is not directly geared towards the inequality issue, though. (Sweden)

Reducing health inequality is seen as the responsibility of health as well as non-health agencies . . . statements often tend to go further than action, especially in areas where there are obvious conflicts between the interests of health and non-health agencies. The fat content of milk, relative prices of butter and margarine are examples where the interests of agricultural and health agencies are in conflict, resulting in decisions which do not appeal to the health agencies. (Finland)

Non-health policies are discussed in local authority/health authority liaison groups (where these exist): environment, housing, employment, transport. (UK)

1.6 Are policies on health inequality universal or selective?
UK: Universal 1 Selective 1 Both 1
Others: Universal 2 Selective 2 Both 5

Some new measures have been taken to guarantee access to care to those unemployed without benefits. Therefore a move to selective rather than universal policies can be identified. Unlike Britain it should be noted that there is a poor tradition of means-tested benefits (or even of social benefits). Therefore the selective measures taken by the present government can be felt as progressive steps by some strata of the population. (Spain)

They are both. Examples of universal policies are those related to the emphasis on primary health care (redistribution and reallocation of resources). Examples of selective policies are related to chronic illness (for instance, individuals who have thalassaemia have the right to enter university with no examinations), to the provision of health insurance to students, and to the financial support offered to agencies who employ handicapped persons. (Greece)

. . . there is near-total, egalitarian coverage and access for curative health care, irrespective of income. . . . Recently, the disparities in health status between Jewish and Arab Israelis have attracted some attention, with special programmes being set up to focus on improving health services for Arabs. (Israel)

Selective and universal, e.g. improving environment and service delivery in deprived areas; improving levels of immunisation, cardiovascular disease, smoking and alcohol consumption, drug abuse. (UK)

1.7 Do policies distinguish between deprivation and inequality?
UK: Yes 2 No 5
Others: Yes 6 No 1

Yes; over the last few years there has been more emphasis on deprivation and less on inequality, leading to wider disparities. (UK)

Yes, but the stress is on inequality. Even measures taken to ameliorate deprivation are often universalistic in character. (Sweden)

Yes. Measures have been taken for the deprived in relation to health insurance, access to and use of health services. Other policies relate to the reduction of inequality. More emphasis is given to the former. (Greece)

Owing to a lack of Government policy in this area, it is difficult to say whether such minimalist policies as there are distinguish between deprivation and inequality. Broadly speaking it would appear that they are more concerned with deprivation than with inequality. (UK)

Such little attention as the subject receives is concerned with deprivation. Inequality does not cause concern. (UK)

1.8 Is multiple deprivation a target of policy?
UK: Yes 6 No 1
Others: Yes 7 No 1

Sometimes, e.g. for the young uneducated unemployed and for single mothers. (Denmark)

Multiple deprivation was of particular interest in the 60s, both in terms of individuals or families and regions or areas with heavy disadvantages. An attempt was made to develop a social ?work repertoire at the individual level and state subsidies to industries and local government and active labour market policies were tried in the disadvantaged regions. Local government subsidies were even given to scarce personnel categories like medical doctors in those areas.
Interest in dealing with this form of clustered problems has diminished, I would say, both at the individual and regional levels. The rather non-precise policies attempted in the 1960s and early 70s have probably not resulted in any major change in the level of disadvantage. (Sweden)

Yes, it is – for instance, the disadvantages of migrants. Policies are aimed both at individuals and at groups. (Hungary)

In social support services multiple deprivation is strongly emphasised. In other areas of policy the question has received much less attention, especially regarding individuals. Geographical areas with several disadvantages have been more widely discussed. (Finland)

Policies aim to solve the problems of individuals and of groups. . . . An example of deprived groups are the Romes (gypsies) with a traditional orientation to the nomadic way of life. A number of measures taken by the community to change this way of life most frequently remain without success. (Yugoslavia)

Multiple deprivation is a favourite phrase in Britain, I suspect because of its victim-blaming connotations. It is often taken to mean 'undeserving poor' and to justify policies of surveillance and policing, e.g. of attendance at 'preventive' health facilities; or as a reason for non-take-up of preventive services. At the same time, evidence of the physical health problems of prisoners, social work clients etc. does not seem to have been taken on in policy terms, i.e. the improvement of services offered to these groups. So I am sceptical of any reality behind statements about multiple deprivation, in terms of intent to change policy. In Scotland, the SHARE scheme for health service resource allocation may be a bit more successful in diverting resources to multiply-deprived *areas*. (UK)

2. Objective of policy

2.1 To what extent are policies concerned with changing behaviour/improving access/broader policy objectives?

Individual behaviour change: very much so in health education – smoking cessation, dieting, exercise, keeping warm in winter *rather than* taking on tobacco promotion, agricultural subsidies, food policy, heating costs and state benefits. Access to health care: very little. Still designed to suit the providers on the whole, e.g. centralised antenatal clinics. Social and economic policy: not at all. (UK)

They often speak about changing individual behaviour to reduce health *costs*, not health inequality. (Hungary)

Health education at national and local level focuses on changing individual behaviour: diet, exercise, smoking, alcohol and drug consumption are the targets.
Access to services is rarely a problem but policy aims to ensure adequate provision and the location of primary care services in deprived areas . . .
Local authorities endeavour to improve environment, housing, transport. Positive discrimination channels more resources into deprived areas.
. . . Health improvement is normally a positive albeit secondary aim.
National policies are located for the most part in health departments. Economic policies may be inconsistent with health policies, e.g. financial support for Skoal Bandits [tobacco-chewing sachets] factory in Scotland. (UK)

Policies to reduce health inequalities have been concerned mainly with improving access to medical care. This has been the traditional orientation. Broader policy objectives have also been discussed, whereas changing individual behaviour has not generally been seen as a relevant method for reducing health inequalities. (Finland)

2.2 Is there a clear distinction between improving health and reducing health inequality?

UK: Yes 0 No 4
Others: Yes 1 No 8

Which is given greater priority?

UK: Improving health 6 Reducing inequality 0
Others: Improving health 5 Reducing inequality 2

Policies are mainly aimed at improving health, via changes in health practices and lifestyle. Nevertheless it is recognised that the greatest potential for improvement lies in groups with the worst health characteristics. Some groups more readily accept health messages. Efforts to improve service delivery have effected significant improvements in, for instance, perinatal deaths in all social groups, but had little effect on the differentials between them. (UK)

Policies are more or less exclusively aimed at improving health. (UK)

Improving health is given greater priority, similar to the way this has happened in Britain. (Hungary)

No, not a clear distinction. Given our general societal setting today I would say that the overall improvement of health is given greater priority. This standpoint of mine is however based on a knowledge base where there is no evidence of *expanding* health inequalities and very little evidence which can be used to describe existing inequalities as great. If such information existed, the priorities might be different. (Sweden)

Which do you think is more important?

. . . it all depends on what type of progress you wish to make – it doesn't seem very positive to attempt to reduce inequalities in health by a levelling-down process. It might be better to allow them to increase if this happened in the process of major improvements overall. There is no final answer to this one. Only philosophical and ideological ones. (France)

Income redistribution – my favourite policy – does not pose the problem. (UK)

I think improving health is more important than reducing health inequality. The former has impact on the population as a whole or at least a rather big stratum of the population. (Hungary)

For me, inequality-reducing policies are the best way to achieve overall health improvement since they ensure that the most needy are dealt with first. (UK)

In my view, inequality of health should be a policy objective, and I would therefore regard policies developed within an egalitarian framework as being the more desirable. (UK)

My opinion is both. (New Zealand)

I believe that the concept of inequality can be broken down into major components (e.g. cost, access, treatment, outcome). To reduce these inequalities I would support policies of positive discrimination (more to people worse off). This must be done not just in the health sector but in all those sectors influencing people's opportunities, power, information etc. We *must* do this within a policy framework inspired by *universal* policy philosophy, otherwise selective or targeted policies could go hand in hand with cost-containment goals (where the main policy objective could become just that of economising). (Italy)

2.3 Is the reduction of health inequality a realistic policy goal?
UK: Yes 7 No 0
Others: Yes 7 No 3

Depends on economic conditions. Health inequalities are bound to occur with economic inequalities. (Denmark)

Yes – in the sense that societal conditions affect health status and that some of these conditions change and are changeable over time. (Sweden)

There is considerable scope for diminishing health inequality by improving citizenship equalities. My policy priorities would be:
(i)   Making health a political issue by establishing the Health Education

Council as a fully independent body (free of government and medical domination) with much greater resources to carry out research, evaluate existing policies and publicise findings.

(ii)   Much more redistributive tax and benefit system.

(iii) Concerted attack on the normative symbols of civic inequality (public schools, House of Lords etc.) to create an ideological framework which challenges rather than sanctions the idea that social inequality is natural and therefore legitimate. (UK)

The reduction of some forms of health inequality is a realistic policy goal. This applies particularly to *regional* and – to a lesser extent – *social* inequalities in *access to health services. Regional* differences in *morbidity, survival and mortality* should also be possible to reduce considerably. *Socioeconomic morbidity and mortality differences* can be reduced but not abolished. (Finland)

It is not realistic but it must always be there as a goal and go as far as possible, including as many aspects as possible. (Greece)

The reduction of health inequality (concerning underutilisation in the lower classes) is desirable, but politically not realistic, since the aim of health politics presently is to reduce costs. . . . (W. Germany)

Definitely. With an adequate policy, strict implementation in practice of planned measures, and the engagement of the community as a whole, inequalities could be reduced to a great extent. (Yugoslavia)

Yes. Only relatively modestly in capitalist societies – though a continuing gradualist approach involving intersectoral policies relevant to health (economic, housing, agriculture, transport) could go a long way. (UK)

Reducing health inequalities is the major public health task now facing most industrialised societies, similar to the control of infectious diseases in the 19th century. It would be a major opportunity to attempt the application of scientific and social–scientific knowledge in an area of social planning where a clear outcome measure can be designated. It would seem to me an area where a nation might achieve major advances, with implications far beyond the health field. (UK)

It should be a goal with the understanding that it will be an unattainable objective. (New Zealand)

The only limit to the reduction of inequality is the political will. (UK)

Of course the reduction of health inequality is a realistic policy goal. . . . It must not be seen just as a health policy goal but as a moral goal. . . . It would be impossible to eliminate *differences* in health status which can be explained by physiological reasons . . . but we can drastically reduce *inequalities* in health. (Italy)

3. The policy process
3.1 Is health policy treated entirely separately from other aspects of social policy?
UK: Yes 6 No 1

Others: Yes 1 No 6

There is no linkage made between health policies and policies in other areas of life. (Israel)

The aim of health policy is to add years to life, health to life and life to years. This requires that more attention be given to the promotion of health and to the health approach in general social policy. (Health Policy Report 1985) (Finland)

3.2 What is the role of non-governmental agencies in reducing health inequalities?

There is no such institution. All institutions and all activities concerned with the way of life and conditions of work, and the health of the population in general, belong to the social system. (Yugoslavia)

It depends on the government. Trade unions are important under Labour governments; voluntary organisations are to some extent under the Conservatives. At present all such agencies are merely exhortatory since the government is not interested in reducing inequality. (UK)

Generally speaking voluntary organisations, community groups, trade unions and political parties outside Government have shown little interest in reducing health inequalities. However, in recent years, some UK community groups and some opposition political parties have begun to give priority to thinking in this area. (UK)

Considerable, and with political/public blessings. (New Zealand)

They haven't any role, unfortunately. (Hungary)

Voluntary organisations and community groups help pick up the pieces. Trade unions and political parties act as pressure goups. (UK)

Non-governmental agencies such as trade unions, academics, political parties and groups within the National Health Service are important as pressure groups. (UK)

The role of NGOs is very important as lobby groups in the policy-creating process but very minor in service delivery . . . (Sweden)

I think that they have a considerable importance, but there are also plenty of non-governmental interests and groups which operate in the opposite direction to reinforce health inequalities (tobacco interests, dairy industry etc). (UK)

Governmental agencies clearly play a more important role in reducing health inequalities. Perhaps the most significant exception to this concerns developments in occupational health where trade unions have been very active. (Finland)

Apart from being lobby groups, they participate by making proposals to official agencies, sensitise people by making widely known aspects which have not been considered, organise self-help groups etc. (Greece)

4. Policy implications of health inequality

4.1 Which areas of health inequality require further research before the policy implications become clear?

The fact that the concept (of inequality of access) appears so often in governmental documents and elsewhere indicates its importance as an objective for social policy in the health field; but its imprecision means that it offers little by way of clear implications for that policy.

. . . it seems necessary to use large samples to establish on a statistical basis what are the principal factors in the socio-economic environment that affect health. . . . Much of the data necessary to resolve (policy) issues is likely only to be available from longitudinal studies . . . once the basic statistical relationships have been established, it will be desirable to explore in depth, necessarily using a much smaller sample, exactly the way in which the factors indicated operate.

. . . it seems important to establish the relative importance of medical care as an influence on health states . . .

. . . there has been no overall study of the reasons for differences between social classes in their utilisation of health care services . . .

Obvious issues . . . concerning (the effects of) inequalities in *health* include (their effect) on employment, income, quality of life and other aspects of living. The impact of inequalities in health on attitudinal differences between groups also seems a potentially fruitful area. The principal issue so far as *health care* is concerned is presumably the extent to which inequalities in health give rise to different needs for health care and inequalities in health care contribute to inequalities in health.

. . . extensive research on the effects of different institutional structures on inequalities in health and health care [is needed]. In this connection, international comparisons are likely to be very useful.

Another more specific proposal is an investigation of the effects of the recommendations of RAWP . . . it would be of interest to explore the effects both on the reallocation of health care resources and on the variables that the reallocation was intended to affect (such as mortality rates).

. . . what is the impact on inequalities in health of social policy directed at other ends (for instance, pensions policy)? .. . what is the impact of health policy directed at other ends on inequalities in health (e.g. anti-smoking campaigns that have a greater impact on the better off and hence actually widen health inequalities)? . . . what are the political and other impediments to policy-making in this general area? (Le Grand, 1986). (UK)

. . . interest seems to be focusing on the size of (particularly class) differentials and the direction of change as regards these differentials. Such data don't exist at present. (Sweden)

. . . I belive enough is understood now of the most significant causal mechanisms to design policies to counter health inequality. In general I feel the most important goal for research in this area is to reveal the truly *social* nature of health and personal welfare. This must also involve research to demystify the contribution of medicine to health in the contemporary world. (UK)

Time trends in inequalities; inequalities in survival (rather than only in incidence); the process whereby inequalities emerge and their social determination from one generation to the next; action research. (Finland)

Relation of level of education to health. Relation of mortality to occupation. Relation of personality, social and cultural characteristics to health behaviour and to the demand for health services. (Greece)

The assumption that egalitarian access to services is the decisive factor in determining health status is widespread. Not until this assumption is analysed is there likely to be research, debate or action on the level of national consciousness. (Israel)

Inequalities between men and women, especially as this applies to work-related conditions. (UK)

The most pressing area for further research concerns the significance of work for health expectations. By this I mean to include not only unemployment, but also working conditions, working practices, and job satisfaction. (UK)

It is doubtful if much further research is required to establish the facts. There is considerable scope for the application of present knowledge. (UK)

The input and output elements of various policy options; exploration of and research on methodologically sound policy-making approaches to introduce change and innovation in health-related sectors with the aim of reducing health inequality. (Italy)

4.2 What are the major non-health areas where policy actions could reduce health inequality?

Impossible to say without talking about the types of inequality. If you're talking about mortality, then it would be those factors which might be the cause of excess mortality: in particular, structural and collective factors – work hazards, income, housing, etc. . . . and in France those which may have contributed to the lowering of alcoholism. (France)

Economic inequalities. (Denmark)

Income distribution and welfare benefits. (UK)

Housing and education. (Finland)

The educational/cultural level. Occupational/economic status. (Greece)

Such areas include education, culture, physical culture, public utility policies, housing policy, food, water supply. (Yugoslavia)

Economic/employment policy, housing, transport, food and agriculture, environmental control (pollution, health and safety), social security. (UK)

Urban planning to reduce accidents to children, which are the major source of class inequality at certain ages. Health and safety at work. The UK should have an active labour market policy, as in Sweden, to avoid the present extreme concentration of unemployment. Care of the chronically ill and disabled. (UK)

Policy action could reduce health inequality in the fields of housing, food production and distribution, a drive against poverty (e.g. by provision of a national minimum wage), alteration in practices throughout industry and commerce (e.g. concerning advertising and publicity for unhealthy products). (UK)

Income policy (redistribution of wealth); employment policy (but with emphasis on the quality of job – I am sceptical about the narrow British objective of full employment *per se*); equal opportunities for education, housing and leisure. I believe that we should pay far more attention to the *ends* of our policies rather than, as often happens, to their *means*! (Italy)

5. Information
What kinds of information are used in making policy on health inequality?
Scientific and official publications concentrate on mortality statistics. (France)

Mortality statistics provide by far the most powerful evidence. (UK)

All examples mentioned in the question; material from ongoing so-called level of living surveys, i.e. self-reported information on health problems and utilisation of health care, has become more important recently. (Sweden)

Studies based on linking census data with death certificate data; surveys concerning diagnosed health impairments, perceived health, opinions about health care etc; other mortality and morbidity studies. (Finland)

Universal directions, for example WHO targets, and political–ideological programmes. Opinion surveys may help to some degree as well as some research results for specific problems. (Greece)

One can have complete equality of access, while social conditions can create considerable inequality in health status. This is most dramatically seen in the data on Israeli/Muslim/Arab infant mortality rates, which are 22.1 compared with 11.6 for Jews. No real socio-economic status data are available. Area differences, other than those which reflect Arab-Jewish differences, show no general patterns. . . . There is work on Jewish ethnic differences, which largely focuses on differential mortality from different diseases. (Israel)

'Mortality, census data, ad hoc health surveys, General Household Survey, National Food Survey, General Practice Morbidity Survey data, ad hoc clinical research with social class data.' (UK)

Mortality statistics, hospital data, surveys, foreign literature. (Hungary)

In Italy the information used is confined to mortality and morbidity data and data on health expenditure and use of services. I believe that in this area we could give more space to subjective indicators. (Italy)

6. Further relevant comments
One of the underlying problems is that you pressume that health policies

are rational. It seems to me that one needs to write quite a lot about why policies are predominantly irrational. (UK)

Official policy and health inequality in England 1980–1986

The views of the 11 respondents from the United Kingdom which are summarised in the previous section give an indication of its recent history and 'policy climate' regarding health inequality. This section covers these issues in more detail, in order to demonstrate more clearly some of the barriers which require to be overcome in order to make progress towards equity in health. Because of differences which exist between the policy mechanisms in the constituent countries of the UK, it refers only to England.

The debate on health inequality during the 1980s has been dominated by the 'Black Report' on Inequalities in Health (*Inequalities in Health*, 1980), which was commissioned in 1978 by a Labour government, but reported in 1980 to a Conservative government which was clearly less sympathetic to the issue than was its predecessor. The report documented substantial UK and international evidence on social and other inequalities in health and health care, and recommended a radical programme of social and economic reforms to address the material inequalities it identified as their primary cause. In his Foreword to this report, the then Secretary of State for Health, Patrick Jenkin, stated:

> It will be seen that the Group has reached the view that the causes of health inequalities are so deep-rooted that only a major and wide-ranging programme of public expenditure is capable of altering the pattern. I must make it clear that additional expenditure on the scale which could result from the report's recommendations – the amount involved could be upwards of £2 billion a year – is quite unrealistic in present or any forseeable economic circumstances, quite apart from any judgement that may be formed on the effectiveness of such expenditure in dealing with the problems identified. I cannot, therefore, endorse the Group's recommendations.

Both this summary dismissal of the report and the manner of its publication (a few hundred photocopied typescript versions were released by the Department of Health) provoked a major public reaction, culminating 2 years later in the publication of a shortened version by a commercial publisher (Townsend and Davidson, 1982) which became an immediate best seller. The introduction to this version, which was co-written by one of the Black Report group's members, contested both the Government's costing of the report's programme and its disregard of the many cost-free recommendations it contained.

The government's response to the controversy created by its rejection of the Black Report was at first to quote research findings, from both Department of Health (Burchell, 1981) and independent researchers (Collins and Klein, 1980), which contradicted some of the report's conclusions (Patrick Jenkin, speech at Cardiff, 13 March 1981). However, no regard was subsequently paid to work which demonstrated the inadequacy of these studies (Scott-Samuel, 1981; Townsend and Davidson, 1982: Studies quoted in Introduction to *Inequalities in Health*). Since this period the offical response has changed relatively little. A Department of Health (DHSS) perspective on the Black Report in 1985 echoes strongly Mr Jenkin's original response:

> . . . many of the recommendations of the Working Group would be immensely expensive, and the Government is not convinced that expenditure on the scale envisaged would necessarily be effective, even if it could be afforded. (DHSS, 1985).

The government's position had perhaps been made most clear by its then two senior health ministers during an earlier parliamentary debate on inequalities in health:

> Overlying all the specific problems mentioned in the Black Report is the central issue of the view taken by the different political parties not only of the needs of the Health Service but of how those needs are to be met. The Government believes that the first essential is to base policy upon an economic strategy, which has resulted in lower inflation, which in itself must aid industrial recovery and which, in its turn, will provide the resources for health care. We reject policies that merely put us back on the road to higher inflation, which will affect the resources that can go to the NHS and the lives of most of those with whom the Black Report is concerned. (Norman Fowler, Secretary of State, House of Commons *Hansard*, 1982, col. 614)

> There are inequalities, there have always been inequalities but there should not be such great inequalities between social classes. (Kenneth Clarke, Minister for Health, House of Commons *Hansard*, 1982, col. 671.)

Despite the paucity of official research and action on health inequality in the 1980s (and partly because of it) many research studies and policy reviews have been undertaken (Scott-Samuel, 1986), often funded by local authorities or voluntary organisations, and the nature of many of the issues is clearer now than when the Black working group's report was published.

The WHO Regional Strategy, to which we referred in the Introduction, has once again placed the issue of inequalities in health on the political agenda. The official reaction has been instructive: the DHSS has stated that 'the UK Government is fully committed to the strategy of achieving Health For All by the Year 2000' in its initial response to WHO (DHSS, 1985). However, this response refers to the fundamental WHO theme of social equity in health only in terms of geographical inequalities in resource allocation. One table of infant mortality by social class is included, but without any commentary. The wealth of information available from successive Decennial Census Occupational Mortality Supplements is entirely excluded. A further DHSS summary of the UK response to the European Regional Strategy, is notable for making no mention whatever of equity in its four pages – despite its claim that 'Differences between UK policies and the strategy relate to differences of emphasis and relative priority between objectives rather than to any fundamental differences of principle' (DHSS, 1986). A possible explanation for this ambivalence is suggested by a *Lancet* correspondent, reporting on the WHO European Regional Committee's first evaluation meeting on the Strategy: 'It is not clear how much [the] publicly cautious stance of officials acting for uninterested Ministers and an even less enthusiastic Government differs from the officials' own enthusiasm for action (Turner, 1985).

The publication in July 1986 of the Occupational Mortality Supplement to the 1981 Census (OPCS, 1986) has further fuelled the debate. For the first time, virtually all of the data on social class are available only on microfiche (and thus inaccessible to the general reader), with only a brief commentary in the main report. This is attributed to weaknesses in the data (especially those for social class 5) resulting from changes in the Registrar-General's Classification of Occupations. But such changes have never in the past prevented the publication of social class data – accompanied by 'bridge-coding' exercises to demonstrate the effects of the new classification. Furthermore, some indication of the trends in social class mortality differentials could have been given by combining data for social classes 1+2 and 4+5 (Anon, 1986), or for all non-manual and all manual workers (Anon, 1986; Marmot and McDowall, 1986). The facts that such exercises demonstrate widening class inequalities, and that one such exercise was published elsewhere simultaneously with the Occupational Mortality Supplement, by its chief author (Marmot and McDowall, 1986), have added to the suspicion that the data were effectively suppressed because their conclusions were unpalatable to government. Indeed, the *British Medical Journal* took the unusual step of publishing some of these allegations in an editorial provocatively titled 'Lies, damned lies and suppressed statistics' (Anon, 1986).

Like the Black Report, publication of the Occupational Mortality Supplement was delayed until the parliamentary recess, thereby limiting the scope for immediate public debate. But in a letter to a Member of Parliament who had asked, prior to the recess, if he would implement the recommendations of the Black Report the then Minister for Health, Mr. Barney Hayhoe, confirmed that 'there is nothing I can usefully add to what my predecessor, Kenneth Clarke had to say on this subject' (Hayhoe, 1986). However, it seems clear that the continuing social inequalities in health will remain a controversial issue of public policy – assisted further by the publication in September 1986 of a report, co-authored by a member of the Black Report Committee, detailing wide inequalities in health and deprivation between the electoral wards of the Northern Health Region (Townsend, Phillimore and Beattie, 1986).

Commentary on the survey

Our aim has been to allow the responses we have presented to 'speak for themselves' in drawing attention to relevant issues of policy, practice and research; nevertheless, some general observations are appropriate.

Reducing health inequality seems to be a policy objective in most of the countries surveyed. Responses were largely concerned with official government policies, reflecting the fact that the areas of social policy perceived as determining health inequality are chiefly influenced by governmental action. An awareness of the importance of non-health policies is clearly seen in many of the countries.

Concepts of health inequality vary from a narrow focus on equalising resource inputs (with the associated implication that equal resources mean equal health outcomes) to a broad aim of equality of health for all (seen typically in the Scandinavian countries).

The debate on *universal or selective policies* seems to some extent to be a function of particular social systems; however, it is clear that economic recession has not entirely prevented the making of policies affecting whole populations. Nonetheless, the identification of health-deprived groups is clearly a popular way for health policymakers to express concern about inequality.

A wide range of *policy approaches* was apparent – though policies dependent on individual behaviour change were much the commonest, reflecting the predominance of the medical model of health care. This clearly has implications for the ability of countries in which such approaches predominate to seriously tackle health inequalities rooted in broader social/economic inequalities. Even countries with a more sensitive appreciation of the roots of inequality did not appear to make a clear distinction between health policy and health inequalities policy, however. The actions of WHO in attempting to clarify these issues (*Social Justice and Equity in Health*, 1986) are clearly of importance.

Equity in health was seen as a *realistic aim*, albeit one crucially dependent on the political will. Economic inequality was the barrier most frequently identified (with redistributive policies most often mentioned as the means to overcoming it).

Despite the major potential role of governments in promoting equality, there was clearly an important role in many countries for *non-governmental organisations* – particularly as pressure groups, but also in initiating action themselves.

Although the *research* needs posed by health inequality are many, varied and interesting, both specific comments and the general content of responses to the overall questionnaire show that action to reduce inequalities does not need to await their outcome. Enough is known at the level of broad policy to attack inequality here and now, given the political commitment. A consensus clearly exists around the non-health areas where action is required.

Information is a key issue both in identifying and monitoring areas for policy action. A commitment to achieving equity in health is a prerequisite to researching and developing the necessary information systems, and to publicising widely their output in order to stimulate debate directed towards further policy development.

Some concluding observations

In concluding, we return inevitably to our introductory comment that all scientific research takes place in a context of socially constructed values. The problems that some participants found in responding to our survey are in themselves a criticism of science (and especially of medical science) that seeks to divorce itself from its social context. Hand in hand with policies to achieve equality in health must go the development of a social epidemiology that acknowledges, examines and explicitly reflects the values that determine it. The WHO strategy for social equity in health is one means to achieving this, and its universal endorsement by European governments, although clearly only a tentative first step (Illsley and Svensson, 1986) must give us major cause for hope. Ultimately these governments must acknowledge the radical social reforms and genuine public participation in policymaking to which they have committed themselves. It is appropriate to conclude with the words of one such government which has already commenced this process:

> Economic and other social policy aimed at increasing social security and reducing inequality works in the same direction as the goals of health policy. The great differences in health between social groups in Finland call for active social and health policy to level out these differences (Health Policy Report, 1985).

References

Anonymous (1986), 'Lies, damned lies, and suppressed statistics', *British Medical Journal*, **293**, pp. 349–50.
Burchell, A. (1981), 'Inequalities in Health: analysis of the 1976 General Household

Survey', Government Economic Service Working Paper no. 48, Economic Adviser's Office, DHSS.

Collins, E. and Klein, R. (1980), 'Equity and the NHS: self-reported morbidity, access and primary care', *British Medical Journal*, 281, pp. 1111–15.

DHSS (1985a), Reply to AGM Resolution on Black Report, *Community Health News*, no. 11, London: Association of Community Health Councils in England and Wales.

DHSS (1985b), 'United Kingdom's Evaluation Report of the Strategies for Health for All by the Year 2000', (unpublished).

DHSS (1986), 'The European Regional Strategy and the UK', Paper given at meeting on 'Health for All by the Year 2000 – Implementation of Strategies at Local Level', Leeds.

Hayhoe, B. (1986), Letter to Laurie Pavitt MP, 4 August.

Health Policy Report by the Government to Parliament (1985), Helsinki: Ministry of Social Affairs and Health.

House of Commons Hansard, 6 December 1982, col. 614.

House of Commons Hansard, 6 December 1982, col. 671.

Illsley, R. and Svensson, P–G. (eds) (1986), 'The Health Burden of Social Inequities', Report based on the proceedings of a WHO meeting, Copenhagen, 5–7 December 1984, Copenhagen: WHO Regional Office for Europe.

Inequalities in Health (1980), Report of a Research Working Group, DHSS (Black Report).

Le Grand, J. (1986), 'Inequalities in health care – a research agenda' in R.G. Wilkinson (ed.), *Class and Health: Research and Longitudinal Data*, London: Tavistock Publications.

Marmot, M.G. and Mcdowall, M.E. (1986), 'Mortality decline and widening social inequalities', *Lancet*, 2, pp. 274–6.

Office of Population Censuses and Surveys (1986), *Occupational Mortality Decennial Supplement, 1979–80, 1982–83*. Part 1: Commentary. Part 2: Microfiche tables. London: HMSO.

Scott-Samuel, A. (1981), 'Social class inequality in access to primary care: a critique of recent research', *British Medical Journal*, 283, pp. 510–11.

Scott-Samuel, A. (1986), 'Social inequalities in health: back on the agenda', *Lancet*, 1, pp. 1084–5.

Social Justice and Equity in Health (1986), Report on a WHO meeting, Leeds, 22–26 July 1985, Copenhagen: WHO Regional Office for Europe.

Szalai, J. (1986), 'Inequalities in access to health care in Hungary', *Social Science Medicine*, 22, pp. 135–40.

Targets for Health for All (1985), Copenhagen: World Health Organisation Regional Office for Europe.

Townsend, P. and Davidson, N. (eds) (1982), *Inequalities in Health*, The Black Report, Penguin.

Townsend, P. and Davidson, N. (eds) (1982), Studies quoted in Introduction to *Inequalities in Health*, The Black Report, Penguin.

Townsend, P., Phillimore, P. and Beattie, A. (1986), *Inequalities in Health in the Northern Region*, Newcastle: University of Bristol and Northern Regional Health Authority.

Turner, J. (1985), 'Europe's objectives', *Lancet*, 2, pp. 734–5.

Appendix 3A   European Science Foundation Workshops On Inequalities in Health: Survey On Policy And Health Inequality

Please answer all questions from the specific position of your country

1. Concepts of health inequality in policy

1.1   Is the reduction of health inequality a policy objective in your country?

1.2   It is seen as the responsibility solely of health agencies? (For instance, Government Health Department; Local Health Authorities.) What other agencies also share this responsibility? Please list all health and non-health agencies which have the reduction of health inequality as a policy objective.

1.3   How is health inequality conceptualised in the policies of the agencies listed in 1.2?

1.4   What dimensions of health inequality are considered in policy debate in your country?

1.5   Do policies aimed at reducing health inequality explicity consider the influence of non-health policies? (For example, economic, housing, transport, food/agricultural policies.) If so, which non-health policies are considered? How are they considered?

1.6   Are policies on health inequality *universal* or *selective?* What arguments are used for and against each of these principles? Please give examples from the last 5 years.

1.7   Do policies distinguish between *deprivation* (improving the lot of those 'at the bottom of the scale') and *inequality* (equalising the position of all)?

1.8   Is 'multiple deprivation' (the combination of several specified disadvantages) a target of policy? Please state which particular disadvantages are considered. What is the policy response to multiple deprivation? (For example, are policies aimed at *individuals* with several disadvantages or at *areas* where several disadvantages are known to be prevalent?)

2. Objectives of policy

2.1   To what extent are policies to reduce health inequality concerned with:

  (i)   Changing individual behaviour?
  (ii) Improving access to health care?
  (iii) Broader social/economic/other policy objectives?
  Please illustrate your answers with examples.

2.2 Is there a clear distinction between policy aimed at *improving health* and at *reducing health inequality*? Please give examples if possible. Which is given greater priority? (For example, in Britain the first of these goals has greater priority in relation to smoking, where health education has reduced overall morbidity-/mortality while increasing inequality, since there is a direct relationship between cessation and social class.)
  Which of these goals do *you* think is more important? Why?

2.3 Do you think that the reduction of health inequality is a realistic policy goal? If so, how far do you think that inequality can be reduced?

3. The policy process

3.1 Is health policy generally treated entirely separately from other aspects of social policy?

3.2 What is the role of non-governmental agencies in reducing health inequalities? (For example, voluntary organisations, community groups, trade unions, political parties outside government.)

4. Policy implications of health inequality

4.1 Which areas of health inequality require further research before the policy implications become clear?

4.2 What do you consider to be the major non-health areas where policy actions could reduce health inequality?

5. Information

What kinds of evidence/information are used in debating/formulating policy on health inequality? (For example, mortality statistics; opinion surveys; census data.)

6. Please add any further relevant comments you may have.

Thank you for answering this questionaire
Dr Julia Szalai, Dr Alex Scott-Samuel

PART II
DIFFERENCES IN
MORTALITY

4 An international comparison of distributions of ages-at-death
Julian Le Grand

Demographers, epidemiologists and medical sociologists have long collected mortality data from various countries to engage in international comparisons of mortality of various kinds. These have been generally used to construct mortality rates, or indicators that are functions of mortality rates such as Standardised Mortality Ratios (SMRs). Sometimes SMRs or their equivalents are constructed for different social groups within the countries concerned, in order to assess and to compare the 'social' inequality in mortality (Black, 1980; Preston, Haines and Pamuk, 1981; Pearce *et al.*, 1983; Lynge and Andersen, (Chapter 8).

Here we use the same data to compare variation in the age at death between different countries. The inequality involved is of a rather different kind from the 'social' inequality (that is, the disparities in the mortality experiences of different social groups) measured in the other studies. The methodology is derived from that used, chiefly by economists, in the international comparisons of other dimensions of economic and social inequality, such as income or wealth (see, for example: Ahluwalia, 1974; Wiles, 1974; Sawyer, 1976; UK Royal Commission on the Distribution of Income and Wealth, 1977; Morrison, 1984; Quan and Koo, 1985).

The paper begins with a brief description of the methodology. Then the results of applying the methodology to 32 developed countries are presented and some of their implications discussed. Finally, some observations are offered on the differences between this approach to measuring inequality in mortality and some of the other approaches.

Individually-based inequality measurement
The choice of age at death reflects our desire to select an indicator of mortality that can be attached to individuals, in a way that, for instance, income or wealth holdings can be attached and for which a distribution can be constructed. Our interest is then to look at the spread of this indicator across the community.

To illustrate the kind of distribution involved, Figure 4.1 shows the distributions of age-at-death in 1982 for England and Wales and Poland. It will be observed that they are rather different in shape from

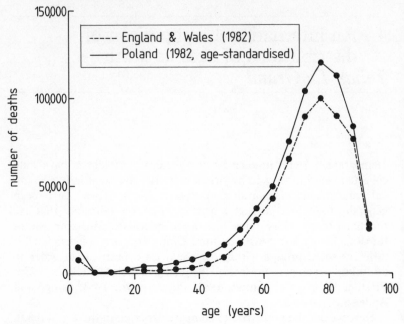

Figure 4.1   Age-at-death distributions

the distributions of other dimensions of inequality, such as income or wealth. In particular, unlike those distributions, these are bimodal, with a low peak at a very early age (representing infant mortality) and a much higher peak in later years. Moreover, each distribution is bounded by biological limits, in a way that has no parallel in income and wealth distributions.

The way in which the information available concerning the distribution of individuals' ages-at-death can be summarised in an inequality measure can be illustrated with reference to a simple example using the most commonly used measure: the Gini coefficient. Consider a population of four individuals, one of whom dies at birth, one who lives for 25 years, one who lives for 50 years and one who lives for 75 years. The total years of life for this population is 150 years. We can therefore draw up a cumulative percentage distribution for this population as in the table below.

From this table we can draw a 'Lorenz' diagram of the type illustrated in Figure 4.2, where the diagonal line represents an equal distribution (everyone dies at the same age) and the curved line, the Lorenz curve, the actual distribution as in the table. The area between the actual distribution line and the diagonal, expressed as a proportion of the total area under the diagonal, is a measure of the divergence

Table 4.1   Cumulative percentage distribution of age-at-death

Individual	Age-at-death	Cumulative percentage of population	Cumulative percentage of population
1	0	25	0
2	25	50	16.7
3	50	75	50
4	75	100	100

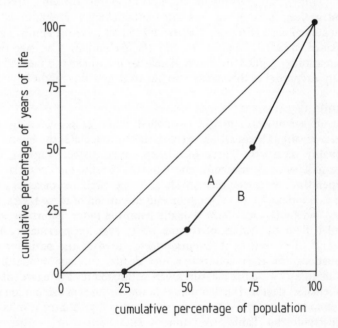

Figure 4.2   A Lorenz curve

from complete equality: this measure (A/[A + B] in the diagram) is the Gini coefficient. As is clear from the diagram, the Gini coefficient can only take on values between zero, corresponding to complete equality (A = O in the diagram), and one, corresponding to 'complete' inequality (B = O). For the particular distribution in Table 4.1, it is 0.417.

The Gini coefficient is, of course, not the only measure that can be constructed using this kind of data and approach. Others include the variance, the coefficient of variation (the variance divided by the mean), the Absolute Mean Difference or AMD (the Gini coefficient multiplied by the mean) and the recently developed class of 'social welfare' measures, such as the Atkinson or Kolm indices (Atkinson, 1970; Kolm, 1976). Each of these measures has different properties, and the choice between them will depend on the properties desired. This is discussed in more detail in Illsley and Le Grand (1987).

This methodology has been applied to the problem of measuring changes in inequalities in mortality within the same country over time (Illsley and Le Grand, 1987; Le Grand and Rabin 1986). There have also been some interesting, although, as explained in Illsley and Le Grand (1987), rather different, attempts to address the same problem by integrating the summary statistic methodology with that based on occupational class (Preston, Haines and Pamuk, 1981; Pamuk, 1985; Koskinen, 1985). However, as yet, the techniques have not been systematically applied to international comparisons; the task of the research reported in this paper is to illustrate how this might be done.

Results

Data on age-at-death for 32 developed countries provided by the World Health Organisation were used to calculate three sets of inequality measures. Three inequality measures were chosen: one 'scale-independent' measure, the Gini coefficient; one 'translation-independent' measure, the AMD; and one 'welfare' measure, the Atkinson index (for an explanation and discussion of these terms, see Illsley and Le Grand, 1987). For the Atkinson index, estimates were calculated for two values of the inequality aversion parameter, 0.75 and 1.25. Two sets of distributions were used as the basis for the calculations for each country: actual deaths and age-standardised deaths. In each case the measures were estimated for aggregate (males plus females) deaths. Further details of the methods of calculation can be found in Appendix 4A, as can the country-by country results for aggregate deaths (Tables 4A.1 and 4A.2).

Table 4.2 summarises the results. It was constructed by ranking the countries according to their AMD value and grouping them into three broad categories; where relevant, footnotes indicate how their categorisation would change if they were ranked according to either of the other measures.

It is notable that the rankings, admittedly in terms of these very broad categorisations, are fairly insensitive to the choice of inequality measure. So far as the actual distributions are concerned, the ranking is invariant for over two-thirds of the countries (23 out of 32) whichever inequality measure is chosen; the Gini coefficient gives the same ranking as the AMD for all but two of the countries; the

Table 4.2 *Mortality inequality, all ages: summary*

Ranking by AMD	Actual		Standardised	
Lowest Third (10)	Austria[1]	GDR	Czechoslovakia[7]	Luxembourg
	Denmark	Luxembourg	Eire	Netherlands
	England & Wales	Norway	England & Wales	N. Ireland
	FRG	Scotland	Finland	Scotland
	Finland[2]	Sweden	GDR	Sweden
Middle Third (11)	Belgium	Hungary	Australia	Iceland[8]
	Bulgaria[3]	Italy	Belgium	Italy[3]
	Czechoslovakia	Netherlands	Bulgaria	Japan[6]
	Eire[3]	N. Ireland	Canada	Norway
	France	Switzerland	Denmark[8]	Switzerland
	Greece[4]		FRG	
Highest Third (11)	Australia	Portugal	Austria[1]	Portugal
	Canada[5]	Romania	France[1]	Romania
	Iceland[1]	Spain	Greece	Spain
	Japan[1]	USA	Hungary	USA
	New Zealand	Yugoslavia	New Zealand	Yugoslavia
	Poland		Poland	

AMD = Absolute Mean Difference
FRG = Federal Republic of Germany
GDR = German Democratic Republic

Notes
1. Middle third by Atkinson Index (e = 0.75, 1.25)
2. Middle third by Gini coefficient
3. Highest third by Atkinson Index (e = 0.75, 1.25)
4. Highest third by Atkinson Index (e = 1.25)
5. Middle third by Atkinson Index (e = 1.25)
6. Lowest third by Gini coefficient and Atkinson Index (e = 0.75, 1.25)
7. Middle third by Gini coefficient and Atkinson Index (e = 0.75, 1.25)
8. Lowest third by Atkinson Index (e = 0.75, 1.25)

Source: Tables 4A.1 and 4A.2.

Atkinson index for e = 0.75 gives the same ranking for three-quarters of the countries, and, for e = 1.25, for two-thirds. For the standardised distributions, again the rankings are insensitive to the choice of inequality measure for nearly two-thirds of the countries (22); the Gini coefficient again gives the same ranking as the AMD for all but two, while the Atkinson index, for both parameter values, gives the same ranking as the AMD for 22 countries.

Looking at the results for specific countries, we can make the following observations. For all three inequality measures, except the Gini coefficient for Finland, the Scandinavian countries are consistently in the lowest third for the actual distributions. However, the standardised estimates for Norway, and, according to the AMD and the Gini, for Denmark and Iceland, puts these countries down a category, suggesting that their relatively low actual inequality was in part due to their age distribution. England and Wales and Scotland appear to have relatively low inequality in both actual and standardised deaths. Standardisation moves both Northern Ireland and Eire from the middle to the lowest category, again with the exception of the standardised Atkinson measure for the former. Of the Benelux countries, Belgium is the only one not to appear in the lowest category. The two Germanies are both in the low category for the actual distributions, but standardisation suggests that, for the FRG, this was in part due to its age distribution. Standardisation moves Czechoslovakia from the middle to the lowest category; Bulgaria remains in the middle category, as does Italy; standardisation moves Greece into the highest category.

Looking nearer the bottom of the table, New Zealand, Portugal, Romania, Spain, the United States and Yugoslavia exhibit relatively high inequality, regardless of inequality measure or standardisation. In New Zealand's case this may be due to the relatively high infant and child mortality that characterises the Maori minority. Standardisation shifts Hungary and France (except according to the Atkinson index) from the middle to the highest category, while the reverse is true for Australia and Canada. Standardisation moves Austria from the lowest to the highest category (except according to the Atkinson index); the reverse is true for Japan, at least according to the Gini coefficient.

It is of interest to examine the extent to which these differences arise because of differences in mortality at different ages. In particular, since these measures of disperson are likely to be particularly sensitive to infant and child mortality, it is important to ascertain the extent to which a country's relative position depends on these factors.

Accordingly, the same inequality measures were calculated for each country, first, excluding infant (0–1) deaths, thus measuring non-infant inequality and, second, excluding all deaths at age twenty and below, thus measuring adult inequality. The results are given in Table 4A.3 in the Appendix. Table 4.3 summarises those for the AMD.

Perhaps the most striking feature of Table 4.3 is how few differences there are between the rankings and those for the standardised AMDs in Table 4.2. Two-thirds of the countries remain in the same category for all three types of inequality. For these countries, it would appear that infant or child mortality are not among the principal factors determining their position in terms of relative inequality.

Table 4.3 Mortality inequality, non-infant and adult: summaries

Ranking by AMD	Non-Infant		Adult	
Lowest Third	Czechoslovakia Eire Eng. and Wales GDR Greece	Luxembourg Netherlands N. Ireland Scotland Sweden	Bulgaria Czechoslovakia Eire Eng. and Wales GDR	Greece Luxembourg Netherlands N. Ireland Scotland
Middle Third	Belgium Bulgaria FDG Hungary	Italy Japan Norway Spain Yugoslavia	Australia Belgium FRG Norway Italy	Japan Portugal Spain Sweden Yugoslavia
Highest Third	[Denmark, Finland, New Zealand][1]			
	Australia Austria Canada France Iceland	Poland Romania Switzerland Portugal USA	Austria Canada France Iceland	Hungary Poland Romania Switzerland USA

AMD = Absolute Mean Difference
FRG = Federal Republic of Germany
GDR = German Democratic Republic

Note 1. These three had the same AMD value for non-infant mortality, above those in the middle category and below those in the highest category.

Source: Table 4A.3.

Of the remainder, the major differences concern the Southern European and Scandinavian countries. More specifically, the position of the Southern European countries markedly improves in Table 4.3 relative to Table 4.2. Greece moves from the bottom third to the top third in both cases, suggesting that its high overall inequality is due very largely to high infant mortality. Yugoslavia and Spain move from the bottom third to the middle category, again indicating the influence of infant mortality on their overall inequality.

So far as the Scandinavian countries are concerned, Finland drops from the top group and joins Denmark and Norway in the second group for both non-infant and adult inequality; for adult inequality, Finland and Denmark indeed actually move to the borders of the highest inequality group. Sweden also moves from the first to the second group for adult inequality. This is interesting – and perhaps surprising – given the fact that all four countries were in the lowest group as far as actual aggregate inequality is concerned, and given the apparent egalitarian nature of Scandinavian society in other respects. It suggests that the reasons for their relatively low actual inequality include both their age structure and their relatively low infant and child mortality. So far as adult health inequality is concerned, and when differences in their age structure are taken into account, they do not do so well.

Two other points are worthy of note. The first concerns Switzerland, which drops from the second to the third category for both non-infant and adult inequality – again a somewhat surprising outcome given its egalitarian reputation. The second concerns New Zealand. This rises to the borders of the second category for adult inequality, offering some confirmation of the thesis that its high overall inequality is due in part to relatively high child mortality.

The prime aim of this paper has been to examine measures of dispersal. We conclude, however, with a brief discussion of the relationship between these measures and estimates of mean mortality, such as the (standardised) mean age-at-death and the Standardised Mortality Ratio. These are given country-by-country in the Appendix Tables 4A.1 and 4A.2; actual mean age-at-death in 4A.1 and standardised mean age-at-death and the SMR in 4A.2. Their rankings are summarised in Table 4.4 below.

The interesting feature of these sets of rankings is the *difference* between them and the inequality rankings. Comparison of Table 4.4 with Table 4.2 reveals that just over half the countries fall into the same category for the mean and the AMD and only just over a third for the SMR. The extent of dispersion in mortality apparently bears little relationship to mean mortality. Although there is no necessary relationship between the mean and measures of dispersion, this conclusion nonetheless seems rather surprising – not least because in other dimensions of inequality, such as income and wealth, countries with high means tend to have relatively low inequality.

To explore this further, and to examine the relationship between inequality and socio-economic factors, a regression exercise was carried out, the details of which are reported in Le Grand (1987). Standardised AMDs were regressed against the standardised mean age-at-death and a number of socio-economic variables, including per capita GNP, per capita medical expenditures, the proportion of medical expenditures that were publicly funded and a measure of economic inequality. The results confirmed the absence of any significant relationship between mean age-at-death and inequality in mortality. But there was a significant positive relationship between mortality inequality and economic inequality and a significant nega-

Table 4.4:   Mean mortality, all ages: summary

	Mean age-at-death		SMR	
	Eire	Norway	Australia	Japan
	GDR	Portugal	Canada	Netherlands
Highest	Greece	Spain	Greece	Norway
Third	Japan	Sweden	France	Sweden
	Netherlands	Switzerland	Iceland	Switzerland
	Austria	Finland	Austria	Italy
	Czechoslovakia	Iceland	Belgium	Luxembourg
Middle	Belgium	N. Ireland	Denmark	New Zealand
Third	Denmark	Italy	Eng. and Wales	Spain
	Eng. and Wales	Scotland	FRG	USA
	FRG		Finland	
	Australia	New Zealand	Bulgaria	Poland
	Bulgaria	Poland	Czechoslovakia	Portugal
Lowest	Canada	Romania	Eire	Romania
Third	France	USA	GDR	Scotland
	Hungary	Yugoslavia	Hungary	Yugoslavia
	Luxembourg		N. Ireland	

SMR = Standardised Mortality Ratio
FRG = Federal Republic of Germany
GDR = German Democratic Republic

tive relationship between GNP per head and mortality inequality, suggesting that richer and more equal countries economically are also more equal in terms of mortality. Perhaps more surprisingly, there was a positive significant relationship between mortality inequality and per capita medical expenditures; but there was no significant relationship with the proportion that was publicly funded.

The limitations of the data and the absence of a systematic explanatory framework mean that too much should not be made of the results. However, they are suggestive and, at the least, offer interesting guidelines for future research into determinants of inequality.

Conclusion: Some general issues

Perhaps the best way to appreciate the advantages and disadvantages of this approach to measuring inequalities in mortality is to understand what it does and does not do. What it *does* is to measure the variation in mortality within the population as a whole. What it *does not do* is measure differences in mortality between sub-groups of the population: between social classes, between genders, between regions, etc. (It can, of course be used to measure inequality *within* these sub-groups, but that is a different question.) This has the advantage that the method of measurement is therefore independent of the definitions of these groups; an advantage that is particularly acute in the context of international comparisons. However, it carries with a number of features that some might find less attractive.*

One set of criticisms relates to the issue of causality. It could be argued that, unlike, say, comparisons between social classes, the approach offers no insight into determinants of inequality in health. The inequality measured could be caused by genetic, social, economic or demographic factors; all are embraced within the measure. Carr-Hill (1986) has gone further and argued that the approach actually supports a genetic view of the determinants of inequality, presumably because of the absence of any reference in the calculations to class or other socio-economic factors.

But here a number of points arise. First, it seems better in general to separate the question of causality from the question of measurement. Measurement is, after all, only a form of description; and it could be argued that it is more scientific to describe the phenomenon to be explained before attempting the explanation itself. Second, the fact that inequalities in health as measured this way may in part be genetically determined does not imply that they are wholly or largely so determined, any more than the comparison of different gender mortality rates (another form of measuring inequality)implies that the inequalities so revealed are solely genetic. In fact, the approach is completely neutral towards the relative importance of different determinants – a point reinforced by the fact in the extensive controversy surrounding the extent to which inequality in earnings was genetically or environmentally determined, the use of summary statistics as a method of measuring that inequality was never at issue (see Goldberger, 1979, for a useful summary of the literature, as well as a powerful refutation of the geneticists' case).

Third, although the measures themselves offer no direct indication of causality, there are ways in which they can be used to illuminate the question. Certain inequality measures can be 'decomposed' to provide an analysis of inequality within and between groups in the population. Illsley and Le Grand (1987), for example, use the technique to explore inequalities in deaths from different causes. Another possibility would be to use the measures to ascertain how much overall population inequality was due to inequality within the social classes, and how much between them.

Yet another way that measures could be used to indicate causality is to compare changes or differences when some key factors are held

*This section has benefited from, and is partly in response to, extensive discussions with participants at the European Science Foundation Workshops on Inequalities in Health, and comments published in issue no. 35 of the *Radical Statistics Newsletter*.

constant. For instance, if we observe declining population inequality in mortality over, say, a 40-year period, during which time there was little population emigration or immigration, it would seem reasonable to suppose that the decline is due to socio-economic changes rather than to genetic ones. Or, if there are substantial differences in population inequality between countries of broadly similar ethnic composition, again it seems likely that the causes of those differences are socio-economic rather than genetic.

Another criticism of the approach is that it treats all individuals identically, without regard to class origins. This has the implication that certain, socially relevant changes in health patterns may not be reflected in the figures. For instance, a class reversal with fewer people in Social Class I, dying of a particular disease but with more in Social Class V, while the population mean age-at-death and the population dispersion around the mean unchanged could (if the numbers involved were the same) leave a summary statistic measured over age-at-death unchanged.

It is true these measures will be insensitive to changes of this kind. This is because, at least as conventionally used, they do not weight individuals differently according to their social origins. This does not seem, *ipso facto*, necessarily undesirable; a respectable case can be made for treating individuals identically. Moreover, even if it were considered desirable to 'weight' certain individuals more than others, there are possibilities for development; if suitable weights could be devised, they could be applied to each individual's age-at-death before it was entered into the calculation.

A final possible area of objection, related in part to some of the points already made, concerns the policy objective 'implicit' in the measures. It might be argued that the use of these measures implies that the policy aim is to achieve full equality of age-at-death, an aim that, given inevitable stochastic variation, is obviously quite impractical. A more appropriate aim, it could be said, is to give each individual an equal *chance* of dying at any particular age, regardless of economic or social circumstance, an aim that is implicit in the social class approach.

This is part of a wider philosophical debate concerning the relative merits of equality of outcome versus equality of opportunity, and, as such, it cannot be resolved here. Suffice it to say that, whether or not greater equality of outcome is an important social aim, it is likely still to be of interest to know the extent to which it has been achieved – if only to ascertain the desirability of simply relying on equality of opportunity as an objective.

By way of summary we may say the following. The methodology suggested here does not directly answer several questions concerning mortality inequalities that are of interest, notably those dealing with issues of causality. However, it can be used as part of a process for addressing such questions. One way in which this may be done is illustrated by the analysis of inequalities in causes of death by Illsley and Le Grand (1987); another can be found in the regression analysis presented in Le Grand (1987). As such, they can provide a useful complement to measurement techniques that directly incorporate indicators of causation, such as those based on social class.

But there is another purpose to the use of the methodology. The techniques employed are methods of measuring a particular form of inequality: that in individuals' lengths of life. Although this is clearly not the only dimension of inequality that is of social concern, equally clearly it is one of those dimensions. Prematurely to be deprived of life is obviously an acute form of relative deprivation; indeed, arguably more so than other forms of relative deprivation such as income or wealth. As Arrow has argued (1963, p. 75): 'the desire for the prolongation of life . . . we may take to be one of the most universal of all human motives'.

Acknowledgements

This research was supported under the Welfare State Programme at the Suntory-Toyota International Centre for Economic and Related Disciplines at the London School of Economics.

I am very grateful to Maria Evandrou and Ray Kobs for their tireless programming assistance. Fiona Coulter's help in producing the inequality estimates was indispensable; she also made several suggestions that significantly improved the paper. Many thanks are also due to Frank Cowell for the use of his inequality analysis package. I have also had several helpful discussions on earlier versions of some of the material in this paper with A.B. Atkinson, John Fox, Raymond Illsley, Richard Wilkinson and David Winter. John Fox was particularly important in helping me obtain the data in the first place and in making substantive editorial comments on earlier drafts. The basic data were provided by the World Health Organisation. I alone, of course, am responsible for the paper's contents.

References

Ahluwalia, M.S. (1974), 'Income inequality: some dimensions of the problem' in H Chenery, M.A. Ahluwalia, C.L.G. Bell, John H. Duloy and Richard Jolly, *Redistribution With Growth*, Oxford: Oxford University Press.

Arrow, K.J. (1963), *Social Choice and Individual Values*, 2nd ed. New York: Wiley.

Atkinson, A.B. (1970), 'On the measurement of inequality', *Journal of Economic Theory*, 2, pp. 244–63. Reprinted with non-mathematical summary in Atkinson (1980), Reading 3.

Atkinson, A.B. (1980), (ed.) *Wealth, Income and Inequality*, 2nd edn, Oxford: Oxford University Press.

Black, D. (1980), *Inequality in Health*, report of a research working group chaired by Sir Douglas Black, London: Department of Health and Social Security.

Carr-Hill, R. (1986), 'Distribution in or inequality in health', *Radical Statistics Newsletter*, No. (34).

Goldberger, A.S. (1979), 'Heritability', *Economica*, 46, pp. 327–47.

Kolm, S.C. (1976), 'Unequal inequalities', *Journal of Economic Theory*, 12, pp. 416–22; 13, pp. 82–111.

Koskinen, S. (1985), 'Time trends in case-specific mortality in England and Wales – An exploratory study'. Prepared for the IUSSP XX General Conference, 5–12 June, Florence, Italy.

Illsley, R. and Le Grand, J. (1987), 'The measurement of inequality in health' in A Williams (ed.) *Economics and Health*, London: Macmillan.

Le Grand, J. (1987), 'Inequality in health: some international comparisons', *European Economic Review*, 31, pp. 182–91.

Le Grand, J. and Rabin, M. (1986), 'Trends in British health inequality, 1931–1983' in A.J. Culyer and B. Jönsson (eds), *Public and Private Health Services*; Oxford: Basil Blackwell.

Morrison, C. (1984), 'Income distribution in East European and Western countries', *Journal of Comparative Economics*, 8, pp. 121–38.

Pamuk, E. (1985), 'Social class inequality in mortality from 1921 to 1972 in England and Wales', *Population Studies*, 39, pp. 17–31.

Pearce, N.E., Davis P. B., Smith, A. H. and Foster, F. (1983), 'Mortality and social class in New Zealand I: overall male mortality', *New Zealand Medical Journal*, 96, pp. 281–5.

Preston, S.H., Haines, M.R. and Pamuk, E. (1981), 'Effects of industrialization and urbanization on mortality in developed countries' in International Union for the Scientific Study of Population, 19th International Population Conference, Manila, 1981. *Selected papers*, Volume II. Liege.

Quan, N. T. and Koo, A. Y. C. (1985), 'Land holdings concentration', *Journal of Development economics*, 18, pp. 101–17.

Sawyer, M. (1976), *Income Distribution in OECD Countries*. Paris: OECD.

UK Royal Commission on the Distribution of Income and Wealth (1977), *Report No. 5*, Cmnd 7595, London: HMSO.

Wiles, P. (1974), *Distribution of Incomes East and West*, Amsterdam: North Holland.

Appendix 4A

Country-by-country results are provided in Tables 4A.1, 4A.2 and 4A.3. The data for each country were for the most recent year available at the time of the calculations. The data were grouped in age ranges; it was assumed that the average age-at-death was in the middle of the age-range. The last range (85+) was open-ended; it was assumed that it 'closed' at 100. Except for the Atkinson index, two grouping assumptions were used. One, the upper bound, assumed that deaths were divided equally between the upper and lower ends of each age range; the other, the lower bound, assumed that all deaths took place at the middle of the range. The mean of the two was taken as the final figure. The upper bound calculation is not appropriate for the Atkinson index, because the procedure would generate observations of value zero for the lowest age-range. Hence only the lower bound calculation was used.

The age-standardisation procedure was to calculate the deaths that would have occurred at each age for a particular country if its own age-specific mortality rates were applied to the population distribution of England and Wales. The resulting distribution gives the number of deaths that would have occurred at each age in the country concerned, if it had had the same population distribution as England and Wales.

Table 4A.1   Aggregate inequality in age-at-death: all ages, actual

Country	Year	Mean	AMD	Gini	Atkinson 0.75	1.25
Australia	1981	68.79	10.60	0.154	0.074	0.226
Austria	1981	72.77	8.99	0.124	0.045	0.140
Belgium	1978	72.42	9.03	0.125	0.046	0.144
Bulgaria	1981	68.69	9.71	0.141	0.070	0.227
Canada	1982	69.22	10.75	0.155	0.070	0.210
Czechoslovakia	1981	69.67	9.23	0.132	0.046	0.150
Denmark	1982	72.84	8.83	0.121	0.037	0.108
Eire	1979	70.40	9.76	0.139	0.073	0.240
England & Wales	1982	72.82	8.54	0.117	0.042	0.138
Finland	1981	70.08	9.00	0.128	0.042	0.122
FRG	1982	72.66	8.68	0.120	0.040	0.121
France	1981	72.66	9.89	0.136	0.055	0.168
GDR	1983	73.28	8.51	0.116	0.043	0.135
Greece	1981	71.98	9.72	0.135	0.069	0.229
Hungary	1982	68.99	9.43	0.137	0.058	0.188
Iceland	1979	71.78	10.62	0.148	0.068	0.210
Italy	1979	71.30	9.40	0.131	0.056	0.181
Japan	1982	70.10	9.94	0.142	0.055	0.163
Luxembourg	1982	71.96	8.88	0.123	0.043	0.130
Netherlands	1982	72.58	9.31	0.128	0.049	0.150
New Zealand	1982	68.26	10.80	0.158	0.081	0.248
N. Ireland	1982	70.47	9.58	0.136	0.067	0.219
Norway	1982	73.67	8.76	0.119	0.041	0.128
Poland	1982	65.48	11.36	0.174	0.109	0.341
Portugal	1979	66.62	11.81	0.177	0.121	0.371
Romania	1982	65.07	11.73	0.180	0.120	0.364
Scotland	1982	71.35	8.64	0.121	0.044	0.139
Spain	1979	69.13	10.68	0.154	0.087	0.277
Sweden	1981	74.55	8.26	0.111	0.032	0.095
Switzerland	1981	73.39	9.19	0.125	0.043	0.128
United States	1982	68.67	11.02	0.161	0.077	0.236
Yugoslavia	1980	64.73	11.97	0.185	0.135	0.413

AMD = Absolute Mean Difference
FRG = Federal Republic of Germany
GDR = German Democratic Republic

Table 4A.2   Aggregate   inequality   in   age-at-death: all   ages,
standardised

Country	Year	Mean	AMD	Gini	Atkinson 0.75	1.25	SMR
Australia	1981	72.09	9.02	0.125	0.047	0.146	91.97
Austria	1981	72.63	9.12	0.126	0.046	0.144	106.35
Belgium	1978	72.59	8.91	0.123	0.045	0.141	102.01
Bulgaria	1981	72.05	9.04	0.125	0.055	0.179	123.16
Canada	1982	71.99	9.01	0.125	0.045	0.139	88.67
Czechoslovakia	1981	72.39	8.68	0.120	0.046	0.150	130.17
Denmark	1982	72.27	8.75	0.121	0.040	0.121	93.54
Eire	1979	72.18	8.38	0.115	0.039	0.126	118.54
England & Wales	1982	72.82	8.54	0.117	0.042	0.138	100.00
Finland	1981	72.46	8.58	0.118	0.034	0.100	100.12
FRG	1982	72.72	8.91	0.123	0.045	0.142	96.71
France	1981	71.80	9.53	0.133	0.055	0.168	89.34
GDR	1983	73.28	8.56	0.117	0.040	0.126	117.29
Greece	1981	73.19	9.20	0.126	0.058	0.194	85.19
Hungary	1982	71.12	9.19	0.129	0.052	0.168	136.48
Iceland	1979	72.56	8.94	0.123	0.041	0.126	78.03
Italy	1979	72.63	9.06	0.125	0.052	0.170	96.52
Japan	1982	73.92	8.71	0.118	0.040	0.120	76.94
Luxembourg	1982	71.56	7.66	0.107	0.038	0.122	97.05
Netherlands	1982	73.18	8.57	0.117	0.041	0.129	85.68
New Zealand	1982	71.63	9.19	0.128	0.050	0.157	100.57
N. Ireland	1982	72.31	8.59	0.119	0.045	0.145	111.81
Norway	1982	72.97	8.77	0.120	0.042	0.131	85.29
Poland	1982	70.92	9.51	0.134	0.060	0.194	127.00
Portugal	1979	73.13	9.56	0.130	0.063	0.209	127.05
Romania	1982	71.53	10.08	0.141	0.072	0.234	124.68
Scotland	1982	72.13	8.51	0.118	0.040	0.128	128.89
Spain	1979	72.88	9.24	0.127	0.055	0.179	115.76
Sweden	1981	73.63	8.53	0.116	0.037	0.112	92.46
Switzerland	1981	73.32	9.03	0.123	0.043	0.130	85.14
United States	1982	70.22	9.67	0.138	0.056	0.172	85.21
Yugoslavia	1980	71.68	9.69	0.135	0.072	0.242	93.87

AMD = Absolute Mean Difference
SMR = Standardised Mortality Ratio. England and Wales = 100
FRG = Federal Republic of Germany
GDR = German Democratic Republic

Table 4A.3 *Aggregate inequality in non-infant and adult age-at-death standardised*

Country	Non-Infant		Adult	
	Mean	AMD	Mean	AMD
Australia	72.98	8.34	73.75	7.77
Austria	73.52	8.45	74.23	7.93
Belgium	73.45	8.26	74.13	7.76
Bulgaria	73.25	8.12	74.05	7.52
Canada	72.82	8.38	73.55	7.85
Czechoslovakia	73.40	7.91	73.91	7.52
Denmark	72.96	8.22	73.50	7.82
Eire	73.94	7.79	74.51	7.35
England & Wales	73.71	7.84	74.29	7.41
FRG	73.60	8.24	74.28	7.73
Finland	72.98	8.19	73.48	7.82
France	72.68	8.88	73.50	8.29
GDR	74.03	7.98	74.62	7.53
Greece	74.64	8.09	73.34	7.56
Hungary	72.28	8.32	72.80	7.93
Iceland	73.28	8.38	73.92	7.92
Italy	73.79	8.17	74.52	7.62
Japan	74.57	8.21	75.25	7.69
Luxembourg	72.32	7.06	72.80	6.69
Netherlands	73.95	7.98	74.60	7.49
New Zealand	72.58	8.47	73.47	7.82
N. Ireland	73.25	7.88	73.83	7.44
Norway	73.74	8.18	74.48	7.63
Poland	72.79	8.49	72.91	8.01
Portugal	72.29	8.49	75.60	7.70
Romania	73.21	8.84	74.29	8.04
Scotland	72.93	7.88	73.42	7.52
Spain	74.09	8.32	74.91	7.71
Sweden	74.27	8.02	74.75	7.67
Switzerland	74.03	8.48	74.81	7.91
United States	71.30	8.87	72.17	8.25
Yugoslavia	73.59	8.26	74.33	7.70

AMD = Absolute Mean Difference
FRG = Federal Republic of Germany
GDR = German Democratic Republic

5 Differential mortality by cause of death: comparison between selected European countries

Annette Leclerc

The objective of this paper is to compare different European countries, concerning the causes of death responsible for the high rate of mortality observed in the lower social classes of the adult population of each country. This could throw some light on the origin of socio-economic gradients, since risk factors and etiology of diseases responsible for death are, at least partially, known for the main causes of death considered in this paper.

Another reason for making the comparison was to highlight the fact that, in each country, a large number of deaths occurring in the lower social classes could be avoided if only some specific mortality rates could equal the mortality rates of another country.

Material and method

In order to make the comparison, we restricted ourselves to comparable data: we focused on the group of male unskilled workers, defined in each country in the most similar way, and consisting (as far as possible) of the same percentage of the active male population.

Similar sources of data (partly unpublished) could be used for England and Wales, Finland, Norway, Denmark and France, for the period 1970–80. Danmarks Statistik, 1979; Fox and Goldblatt, 1982; Lynge and Jeune, 1983; Valkonen, 1983; Andersen, 1984; Desplanques, 1984 (a); Desplanques 1984(b); Desplanques, 1984(c).

In each case, mortality figures came from a cohort study on mortality, based upon a census. Persons registered at a census (or a sample of them) were followed from the census date until death, emigration or end of follow-up, 10 years after the census (5 years in France).

Details on those cohort studies, and data used for comparison are given in Table 5.1. Men only were compared, because data concerning women are difficult to interpret, even if the occupation is well recorded. Health status of women must be related to occupation in a very complex way since a large part of them have no paid work (Bouvier Colle, 1983).

Concerning the socio-economic groups used for comparison, causes

Table 5.1 Sources of data for comparison

	Finland	Norway	Denmark	England and Wales	France
General features of the study		FOLLOW-UP STUDY FROM A CENSUS			
Period of follow-up	1971–80	1970–80	1971–80	1971–80	1975–80
Size of population or sample	3,000,000 (male and female 15–64 years)	1,067,050 men (20–64 years)	2,800,000 (male and female 20–64 years)	187,933 men (15 years and more)	445,000 men (30–64 years) restricted to: French Nationality born in France
Number of deaths (only men: same age group as above)	129,183	82,742	112,910	8,442	14,722
Source of information on cause of death and occupation	Individual matching procedure: occupation = occupation at the census. Cause of death comes from the death certificate				General mortality: individual matching. Mortality by cause of death: indirect procedure
Mortality figures available	For each sub-group (age group at census and socio-economic status), number of deaths, by cause of death, and number of person years	As in Finland	For each sub-group (age group at census and socio-economic status) mortality rate ratio; rates are based on number of person-years standard = all occupied	Number of death and death rate, by cause of death, age and socio-economic status (age=age at death)	Annual risk of death, by age and socio-economic class. The risk is exact (observed) or adjusted, according to a model if the number of death is small

Table 5.1 *continued*

	Finland	Norway	Denmark	England and Wales	France
Coding of social class	8 socio-economic classes including active persons	7 socio-economic classes including active persons	4 social classes	5 social classes	13 socio-economic classes (active)
Men classified in a group including active persons	Economically active and formerly economically active in 1970	Economically active in 1970	Economically active in 1970	Occupied and retired at the census	Active men at the census (including unemployed, but not retired)
Percentage of not classified men by age	10% (45–54 years) 29% (55–64 years)	7% (45–54 years) 16% (55–64 years)	5% (45–54 years) 14% (55–64 years)	2% (45–54 years) 5% (55–64 years)	7% (45–54 years) 49% (55–64 years)
Socio-economic group taken as 'unskilled workers'	Labourers + farm and forestry workers 11% of all men in 1970	Unskilled workers 32% of all men	Class IV unskilled workers 27% of all men	Social Classes IV + V 22% of all men	*Ouvriers spécialisés* + *salariés agricoles* + *manoeuvres*. (Unskilled workers + farm workers + labourers) 25% of all men

of death, age groups and mortality measures, we tried to adopt the same criteria in each country; however, it was not possible to get exactly comparable data.

Causes of death
The *International Classification of Diseases, 1975 Revision* (WHO, 1977) was used in each country. Broad groups of causes of death were used:
- Cancer (ICD 140–209)
- Cardiovascular diseases (ICD 390–458)
- Accidents (ICD E 800–999)
- Respiratory diseases (ICD 460–519)
- Cirrhosis (ICD 571) or diseases of the digestive system (ICD 520–577) or ulcer + cirrhosis.

Differences in the coding of causes of death between countries are probably not large, since the classification is not detailed (WHO, 1973; Kelson and Heller, 1983). Moreover, death occurring over the age of 65 years, for which coding of cause of death could be less reliable, are not included in the comparisons.

Socio-occupational groups
Social classes IV + V in England and Wales, Social class IV in Norway, 'unskilled workers' in Denmark, labourers and farm and forestry workers in Finland, formed the group of unskilled workers. For France the group was *'ouvriers spécialisés'* (unskilled workers), *'manoeuvres'* (labourers), and *'salariés agricoles'* (agricultural labourers).

These choices were based on the fact that authors from the respective countries considered that they were comparable groups (Lynge and Jeune, 1983; Valkonen, 1983), and that they included people having roughly the same occupation. There were slight differences but the discordances occurred only for a very small part of each group.

It was planned to define groups accounting for the same percentage of the population. This was not possible for Finland nor for Norway. The group of unskilled workers in Finland constitutes only 11 per cent of men, compared to 22–27 per cent in England and Wales, Denmark and France. The Finnish group could be compared to *'salariés agricoles'* + *'manoeuvres'* in France (9 per cent of all men). In Norway, on the contrary, the group of unskilled workers (class IV) is larger, accounting for 32 per cent of men.

Large differences between countries were observed in the percentage of persons of each age group classified according to socio-economic group. The most striking difference was observed in France at 55–64 years: 49 per cent of men of this age do not work any more (most of them are prematurely retired). Since inactive persons have a higher mortality, we had to pay attention to the possibility of a healthy worker effect, more or less important in each country. For this reason two comparison groups – 'all men' and 'all occupied' – were taken for a part of the study, and we paid attention to possible differences between age groups.

Immigrant population
The immigrant population was included in only some of the studies. This could have an effect on the results. However, when it was possible to make comparison (Office of Population Censuses and Surveys, 1978; Brahimi, 1980), including or leaving out immigrant population, this had only limited effects on social gradients.

Age-groups and mortality measures
Mortality figures were given by 10- or 5-year age groups, from 25 or 35 years to 65 years.

A death was assigned to the age-group the person belonged to at the time of the census, or to the age-at-death. For comparison, we took the age at death, or the age in the middle of the observation period; these different ways of taking age into account were linked to slight differences in mortality measures. We considered that different measures were comparable, since the total number of deaths was small, in comparison to the population, and the follow-up period was not very long.

Length of follow-up
The length of follow-up was 10 years in every country, except in France where it was five years. This could have some effect on the results since differences between groups are less pronounced in the first years following the census.

Comparison measures
Unskilled workers were compared to the total male population, and to all active men, by measures based on ratios. They were also compared to all active men, by measures based on differences of mortality rates (or risks).

Ratios of mortality according to age were calculated as:

Mortality of unskilled workers/mortality of all men; or
Mortality of unskilled workers/ mortality of all active men.

The ratios were calculated for general mortality.

Table 5.2   *Mortality ratio (overall mortality); unskilled workers/all men,*
or all occupied

	Reference group = all men								Reference group = all occupied							
	25– 29	30– 34	35– 39	40– 44	45– 49	50– 54	55– 59	60– 64	25– 29	30– 34	35– 39	40– 44	45– 49	50– 54	55– 59	60– 64
Finland	149	174	175	153	135	119	103	94	155	186	193	171	151	139	123	119
Norway	118	119	119	111	102	99	92	89	122	127	130	123	113	111	105	103
Denmark									139	140	142	129	122	116	111	106
England & Wales	119	129	126	121	118	113	108	101	129	133	136	126	124	118	113	108
France			150		121		98				162		143		127	

Age = age in the middle of the observation period, or age-at-death

Differences of mortality according to age and cause of death, were
calculated as: mortality of unskilled workers – mortality of all active
men (per 100,000).

Differences by age group were aggregated, taking the same age
distribution in each country (direct method of standardisation). The
age distribution used for standardisation consisted in taking 5-year age
groups of equal size, from 35 to 65. These standardised differences
can be interpreted as a number of 'avoidable deaths' in a group of
100,000 unskilled workers, with a given age structure; these deaths
would be avoided if the mortality in the group was equal to the
mortality of the reference group (all active men in the same country).

The two methods of comparison (ratios by age, and differences)
threw complementary light on the subject: ratios are more frequently
used in epidemiology; differences or 'avoidable deaths' could be
preferred in a public health approach.

Results
Mortality ratios by age
Unskilled workers were compared with 'all men' and 'all active'.

The most reliable comparisons could be made between England and
Wales, Denmark and France, where the groups of unskilled workers
were more comparable.

In every country studied, mortality ratios decreased with age.

Differences between younger men and older men, between compar-

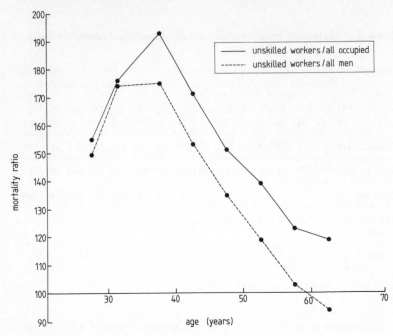

Figure 5.1   Mortality ratios – Finland

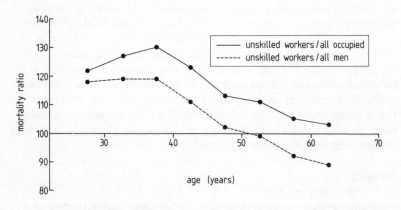

Figure 5.2   Mortality ratios – Norway

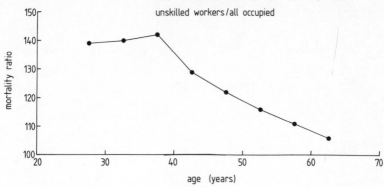

Figure 5.3   Mortality ratios – Denmark

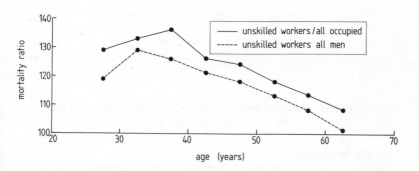

Figure 5.4   Mortality ratios – England and Wales

isons with 'all active' or 'all men' are partly dependent on whether or not unskilled workers remain active when they get older.

The situation of older unskilled workers compared to all men seemed to be comparably better in Scandinavian countries than in England and Wales. This could be related to the fact that in England and Wales only 5 per cent of the age group 55–64 years is not classified in a social class; selection effects, by exclusion from the social classification could be smaller than in other countries. This could have effects on comparison figures. The French situation was particular: a large proportion of men over 55 years are no longer classified in a socio-economic group. However, this possibility of stopping work has only a limited effect on health selection, at least for unskilled workers; those who remain at work still have a high risk of death, compared to other categories.

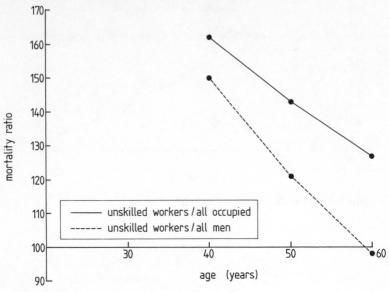

Figure 5.5   Mortality ratios – France

Differences between France and other countries could be even larger if the length of follow-up were the same.

Death in excess
Detailed data on mortality by age and cause of death are given in Tables 5.3 to 5.7.

Figures 5.6 to 5.10 represent the death rates (per 100,000) by cause of death, in a group of unskilled workers of all ages, and the expected death rates, taking all active men as a reference; the differences (observed – expected, per 100,000) could be interpreted as death in excess, in a group of 100,000 unskilled workers. A direct standardisation of age was performed in order to compare groups having the same age distribution.

Very large differences appeared between countries, as regards the causes responsible for the deaths in excess among unskilled workers; these differences remained when age groups were considered separately (cf. Tables 5.2 to 5.6).

In Denmark and Norway, most deaths in excess are due to accidents. In Finland the same situation is observed, with a higher rate of accident (both among unskilled workers, and among all occupied men).

In England and Wales, reducing the number of fatal accidents would reduce social inequalities only to a limited extent. More deaths

Table 5.3 *Deaths in excess /100,000, and mortality of occupied men –*
Finland

		25–29	30–34	35–39	40–44	45–49	50–54	55–59	60–64
General mortality	(1)	89	164	244	295	362	409	368	427
	(2)	162	190	263	418	707	1046	1563	2275
Cancer	(1)	1	−2	−2	7	29	55	92	116
	(2)	12	19	27	50	111	219	392	611
Dis. circulat. syst.	(1)	4	31	48	89	118	141	69	137
	(2)	14	28	71	165	342	565	864	1283
Accidents	(1)	81	125	170	177	167	158	142	114
	(2)	118	119	131	154	181	159	168	170
Dis. of res. syst.	(1)	0	0	5	9	24	21	43	26
	(2)	1	2	4	7	15	28	50	82
Cirrhosis + Ulcer (stomach, duodenum)	(1)	1	3	3	−2	1	10	6	7
	(2)	2	5	7	12	18	21	24	29

Age: age in the middle of the observation period
(1): mortality of unskilled workers – mortality of all occupied
(2): mortality of all occupied (per 100,000)
(1) + (2): mortality of unskilled workers

in excess are due to cardiovascular diseases, cancer, or respiratory diseases.

France differs from England in that fewer deaths and fewer excess deaths, are observed for cardiovascular or respiratory diseases.

On the other hand, a very large number of excess deaths are due to cancer, cirrhosis, accidents, or 'other'. Among excess cancer deaths, a large part is due to upper respiratory and digestive tract cancer (mouth, pharynx, larynx). The situation is not the same in other countries, where cancer deaths in excess are mainly lung cancer cases.

Discussion

The data we used had the advantage of being comparable, with regard to the type of study and the coding of causes of death. However, we

Table 5.4   Deaths in excess /100,000, and mortality of occupied men –
          Norway

		25–29	30–34	35–39	40–44	45–49	50–54	55–59	60–64
General mortality	(1)	23	31	50	58	55	74	53	45
	(2)	106	115	165	255	419	678	1066	1675
Cancer	(1)	0	2	2	9	13	22	15	17
	(2)	13	20	28	48	90	173	289	459
Dis. circulat. syst.	(1)	0	−1	12	16	16	24	2	−4
	(2)	7	12	36	81	175	311	532	862
Accidents	(1)	22	27	25	25	19	14	12	11
	(2)	73	64	69	76	78	78	79	85
Dis. of resp. syst.	(1)	0	1	2	1	4	1	8	7
	(2)	1	1	3	5	9	15	29	53
Dis. of dig. syst.	(1)	0	0	1	3	3	2	−5	2
	(2)	2	3	4	9	14	18	25	38

Age: age in the middle of the observation period
(1): mortality of unskilled workers – mortality of all occupied
(2): mortality of all occupied (per 100,000)
(1) + (2): mortality of unskilled workers

could not find comparable groups of unskilled workers in all five
countries.

Other difficulties in comparison arose from the fact that being an
unskilled worker, at a given age, is the result of a dynamic process
which includes the possibility of changing one's occupation, early
retirement, or becoming a pensioner. Some of the results were clearly
sensitive to the percentage of people who are not classified in a social
group. Differences according to age were important too.

For this reason it seems to be important to compare data using
methods which are not too sensitive to the age structures of the
compared groups.

Nevertheless, when causes of death are taken into account, some
differences between countries can be stressed: England and Wales
were in a better situation than other countries, in regard to the

Table 5.5   **Deaths in excess /100,000, and mortality of occupied men –**
Denmark

		25–29	30–34	35–39	40–44	45–49	50–54	55–59	60–64
General mortality	(1)	41	48	73	83	103	129	132	120
	(2)	106	120	175	282	470	786	1223	1877
Cancer	(1)	0	4	5	9	17	30	32	21
	(2)	14	18	33	60	120	229	372	607
Dis. circulat. syst.	(1)	1	6	12	14	30	32	25	15
	(2)	5	14	31	83	171	323	550	875
Accidents	(1)	34	28	33	31	31	26	26	27
	(2)	70	62	72	78	88	91	101	107
Dis. of resp. syst.	(1)	0	0	2	5	7	11	21	29
	(2)	1	1	3	6	13	27	50	93
Dis. of dig. syst.	(1)	0	4	7	6	8	13	14	10
	(2)	2	6	11	17	27	38	48	56

Age: age in the middle of the observation period
(1): mortality of unskilled workers – mortality of all occupied
(2): mortality of all occupied (per 100,000)
(1) + (2): mortality of unskilled workers

importance of accidents as a cause of social inequalities. This
contributed to a reduction of social inequalities for younger ages,
compared to other countries.

On the other hand, more deaths in excess from cardiovascular
diseases were found among English unskilled workers than in any
other country. It is difficult to know whether this would remain if
fewer people remained classified in the upper age group, where deaths
from cardiovascular diseases are numerous.

In Scandinavian countries it seems that most of the deaths in excess
are due to accidents; but comparisons with other countries are
difficult for Finland and Norway due to the lack of comparability of
the group taken as 'unskilled workers'.

In France, large numbers of deaths in excess were observed for all
main causes of death, even if the situation was relatively better for

Table 5.6   Deaths in excess /100,000, and mortality of occupied men –
England and Wales

		25–29	30–34	35–39	40–44	45–49	50–54	55–59	60–64
General mortality	(1)	22	30	49	64	109	148	184	178
	(2)	75	93	137	248	457	820	1388	2226
Cancer	(1)	−6	9	23	−13	24	41	50	91
	(2)	9	17	27	54	120	254	427	720
Dis. circulat. syst.	(1)	0	5	7	42	51	19	64	34
	(2)	9	18	47	117	236	425	732	1123
Accidents	(1)	16	−2	10	8	10	12	24	7
	(2)	42	40	44	39	44	42	40	54
Dis. of resp. syst.	(1)	2	6	7	6	8	37	27	50
	(2)	4	6	5	10	22	47	94	192
Other	(1)	10	12	2	20	−6	5	20	−5
	(2)	12	11	14	27	36	52	96	137

(1): mortality of unskilled workers – mortality of all occupied
(2): mortality of all occupied (per 100,000)
(1) + (2): mortality of unskilled workers

cardiovascular and respiratory diseases. The high number of deaths due to certain causes of deaths – cirrhosis, upper respiratory and digestive tract cancer – suggests that alcohol consumption could play an important role in social inequalities.

The data demonstrate to what extent the national context, including social risk factors such as tobacco and alcohol consumption, is an important determinant of mortality. The probability of dying from one given cause of death can probably be more accurately predicted by the country where the person lives, than by whether or not he belongs to a given social class.

Acknowledgements
I am indebted to Elsebeth Lynge (Denmark), Hannele Sauli and Tapani Valkonen (Finland), Gerd Skoe Lettenstrom (Norway) and

*Table 5.7   Deaths in excess /100,000, and mortality of occupied men –
France*

		35–44	45–54	55–64
General mortality	(1)	199	296	400
	(2)	319	689	1489
Cancer	(1)	30	93	106
	(2)	72	245	577
Dis. circulat. syst.	(1)	18	27	38
	(2)	55	155	416
Accidents	(1)	51	47	57
	(2)	63	66	84
Dis. of resp. syst.	(1)	8	11	18
	(2)	7	21	57
Cirrhosis	(1)	27	40	68
	(2)	24	63	110

(1): mortality of unskilled workers – mortality of all occupied
(2): mortality of all occupied (per 100,000)
(1) + (2): mortality of unskilled workers

John Fox (England) who kindly provided unpublished tables adapted
to this comparative study.

References

Anderson, O. (1984), 'The Danish model of census-linked mortality studies and the
  future plans', *Scandinavian Population Studies*, 6 (3) pp. 49–60.
Bouvier Colle, M.H. (1983), 'Mortalité et activité professionnelle chez les femmes',
  Population, 1, pp. 107–36.
Brahimi, M. (1980), 'La mortalité des étrangers en France', *Population*, 3, pp. 603–22.
Danmarks Statistik (1979), 'Dodelighed og erhevern 1970–1975', *Statistiske Underso-
  gelser*, (37).
Desplanques, G. (1984a), 'L'inégalité sociale devant la mort'. *Economie et Statistique*,
  162, pp. 29–50.
Desplanques, G. (1984b), 'La mortalité masculine selon le milieu social', *Données
  Sociales*, pp. 348–58.
Desplanques, G. (1984c), 'La mortalité des adultes', *Les Collections de l'INSEE*, 102 D,
  212 p.
Fox, A.J., Goldblatt, P. (1982), *Longitudinal Study: Socio-Demographic Mortality*

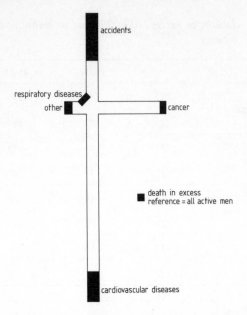

Figure 5.6   Death rates of unskilled workers 35–64 years – Finland

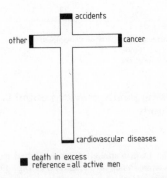

Figure 5.7   Death rates of unskilled workers 35–64 years – Norway

Differentials 1971–1975, Office of Population Censuses and Surveys, series LS No 1, London: HMSO.

Kelson, M.C. and Heller, R.F. (1983), 'The effect of death codification and coding practices on observed differences in respiratory disease mortality in 8 E.E.C. countries', *Revue Epidemologie et Santé Publique.*, 31, pp. 423–32.

Lynge, E. and Jeune, B. (1983), 'Excess mortality among male unskilled and semi-skilled workers, *Scandinavian Journal of Social Medicine* 11, pp. 37–40.

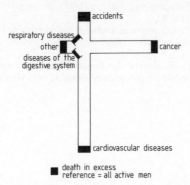

Figure 5.8   Death rates of unskilled workers 35–64 years – Denmark

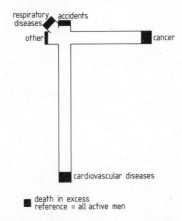

Figure 5.9   Death rates of unskilled workers 35–64 years – England and Wales

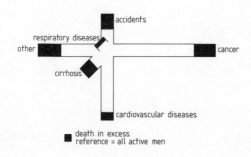

Figure 5.10   Death rates of unskilled workers 35–64 years – France

Office of Population Censuses and Surveys (1978), *Decennial Supplement 1970–1972*, Series DS No. 1, HMSO.

Valkonen, T. (1983), 'Socio-economic mortality differentials in Finland. Health for all in Scandinavia by the Year 2000', *The Nordic School of Public Health Rapport NHV*, 1.

WHO, Copenhagen (1973), *Medical Certification of Causes of Death*: Report on a Study.

WHO, (1977), *International Classification of Diseases, 1975 Revision*, Geneva.

6 Sex, gender and survival: inequalities of life chances between European men and women
Nicky Hart

Sex mortality differences and the modern rise of population
The last two centuries have been a period of demographic revolution in Europe; birth and death rates have been slashed, life expectancy at birth has almost doubled, the size of population has been greatly expanded and a continuous trend of rural/urban migration has seen virtually the whole continent transformed from a predominantly rural/agrarian way of life to an urban/industrial mode of existence. Europe's population boom probably began sometime in the eighteenth century. It was a continental wide phenomenon and during the nineteenth century the numbers of people living in most European nations doubled or trebled. The largest percentage increase was in Britain where the population rose by a factor of almost four in the period between 1800 and 1910. The increase is all the more remarkable when one considers that, throughout this period, there was substantial emigration by people of childbearing age from Europe to North America and Australia.

The demographic revolutions of the nineteenth and twentieth centuries add up to nothing less than a transformation of the conditions of human life. The process involved a massive expansion of life chances, with opportunities for human life improving in two distinctive ways (Hart, forthcoming). The first was a large increase in the numbers of infants born with decent prospects of survival to adult life. In other words, the starting line for the human 'race' was widely extended through a substantial reduction in the risk of premature death for infants and children. The second comprised a true lengthening of adult existence itself. Young adults of 15 years could look forward to four additional decades of existence in 1850. One hundred years later, the figure rose to five or six. This latter change is the result of a decline in mortality risk among adults of all ages.

One feature of declining mortality in industrial societies is a growing divergence in the average length of male and female lifetimes. In the first half of the nineteenth century, male and female life expectancy was roughly equal. Today the average woman can expect to live for a further six years beyond the average male of the same birth date. The bulk of this differential is accounted for by the higher mortality of men of mature age. It is an example of a difference in life chances in the second sense of the term identified above. While the male of the species has shared in general improvements in life expectancy, he has failed to match the success of the female in prolonging the length of adult life.

The width of the gap between the sexes appears to be influenced by rural/urban differences, by marital status and by occupational class. In general, life chances are more equally distributed between the sexes in rural areas. This may explain why Eire in the 1920s was the only European society to reveal a female excess of mortality over quite an appreciable age range and why the gap between the sexes generally widens as societies become more industrialised and urbanised. In Sweden where industrialisation took a rural form, sex mortality differentials appeared much later than in England and Wales where industrialisation originated as an urban phenomenon. Being married also seems to confer some advantage to male longevity. A classic study written at the turn of the century by one the founding fathers of sociology, Emile Durkheim, introduced the coefficient of preservation as a means of measuring the survival advantage attached to conjugal life (Durkheim, 1897). Durkheim argued, that the rate of suicide varied with the level of regulation in social life. Married couples leading a well ordered existence with their behaviour governed by clear rules and expectations seemed to exhibit the strongest instinct for survival, a fact demonstrated by their infrequent resort to suicide (cf. Hart, 1976). In a more recent study, Gove (1973) applied the concept of the coefficient of preservation to causes of death involving psychological stress and found, like Durkheim, that marriage carried even greater advantages for men than women.

Martin (1956) identified an inverse relationship between social class and the sex differential for England and Wales in 1930. Using the *Decennial Supplement of Occupational Mortality* for 1931, he found more inequality among men and women in social class I (professional occupations) than in social class V (unskilled occupations). By the early 1970s this pattern was still evident in every age group over 35. Since then the pattern of sex differentials has shown a number of changes by sex and age.

Over the last two decades in England and Wales, the sex mortality differential below the age of 54 appears to have narrowed in the non-manual class and to have widened among manual workers and their wives. Among older people, the widening trend is evident in both classes. The increasing class gradient in smoking in Britain may underlie current trends in life chances by sex and class (see below).

*Table 6.1   Excess male mortality (%) by social class 1971 and 1981:
England and Wales*

Age	Manual		Non-Manual	
	1970–72	1979–83	1970–72	1979–83
>35	208	244	198	192
36–44	149	163	151	145
45–54	157	168	178	166
55–64	207	248	214	247

Source: *Decennial Supplements of Occupational Mortality 1970–72 and 1979–83* (1978 1986),
London: OPCS, Male death rates expressed as a percentage of female rates. Women:
married and classified by their husband's occupation.

European variations in the sex mortality differential

The emergence of a marked sex differential in the twentieth century is
a European phenomenon. Figure 6.1 charts post-war trends in excess
male mortality from birth to very old age for Europe as a whole by
expressing the death rate for males as a percentage of that of females.
At every age, the trend is upwards. The most spectacular increase is
found in the age range 10–30 where, over the course of 25 years, the
ratio of male to female deaths has virtually doubled. The result: in
1950 the ratio of male to female mortality among young adults was
3:2; by 1975 it was almost 6:2. In mid-life the gradient dips, peaking
once again but at a lower level, in the decade surrounding retirement
age where the post-war era saw an increase of about 50 per cent. Sex
differences in mortality risk achieve their lowest level in the first and
final years of life and, for these age groups, there have been few
changes in recent decades. The male excess has been relatively stable
at about 30 per cent or less.

Within Europe sex mortality gradients vary substantially between
different societies. These variations converge in three fairly distinctive
tendencies. The first, a clear bimodal pattern, is exemplified by the
gradient for England and Wales depicted in Figure 6.2. The sex
mortality differential has two peaks: in the decade around age 20 (the
transition to adulthood) and in the two decades each side of retirement
age (65 years). In the three age bands separating these two peaks,
infancy, mid-life (30–50) and very old age, only slight increases have
been registered in the post-war era. This first form of gradient (type 1)
also tends to be found in Denmark, Holland, Belgium and Scotland.*

*Type 1 is also the tendency in most of the English-speaking non-European societies:
USA, Australia and New Zealand.

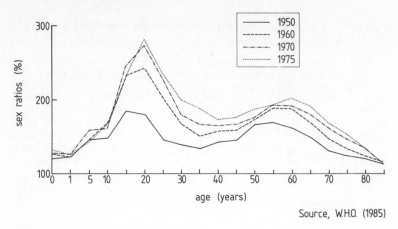

Source, W.H.O. (1985)

Figure 6.1   The sex mortality differential in Europe (male death rates expressed as a percentage of female rates)

The second distinctive pattern, type two, illustrated by the French gradient in Figure 6.2 takes the form of a kind of plateau bounded by two peaks. Once again it is around the age of maturity (18–25) that the largest excess is found but unlike type one, the excess remains very marked throughout the remainder of pre-retirement life, peaking only slightly at the point of exit from the labour market and thereafter descending fairly rapidly among the elderly. Type two is more numerous among continental Western European societies, being found in Austria, Finland, East and West Germany, Italy, Northern Ireland, Norway, Sweden and Switzerland. The pattern for Europe as a whole is also closer to the type two profile.

The third type of sex mortality gradient is illustrated in Figure 6.2 by Hungary. Once again the deviance is found after the age of 25 rather than before it. During childhood and adolescence, excess male mortality climbs rapidly to a pinnacle at age 20, and descends gradually over the remaining decades of lifetime. The peak at retirement age is less marked than in the other types identified. Type 3 has a certain geographical, if not a politico-economic, clustering. It predominates in Eastern and Southern Europe (Bulgaria, Czechoslovakia, Greece, Hungary, Poland, Portugal and Yugoslavia).

Between the three societies chosen to represent the three types of sex mortality differential there is relatively little difference in the immediate post-war period. Twenty-five years later the gradients are transformed. In both periods, there is a remarkable uniformity in the first two decades of life in all three societies but considerable deviance after. Overall type 2 males – in our example, the manhood of France –

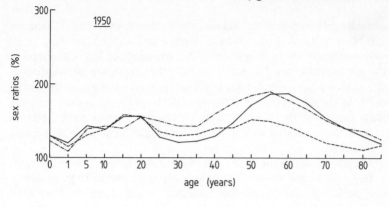

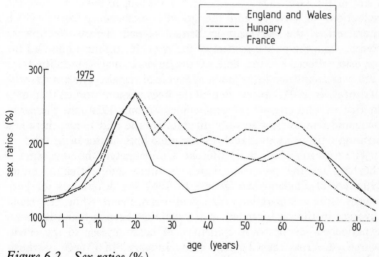

Figure 6.2   Sex ratios (%)

maintains the highest percentage of excess deaths throughout the entire age range. In the middle of the lifetime the lowest excess is registered in England and Wales but thereafter it is our type 3 example, Hungary, where both in 1950 and 25 years later, excess male deaths show the sharpest tendency to fall away.

The causes which account for the wastage of male life vary over the lifetime. Before the age of 40, the lives of young European men are most likely to be forfeited through accidental and violent means. This is equally true in types 1, 2 and 3 although the volume varies considerably between the representative societies. Type 1 societies exhibit a reduced tendency to accidental and violent mortality at all ages and particularly in mid-life. This explains the bimodal shape of the gradient. In type 2 societies, on the other hand, sex differentials in the risk of violent death remain relatively high throughout the prime of life as they do in type 3. After age 40, the principal causes of excess male mortality are cancer and cardiovascular disease with cirrhosis and accidents playing an important complementary role in type 2 and 3 societies.

Figure 6.3 charts the pattern of these causes in the post-war period.

In England and Wales, our type 1 example, mortality from cancer and cardiovascular disease has increased steadily from the beginning of the century among men while showing a fluctuating though overall reducing set of rates for females. The major disturbances in the trends for cardiovascular causes seem to be linked chronologically to the World Wars with a peak in the intervening interval which spanned the years of the Great Depression. It is tempting to conclude that the reductions of poverty and the growth of social solidarity which characterised the war years in Britain helped depress the upward trend, while the public neglect of the poor during the 1930s had the opposite effect. By the end of the period, male mortality from cardiovascular causes was much in excess of female. The same is true of cancer. In 1901, cancer claimed the lives of more women than men in Britain; the cross-over point comes around 1920 and thereafter male and female rates steadily diverge. By the mid-1960s, there is a striking uniformity in sexual divisions for both causes in Britain.

The pattern in France is different. Unfortunately the time series is shorter, but the post-war picture is quite unlike that of either Hungary or England and Wales. In 1941 sex differences for both causes were comparatively small in France and while the trend diverges in the post-war era, it is clear that French males have not experienced the post-war epidemics of heart disease to the extent witnessed across the Channel or in Hungary. In France, cirrhosis occupies the role that cardiovascular disease plays in depressing the survival prospects of men in type 1 and 3 societies. Cardiovascular rates for French women have fallen rapidly over the period to a level well below that of the other countries being compared. This together with the persistently high incidence of accidental causes explains why the sex mortality differential remains high at the mid-point of life in France. The widening gap in mortality from cancer seems to be a post-war phenomenon with the cross-over point occurring 20 years after the same event in Britain.

In Hungary we find yet another set of trends. Compared with British men, rates of mortality from cardiovasular causes are lower,

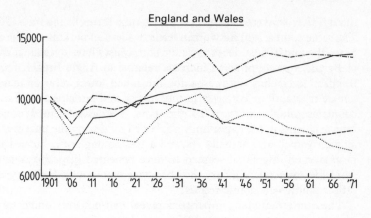

England and Wales

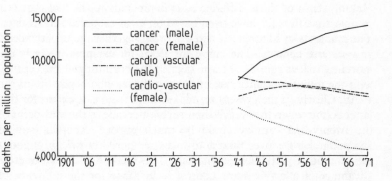

France

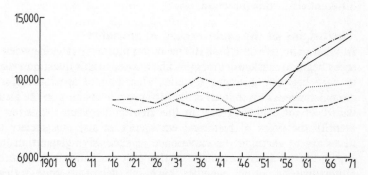

Hungary

Figure 6.3 *Trends in cancer and cardiovascular disease: England and Wales, France, Hungary.*
Source: Alderson, 1981, SMRs.

though they converge at the end of the time series in the mid-1960s. The same comparison for women leads to a less favourable conclusion. Since the mid-1950s, death rates for both causes have overtaken those of Britain and continue to increase relative to Anglo-French female trends. Herein lies the reason for the much lower ratio of male to female mortality in Hungary in middle age and perhaps also in other countries which conform to the type 3 gradient. In Hungary, improvements in life expectancy slackened off during the post-war era among women and actually showed a loss among men. Since European women in general seemed to have benefited disproportionately from life expectancy gains, the shallower gradient in Hungary may reflect politico-economic trends.

These international comparisons reveal that however universal the picture of excess male mortality across the continent of Europe, the shape of the gradient and its constituent elements vary considerably. Making sense of these differences is hampered by the fact that our comparisons thus far have been based on cross-sectional sets of data. The gradients in Figures 6.1 and 6.2 bring together the experience of very diverse cohorts. The curve for 1975, for example, records the mortality risk at age 75, of those born at the beginning of the century with the infant mortality risk of the generation who began life in the 1970s. Clearly, if the present trends continue, the male excess for this latter cohort when they reach their seventh decade in the mid-point of the twenty-first century could be much greater. Another way of analysing changes over time is to focus on mortality risk throughout the lifetime of particular generations. This method also has the great advantage of allowing some control to be made for the influence of major historical events on the lives of specific cohorts. The next section of this paper will reorient the analysis of sex mortality differentials in this direction.

The origins of the male excess in mortality
At what point over the first 100 years did mortality rates between the sexes begin to markedly diverge? The answer to this question is likely to vary between different societies according to specific historical circumstances. This in itself is likely to provide insights on the general nature of the widening gap in life chances between the sexes. To identify the point of historical emergence in any one society it is necessary to examine the experience of successive generations who began life at given intervals in the past one and half centuries. Unfortunately not all societies have the necessary time series to identify the generations who first revealed an excess of male mortality. Among the societies chosen here to represent the three types of sex mortality gradient only France and England and Wales began the

systematic process of registering births and deaths before 1850 and it is to these societies that we must turn to identify the historical roots of the sex differential in mortality.

In both societies there is evidence of excess male mortality, especially after middle age, for cohorts born in the first half of the nineteenth century. We do not have any earlier data for either England and Wales or France. In Sweden where cohorts can be accurately reconstructed from the closing decades of the eighteenth century there appears to be a quite marked sex differential favouring women in pre-industrial times. During the nineteenth century it narrowed substantially and it is only among cohorts born in early twentieth-century Sweden that the dominant European trend of excess male mortality reasserts itself. Since we do not have equivalent data for France or Britain, we cannot tell how widespread sex mortality differentials were in pre-industrial Europe.

However England and Wales and France share a trend that is different from Sweden in the middle of the nineteenth century. In both societies excess male mortality begins to diverge from its 'normal' level of around 20–30 per cent among earlier cohorts. The generation born in the seventh decade of the last century appears to show the first discernible sign of excess mortality among mature men. Figures 6.4 and 6.5 chart the percentage excess of male over female deaths throughout the lifetime of the respective cohorts born between 1841 and 1921 in England and Wales and France.

The highest levels of excess male mortality are found in France. The peak is an excess of 165 per cent recorded for the 1921 cohort in their late fifties (1982). These French levels are well in excess of those of England and Wales. Comparing the same cohort at the same age across the Channel, we find an excess of only 67 per cent. Moreover, while France still appears to be experiencing a steady widening of the gap in survival between the sexes, in Britain there is some indication that sex differences may be declining in older age groups as the downturn in the gradients for the 1921 cohort seems to indicate.

Inequalities in life chances between the sexes were clearly present in some degree among the earliest Victorian generations. During the last quarter of the nineteenth century, the beginnings of a new trend could be discerned which continued in France up to the present day and which only recently showed any sign of levelling off in England and Wales. The trend may have begun later in Hungary as it did in Sweden; unfortunately we are unable to date the exact point of divergence. Whatever underlies the widening gap in survival between European men and women, it seems to have begun among those who started their lives in the late nineteenth century. To unravel the mystery we must seek to understand any changes that took place in

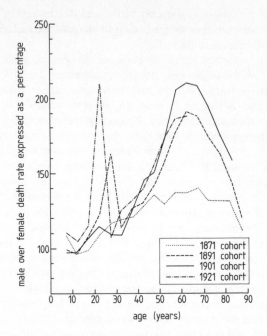

*Figure 6.4   Sex mortality differentials in cohorts born between 1871 and
1921: England and Wales (based on Table 6.3)*

Source: *OPCS*, 1985 (male death rates expressed as a percentage of female rates).

the position of men and women in society from the turn of the century
to the present day.

Sex, gender and life chances in the twentieth century

Why do women live longer than men in the twentieth century? Is it a
matter of sex, or in other words, the outcome of natural biological
differences between males and females? Or does it boil down to
gender; to a socially generated and therefore artificial form of
differentiation which comes about through the roles men and women
play in social and economic life?

The most persuasive evidence for a natural biological explanation is
the higher incidence of foetal and stillbirth mortality in human males
and in other species (cf. Hamilton, 1948). In the advanced industrial
societies male infants are born in the ratio of approximately 106 to 100
females yet their mortality in the first years of life is about 30 per cent
higher. In contemporary times, where efforts to ensure the survival of
all infants regardless of sex are at an all-time high and where scarcity

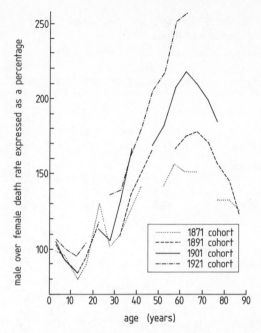

Figure 6.5 Sex mortality differentials in cohorts born between 1871 and 1921: France (based on Table 6.3)

Source: INSEE, 1985 (male death rates expressed as a percentage of female rates)

of food resources seems less of a barrier to survival than ever before, the male is clearly the more vulnerable sex. However, in many, arguably most, societies even today female excess mortality is the norm (Kynch, 1984). Where male longevity is above that of female, the status of, and value accorded to, women tends to be exceptionally low. High wastage of female life is associated with the practice of female infanticide and also with inequalities in the distribution of food (see Sen, 1981). There also appear to be tendencies towards this form of sex discrimination in pre-industrial Europe in the higher mortality of female children which, as we have seen, were found even in late nineteenth century cohorts (cf. Stolnitz, 1956; Wall, 1981). Given contemporary evidence of sex differences in survival at birth and during childhood, the record of reverse trends seems to represent an unmistakable sign of gender discrimination.

In European folk culture, the attribution of these tendencies to food deprivation is in accord with oral history reports that male bread-winners habitually received the lion's share at mealtimes. As living standards rise and food becomes less scarce or even abundant, the populations of the advanced societies have become concerned with

Table 6.2   *Mortality by age, sex and cause: Sweden, France and England and Wales*

Age	Male 5–24	25–44	45–64	65+	Female 5–24	25–44	45–64	65+
Cancer								
Sweden	7.8	22.9	248	1387	5.6	29.6	240	881
France	8.3	35.5	406	1549	5.8	28.9	202	779
England and Wales	8.3	28.9	368	1591	6.3	36.6	301	865
Cardiovascular Disease								
Sweden	—	26.8	481	3732	—	8.8	134	2772
France	—	29.6	313	2737	—	12.4	113	2284
England and Wales	—	43.3	647	3740	—	17.3	246	3071
Accidents								
Sweden	75.8	84.8	118	216	31.9	28.3	—	182
France	116.4	96.9	135	308	26.4	26.6	42	286
England and Wales	60.5	42.8	50	102	17.7	17.1	29	117
Other Causes								
Sweden	14.8	38	161	619	9.9	16.1	80	494
France	27.6	70.9	381	1772	17.8	38.8	162	1420
England and Wales	18.9	26.6	190	611	13.7	21.8	122	552
Respiratory Disease								
Sweden	—	—	—	363	—	—	—	239
France	—	—	—	257	—	—	—	148
England and Wales	—	—	—	1182	—	—	—	757

Source: World Health Organisation (1980).

being overfed rather than undernourished. In the late twentieth century, European women have become diet conscious. Gone are the problems of not getting enough to eat because of scarcity; women today self-consciously deprive themselves of food to control their weight. Could it be that, in circumstances of food abundance, the natural superiority of the female sex is fully revealed? McKeown has argued that improvements in diet in both quantity and quality were the main reason for the decline and ultimate disappearance of infectious diseases (McKeown, 1976). Accounting for 70 per cent of all mortality in earlier centuries, the conquest of infection led to a revolution in the health status of the population of Europe. If we accept the nutrition argument, it follows that food and its social allocation provides one possible key to understanding the distribution of mortality risk between the sexes in times of scarcity and plenty. When scarce, excess female mortality or, as in the case of nineteenth-century Europe, relative equality in the duration of life between men and women is the outcome of unequal distribution of food resources. When plentiful, the greater longevity of women expresses a natural superiority revealed only in conditions of adequate female nutrition.

This explanation can also account for the fact that sex mortality differentials are variable both over time and territory. This variability has served to persuade some observers of the artificiality of greater female longevity (cf. OPCS, 1980). If biological sex is the source of female advantage, why is the greater vulnerability of the male a twentieth-century phenomenon? The plausible answer, given the foregoing account, is that the twentieth century has witnessed a health and living standards revolution which allows the superiority of the female of the human species to be fully revealed for the first time. The thesis is neat but not quite impregnable. If correct, we would expect the transition in the disease profile of the advanced industrial societies to coincide everywhere with a widening of the sex mortality differential. We have already seen that trends in France and Britain were uneven. Working class living standards were higher in late nineteenth-century England and mortality rates fell faster and were below the rates across the Channel. Even so, excess male mortality made an earlier and stronger appearance in France. Comparisons with other societies provide further contrary evidence. Swedish mortality rates fell faster than British rates throughout most of the nineteenth-century. In Sweden, however, male mortality rates remained close to the level of female rates for most cohorts born before the second decade of the twentieth century. In fact male mortality in Sweden in most adult age groups was even below the level of French and English women at a time when mortality from infectious causes was falling rapidly in all three countries.

This picture of national variation suggests that, even if the physiological make-up of the female helps to structure inequalities in life chances at the beginning of the lifetime, it is not a sufficient explanation of the widening gap in longevity in adult life that has ultimately made an appearance in every part of Europe. Equally, our knowledge that excess female mortality is the global norm reinforces the argument that any physiological advantage enjoyed by the fair sex is always mediated by societal forces. These forces might be conceived of as once-off historical events which set off demographic disturbances in some societies but not others. Alternatively, they may be endemic features of the social structure, differences of power, privilege and ideology which differentiate the average lifetime experience of men and women and shape the distribution of life chances between them. These sorts of influences come under the heading of gender. They may be linked to differences which have their origins in nature but they are not indeterminate and should therefore be conceived as an expression of nurture – of the way men and women are treated differently in society, in infancy, adolescence and adult life.

The European trend of excess male mortality is a twentieth-century phenomenon and it follows that any gender influence must share the same periodicity. We have dated the initial appearance of the male disadvantage in France and England in the generations born during the last quarter of the nineteenth century. This must provide the starting-point in the search to identify any possible gender influences on the trend of excess male mortality. What events or processes at the turn of the nineteenth century could have the capacity to alter the balance of advantage in longevity between the sexes so spectacularly? We will consider three possibilities: the role of the Great War acting to discriminate life chances between the sexes via eugenic processes; the decline in fertility and the transformation of motherhood; and lastly, the division of labour between the sexes in the spheres of employment and income generation.

The eugenic consequences of the Great War

The Great War (1914–18) created according to Winter (1982, pp. 105) a 'burnt-out' generation of men depleted by battlefield death and disablement. This is an example of one of the oldest forms of gender differentiation – the expectation that men will be willing and required to risk life and limb in warfare. In the Great War this expectation led to the loss of up to a fifth of the complement of the generations of men born in the closing decade of the nineteenth century. This major event of the early twentieth century has been identified by some as having profound demographic consequences, particularly in the distribution of life chances between the sexes in the mid- to late twentieth century. The War is said to have initiated a eugenic process which depressed the survival prospects of each of the generations who were recruited into the armed services.

The emergence of the trend of excess male mortality seems to make its appearance with the cohorts who fought in the Great War. Among the generations born in mid-century, the survival gap between the sexes is small and relatively static. The cohort born in 1871, gives the first sign of a break with the past. From about age 55, the death rates of males show the tendency which, by 1891, has become quite marked. This was the generation most 'burnt out' by the Great War. The male infants of 1890 were unlucky enough to be born at just the right moment to make the supreme sacrifice. In England and Wales more than 16 per cent of them lost their lives in the 1914–18 war and many of those who returned were chronically disabled. Moreover, these men were not a random selection. They have been literally classified as the fittest examples of British manhood in their age group.

The medical tests which accompanied the process of recruitment in Britain had led to more than 40 per cent of the age group being rejected as unfit for front-line duty (Winter, 1986, pp. 50–65). They were men, selected for their relatively superior physique, stamina and fitness and sent off to the high probability of an early military grave (cf. Winter).

In both France and Britain, substantial numbers of young men were killed in action between 1914–18. In Britain the losses were numbered at over 700,000: 63 deaths for every thousand males in the 15–49 age group. France incurred even greater losses: more than 1,300,000: 133 deaths per thousand in the same age range. Was the male cohort of 1890 in these countries so depleted of its fittest members by the war effort that higher mortality among the survivors of the cohort, many of whom were deemed unfit for trench warfare, was inevitable?

The cohort which suffered the largest loss in the Great War was born about 1890, they were in their early twenties at the outbreak of hostilities. If we compare the sex differential for this cohort in France and Britain with a non-combatant country like Sweden, we get a clear impression that the First World War may have played some part in the growth of excess male mortality in the twentieth century. The nation with the largest excess of deaths among males born in 1890 is France, where the war losses were more than double, in percentage terms, of those of England and Wales. At the same time, the sex mortality differential is more developed in England and Wales than it is in Sweden where there were no war-related deaths (see Hart, forthcoming).

The circumstantial evidence seems to favour a eugenic explanation for the early widening of sex mortality differentials in France and Britain. The same sort of argument has been advanced by Dinkel to explain the recent increase in mortality in the Soviet Union (Dinkel, 1985). The argument in essence is based on 'natural selection'. If some proportion of the fittest members of a cohort are 'lost', the life expectancy of survivors will be correspondingly diminished. It involves the assumption that medical fitness is a relatively fixed attribute of individuals and a principal determinant of the length of life. The loss of a disproportionate number of 'good risks' lowers the survival prospects of the cohort as a whole. This kind of explanation implies that the environment is not the principal determinant of health and welfare and is evidently not thought capable of making up for the loss of 'good risks' by improving the health status of surviving 'bad risks'*.

*The data used to calculate cohort mortality are based on civilian deaths only.

There is one clear sign of possible war-related health selection in Table 6.3 which reproduces the mortality rates of selected British and French cohorts. During 1918–19, an influenza epidemic swept across the world causing more deaths in Britain even than the Great War itself. These deaths appear to have been distributed unevenly between the sexes with more loss of male than female life. The cohort which shows the largest excess of male deaths at this point was born around 1890 and was precisely the cohort which had experienced the greatest mortality in the recent war. But these signs of positive health selection do not persist. Within the space of less than a decade, levels of excess male mortality fall to their pre-war levels and the seemingly inexorable upward trend of excess male mortality is soon re-established. This pattern is brought out clearly by observation of the level of excess male deaths in the 60–64 age band among cohorts born at successive five-year intervals from 1880 to 1905. The percentage excess increases from 64 per cent in the first cohort to 76 per cent, 91 per cent, 102 per cent, 110 per cent and finally 111 per cent (see Table 6.3). The cohort born after the beginning of the twentieth century, too late to be part of the War, records an excess of 111 per cent. In the cohort which contributed the lives of more than 16 per cent of its male members to the war effort, the excess stands at the relatively modest level of 91 per cent. Since the female half of this cohort was not depleted by wartime losses, an imbalance in mortality rates over the remaining lifetime of the cohort might have been anticipated if selection effects were at work. The lack of confirming evidence suggests that selection played no part in shaping the trends in the level of excess male mortality in middle-aged men among the generations born in Britain between 1880 and 1920. Valkonen, reviewing the impact of war on sex mortality differentials in Finland, comes to a similar conclusion (cf. Valkonen, 1985, p. 229).

We can draw even stronger conclusions from this analysis. If the First World War is treated as a kind of social laboratory for testing eugenic theories relating to health and longevity, our conclusion would have to be that 'natural selection' is far less significant than societal forces in shaping the course and length of the human lifetime. Between 1914–18, the political elites of a number of European nations engaged in a conflict which saw large proportions of their medically fittest young men slaughtered. Yet, as we have seen, this wastage of human life seems to have had almost no discernible effect on trends in the level of excess male mortality in England or indeed in France where war losses were even greater. The cohorts who made the greatest sacrifices in the Great War do not markedly deviate from the increasing trend of excess male mortality which has steadily grown during the twentieth century and which achieves its highest level

Table 6.3 *Mortality by sex and age: birth cohorts 1871, 1891, 1921:*
France and England and Wales

Year of birth	1871		1891		1901		1921	
	France	E&W	France	E&W	France	E&W	France	E&W
5–9 %excess	96%	107%	94%	99%	94%	97%	101%	105%
Male	6.4	6.3	4.3	4.1	3.85	3.3	3.0	2.5
Female	6.7	5.9	4.6	4.2	4.1	3.4	3.0	2.3
Current period	1878		1898		1908		1928	
10–14 %excess	80%	97%	84%	96%	84%	97%	96%	115%
Male	4.0	3.2	3.0	2.1	2.3	2.1	1.8	1.4
Female	4.7	3.3	3.5	2.2	2.7	2.1	1.9	1.4
Current year	1883		1903		1913		1933	
15–19 %excess	90%	98%	94%	107%	—	107%	104%	115%
Male	5.7	4.2	4.8	3.0	—	3.9	3.0	2.2
Female	6.4	4.3	5.0	2.8	—	3.7	2.9	1.9
Current year	1888		1908		1918		1938	
20–24 %excess	130%	108%	118%	122%	113%	114%	—	207%
Male	8.7	5.2	6.8	4.0	6.2	3.5	—	5.0
Female	6.7	4.8	5.8	3.3	5.5	3.1	—	2.4
Current year	1893		1913		1923		1943	
25–29 %excess	102%	117%	—	154%	105%	109%	137%	106%
Male	7.7	5.5	—	8.8	5.8	3.5	4.1	1.8
Female	7.5	4.7	—	5.7	5.5	3.2	3.0	1.7
Current year	1898		1918		1928		1948	
30–34 %excess	110%	119%	108%	113%	131%	109%	135%	125%
Male	8.6	6.3	6.7	4.3	6.3	3.5	2.7	1.5
Female	7.8	5.3	6.2	3.8	4.8	3.2	2.0	1.2
Current year	1903		1923		1933		1953	
35–39 %excess	125%	120%	136%	124%	168%	124%	160%	136%
Male	9.8	7.1	7.9	5.2	7.9	4.2	3.2	1.9
Female	7.9	5.9	5.8	4.2	4.7	3.4	2.0	1.4
Current year	1908		1928		1938		1958	
40–44 %excess	141%	128%	149%	129%	—	146%	183%	141%
Male	11.4	9.2	9.7	6.2	—	5.4	4.4	3.1
Female	8.1	7.2	6.5	4.8	—	3.7	2.4	2.2
Current year	1913		1933		1943		1963	
45–49 %excess	—	135%	165%	141%	162%	149%	203%	156%
Male	—	12.0	12.7	8.6	8.6	6.7	6.9	5.3
Female	—	8.9	7.7	6.1	5.3	4.5	3.4	3.4
Current year	1918		1938		1948		1968	
50–54 %excess	142%	129%	—	158%	181%	175%	216%	172%
Male	15.6	13.4	—	12.0	12.5	10.5	9.7	9.1
Female	12.0	10.4	—	7.6	6.9	6.0	4.5	5.3
Current year	1923		1943		1953		1973	

(Table 6.3 cont.)

Year of birth	1871 France	E&W	1891 France	E&W	1901 France	E&W	1921 France	E&W
55–59% excess	157%	138%	167%	174%	207%	206%	252%	186%
Male	23.8	19.7	17.5	17.4	18.0	17.3	14.1	14.5
Female	15.2	14.3	10.5	10.0	8.7	8.4	5.6	7.8
Current year	1928		1948		1958		1978	
60–64% excess	152%	136%	176%	191%	218%	210%	257%	188%
Male	33.6	28.8	26.6	28.5	26.1	28.1	19.3	21.6
Female	22.1	21.1	15.1	14.9	12.0	13.4	7.5	11.5
Current year	1983		1953		1963		1983	
65–69% excess	153%	140%	184%	188%	210%	207%		
Male	49.4	45.8	38.9	43.5	38.2	43.9		
Female	32.6	32.8	21.1	23.1	18.2	21.1		
Current year	1938		1958		1968			
70–74% excess	—	137%	171%	174%	199%	192%		
Male	—	64.3	58.4	67.5	55.0	66.0		
Female	—	46.8	34.2	38.9	27.6	34.4		
Current year	1943		1963		1973			
75–79% excess	133%	132%	158%	162%	184%	176%		
Male	106.8	101.8	88.6	100.8	79.2	97.3		
Female	80.2	76.9	56.1	62.2	43.0	55.3		
Current year	1948		1968		1978			
80–84% excess	133%	132%	145%	146%				
Male	181.3	166.5	129.0	147.9				
Female	136.6	126.3	88.7	101.3				
Current year	1953		1973					
85+	126%	113%	124%	123%				
Male	307.7	239.2	232.2	237.0				
Female	243.4	212.5	187.4	192.8				
Current year	1958		1978					

Death rates per 1,000 population.
% Excess = Male death rate over female death rate X 100.

Sources: England and Wales Office of Population, Censuses and Surveys;
       France Institut National D'Etudes Demographiques: INSEE (1978).

among the generations born in the early decades of the twentieth century, fortunately too late to be part of the mass slaughter of the Great War.

It could of course be argued that the depletion of the 1890 cohort improved the life career prospects for those who survived to 1920. With so many of their age peers gone, male survivors may have experienced better employment and marriage prospects so that the shrinkage of their cohort improved their material prospects despite the appalling economic recession of the inter-war years. If so, then this must indicate a triumph of environment against nature. The 'burnt out' generation overcame its inherent health disadvantage because the circumstances of its social and economic environment improved.

Fertility and female survival

The diverging pattern of excess male mortality in Europe appeared alongside the progressive disappearance of infectious diseases like TB, cholera, typhus and measles. These diseases accounted for more than seven out of ten deaths in the centuries before 1900. Their conquest was associated chronologically with another remarkable demographic change. As the mortality of children and young people fell from 1870 onwards, the beginnings of a substantial decline in birth rates appeared. In the space of six decades the rate of marital fertility was cut by two-thirds. In Britain, the average size of family fell from just over six children for marriages contracted in 1865 to just over three for couples beginning married life at the turn of the century and down to scarcely two for men and women establishing homes during the Great Depression. These changes had far-reaching consequences for married women. The steady descent of childhood and later infant mortality seemed to insure the future survival of infants and this, combined with a contraceptive revolution (based both on technical innovation and a relaxation of moral taboos) turned parenthood into an increasingly rational, planned and purposeful life career decision. The meaning of femininity and character of the female lifetime was correspondingly transformed as motherhood came to absorb a much smaller share of an enlarged timespan. No longer would women need to devote most of their adult lives to procreation and childcare. Motherhood could now become a part-time rather than a full-time preoccupation.

In Britain the shift in the sexual division of labour manifested by this decline is almost perfectly correlated with the rising tide of inequality in survival. Figure 6.6 charts the correspondence between average family size in Britain and the level of excess mortality among 60 year-old men. (This age represents the peak age for excess mortality among British cohorts.)

The generation of British women who began their lives during the first decade of the twentieth century produced fewer children than any other generation before or since. It should be remembered that the marriage prospects of this cohort were in all likelihood restricted by the Great War. Given sex differences in age at marriage, a large proportion of their pool of potential husbands were fated to die between 1914–18. Even so the male members of this cohort, who were

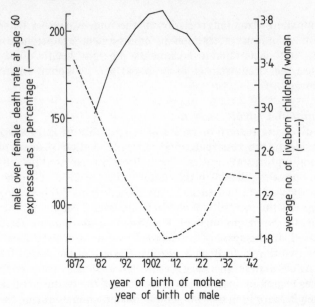

Figure 6.6   Fertility trends and the level of excess male mortality at age 65 among cohorts born between 1872 and 1942: England and Wales

Source: OPCS, 1979; OPCS, 1985.

born too late to be part of the 'lost generations', hold the British record for the sex mortality differential. Their experience appears in Figure 6.6 to be mirrored by the low fertility of their female age peers. Why are these trends linked?

Contrasting the late Victorian mother with her early Edwardian equivalent, we can be certain that the sheer physiological stresses of repeated pregnancy and confinement were halved. This in itself surely had a directly beneficial influence on risks of maternal mortality which rise substantially with the age of the mother and her previous number of confinements. Further less direct, though no less substantial, benefits may have followed. Perhaps the female constitution is inherently stronger because the procreation role is more physiologically demanding. When this is diminished, natural genetic advantage might be realised in improved longevity. This conclusion would fit with the findings of Madigan (1957) who sought to test the hypothesis of natural female superiority by comparing the longevity of Roman Catholic brotherhoods and sisterhoods engaged in educational work. The intention was to control for socio-cultural factors by studying men and women who had opted out of mainstream society. If the sex differential followed the same course as that of the general population in the USA there would be strong grounds for sex as a biological factor rather than gender as a social factor of explanation. His findings were affirmative. Expectation of life for males and females both at 15 and at 45 followed the diverging trajectory of the national population in the USA. The only exception in the picture of female superiority was a male advantage at age 15 in the decade before the First World War, attributable to high tuberculosis mortality among young Catholic sisters (also a feature of national trends). Madigan concluded that socio-cultural factors made only a small contribution to the growing male excess in the national population and that nature itself was by far and away the most important force shaping the survival rates of men and women in the twentieth century.

This sort of conclusion could be readily adapted to account for the somewhat earlier appearance of the trend of excess male mortality in France. During the course of the nineteenth century, the birth rate of France was consistently below that of England and Wales. In 1800 the populations of France and Britain stood at 26.9 and 10.9 million respectively. By 1910 the French population had increased by only 54 per cent to 41.4 million while that of Britain had grown by 274 per cent to 40.8 million. Clearly successive cohorts of French women produced fewer children than their British counterparts during the nineteenth century helping to shape the pro-natalist preoccupations of French social policy in the twentieth. Could French women have been the first to manifest the innate superiority of the female sex by virtue of their avant garde approach to family planning? The answer is not clear-cut. If we restrict ourselves to the nineteenth century, then yes, low fertility goes hand in hand with an increasing female advantage in life chances in the French population. However, when we turn to the twentieth century when the French birth rate is no longer exceptionally low, the trend of increasing excess male mortality maintains its upward climb. Moreover, the mortality rate of French women was higher than their English equivalents up to 1950 suggesting that low fertility itself is not in itself the primary determinant of female vitality and cannot on its own constitute a sufficient explanation for the widening gap between the sexes.

This conclusion is reinforced by Madigan's ingenious attempt to control for the influence of gender as a determinant of longevity. On the face of it, his results add plausibility to the genetic explanation. However, his study leaves one question unresolved: why the divergence in the twentieth century? Unfortunately his observations only go back to 1900 but it does seem that, at this outset, the longevity of men and women opting for a cloistered life was very similar. Moreover, the Catholic sisterhood provides a sample of women who were free from any health risks or benefits associated with procreation and who might therefore have been expected, were fertility to be the critical factor, to record superior longevity well in advance of their age peers in wider society. As childless women, the sisterhood would be subject to a higher risk of some causes such as breast cancer but would be spared the direct risks of maternal mortality as well as any negative long-term influences of repeated pregnancy and childbearing.

With selective emphasis, Madigan's findings can be adapted to either a sex (nature) or a gender (nurture) explanation for excess male mortality. The close correlation between trends for those living 'inside and outside' mainstream society is grist to the mill of the bio-sexual camp while gender theorists can point to the contemporary unique-ness of the phenomenon in Madigan's sample and to the probability that its cause lies in events specific to the relationship of the sexes in the twentieth century. Overall, the correspondence between the survival prospects of the Catholic sisters and the general population of women in the USA suggests that fertility decline cannot be a sufficient explanation for the growth of excess male mortality in the present century. This is reinforced by the knowledge that, among French women who recorded the lowest fertility throughout the nineteenth century, female mortality was in excess of the rates recorded in the much more 'fertile' territory of England and Wales. It would be rash to conclude that reduced risks of maternal mortality and the dramatic fall in the average number of confinements made no difference at all to widening differentials, but at most they can only provide a partial account. This leaves the probability that the close inverse relationship (in Figure 6.6) is spurious or, more likely, indicative of other social changes occurring simultaneously. We have already controlled for the direct influence of the First World War in stratifying the life chances of men and women born around the turn of the century. War-related selection effects are not a useful factor of explanation. So what other possible shifts in gender divisions might have operated to create the largest sex mortality differentials among the cohorts born in the first one and a half decades of the twentieth century?

Sex, gender and the cigarette in the twentieth century
The diseases which contribute most to the widening sex mortality differential in advanced societies, are linked to the consumption of cigarettes. Enterline (1961) calculated that while inequalities in the risk of death between the ages of 15–24 were largely explained by reductions in TB and maternal mortality on the one hand and increases in motor vehicle accidents on the other, reductions in cancer of the uterus and increases in lung cancer and cardiovascular disease played the equivalent role between the ages of 45 and 64 years. Given

that mortality rates for smokers are much higher, that male smokers outnumber female smokers and that smoking has greatly increased since the beginning of the century, Enterline concluded that smoking must have made a substantial contribution to the divergence of male and female life chances since the beginning of this century. This was verified by Retherford (1972), who calculated that smoking accounted for 47 per cent of the sex mortality differential after the age of 40 and was responsible for 75 per cent of the increase between 1910 and 1962. He reached these conclusions by analysing American Cancer Society mortality data which included age, sex, smoking status and ICD cause of death. Cardiovascular diseases and cancer accounted for most of the observed effects of smoking. Similar conclusions were reached by Preston (1976). In a cross-national study of multiple risk factors in excess male mortality he concluded '. . . that a nation's cigarette smoking propensities highly correlate with the amount of *"excess" in its older male death rates*' (1976, pp. 84–5). To complete the case against the cigarette, it also appears that the habit of smoking was the major uncontrolled variable in Madigan's study of Catholic brother- and sisterhoods. While '. . . it had to be admitted . . . ' the males in the sample liked the occasional cigarette, smoking was very rare among females.

The national propensity to cigarette smoking, to use Preston's phrase, has increased steadily over the course of the twentieth century in both England and Wales and France. Unfortunately there are no time series available for Hungary, Austria is included in Figure 6.7 as a rough comparison. As Figure 6.7 reveals, the level of consumption in the United Kingdom has always been well above the level across the Channel and while the Second World War served to depress consumption in France, it led to a dramatic increase in England and Wales.

Of course these per capita figures do not differentiate between the sexes and a good deal of the post-war increase in the UK reflects the rising cigarette consumption of women. In the pre-war period, on the other hand, when cigarette smoking was largely a male preserve, consumption in the UK was two or three times the French level. Even so, as we have seen, excess male mortality in France exceeded that of England and Wales in both absolute and relative terms. This suggests that smoking on its own cannot account for the distinctive national trends in the sex mortality differential charted in Figure 6.2. This fits with the findings of research in Finland whose results are reported by Valkonen (1985). This study estimated the effect of changes in the consumption of cigarettes on death rates and found that even substantial increases in the number of smokers could only have a limited influence on total mortality risk. Such a conclusion is reinforced by the pattern of diseases which makes up the sex mortality

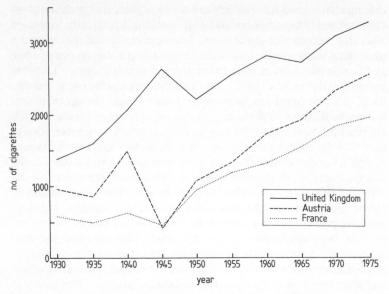

Figure 6.7   Per capita cigarette consumption in European nations 1930–75

Source: Lee, P., 1978.

differential in France where the incidence of smoking-related causes – lung cancer and cardiovasular disease are substantially lower than they are across the Channel. Some part of the lower incidence of cardiovascular disease in France may be explained by the more frequent resort to the category of ill-defined causes in death registration. This residual category is much larger in France and some part of it may include deaths classified under diseases of the circulatory system elsewhere in Europe. However, there is clear evidence that other causes also figure prominently in the sex mortality differential in France. Like Hungary, France records much higher levels of fatal accidents and the incidence of cirrhosis of the liver is extremely high by English standards. These last two causes reflect national variations in alcohol consumption. The French consume more alcohol than any other European nation, approximately 17 litres per head of population per annum – almost double the rate of Hungary and nearly three times that of the UK.

In reviewing the different pattern of diseases which makes up the sex mortality differential in these three societies, what is striking is the universality of excess male mortality despite variations in actual cause of death. In each society the male lifetime is curtailed but the causes of death are highly variable. In large part this explains the shape of the gradients in Figure 6.2. In England and Wales, the contribution of fatal accidents is confined mainly to young people; in France and Hungary, the risk is apparent throughout the lifetime. In all three societies, degenerative disease is the principle reason for inequalities in longevity between the sexes from middle age onwards. Despite variations in the contribution of different causes, one communality unites all three societies. It is the greater male consumption of socially legitimate drugs, alcohol and cigarettes, which appears to underlie the vulnerability of men.

The epidemiological search looks complete. Men die before women because of alcohol and cigarettes. If their consumption could be reduced, sex inequalities in life changes might be eliminated or at least cut to a lower level. How is this to be achieved? Health warnings and tax penalities have some limited power and more rigorous control of advertising would probably be beneficial. In the long run, however, the only foolproof way to eliminate these health risks would be to ban their sale altogether. This involves a degree of state intervention which governments have shrunk away from except at times of national emergency. In France, it took declaration of war with Germany in 1914 for a ban to be made on the production and sale of absinthe, a poisonous but popular beverage of the turn of the century. Likewise, in Britain, effective legislation (of the kind advocated by the Temperance Movement) to curb the production and sale of alcohol was only introduced as part of the Defence of the Realm Act in the same year. If we have to wait for the next war in order to see effective policy initiatives to eliminate the cigarette, the gain in terms of health promotion might be purely notional.

This leaves us with an unexplained question of a kind which a purely epidemiological perspective does not usually seek to address but which appears of critical importance to a sociologist. Why do men drink more than women, smoke more than women and why, moreover, has this sexual division only been associated with a substantial inequality in life chances in the twentieth century? It is this last question which is of principal interest in the present context. While the pipe or snuff box were not toally unknown to women in pre-industrial Europe, their use was far far more prevalent among men. The same is true of alcohol. Taverns, cafes and public houses were the province of men and as tobacco consumption became more widespread, it was typically sold along with beer and spirits in these places of male sociability. In fact the two commodities were closely identified. Early writers linked the craving for drink with that of tobacco and attributed drunkenness as much to the effects of the one as the other (see Corti, 1931). As we view the pattern of excess mortality in France, Hungary and England and Wales we might agree that any similarity in the effect of these drugs in the short term is matched equally by the lethal effects of their long-term use in damaging the physical fabric of the human body. However these effects are only witnessed among cohorts born after the middle of the nineteenth century? Why?

The superficial reason applicable to the United Kingdom, though not to France, was that cigarette consumption increased substantially during the decades when the high-risk cohorts identified earlier reached adult life. As cigarettes became more popular, the sales of other tobacco products, cigars, snuff, pipe tobacco fell back although the total volume of tobacco sold also increased. Over the same period the volume of alcohol consumed in Britain fell dramatically. During the first three decades of the present century per capita alcohol sales fell by almost two-thirds to scarcely four litres per annum in 1930 (Royal College of Physicians 1986). That British men were substituting cigarettes for alcohol over the period seems unmistakable.

The shift from alcohol to tobacco received an enormous boost by the First World War. A number of writers have recognised the role of warfare in promoting the consumption of tobacco (Corti, op. cit.; Sobel, 1978). In 1914, young men recruited into the armed forces were allocated cigarettes as part of their ration. The effect of state-sponsorship was witnessed by the jump in cigarette sales in 1919 when the troops returned home. Between 1900 and 1918, per capita consumption among the civilian population rose at an annual rate of 21 per cent. In 1919 the increase was 202 per cent. The young men who came back from the front were hooked and no wonder. Judging by the number of lives lost and the numbers disabled, it had been a costly war and those lucky enough to survive must have frequently been exposed to mortal danger and grateful for the solace of the cigarette. The appeal of cigarettes grew from the association with young patriotic soldiers gaining a second similar boost from the Second World War, 1939–45. Thereafter British governments continued to make cheap cigarettes a perk of the serviceman's life long after the link with lung cancer had been strongly suggested.

The significance of cigarettes to the war effort should not be underestimated. The use of alcohol in military campaigns to strengthen the will to combat is well known. Rations of gin, vodka, rum or other appropriate national spirits have always been used to build 'Dutch courage' in the face of battle (see Keegan, 1976). That cigarettes could play the same function in a more effective way is evidence in General Pershing's request to Washington during the Great War.

> Tobacco is as indispensable as the daily ration; we must have thousands of tons of it without delay (Corti, 1931, p. 264).

The urgency of these words underlines the fact that cigarettes have a long association with warfare not merely because soldiers and sailors spread the habit via exotic travel, but that the now infamous weed is a powerful narcotic and agent of stress relief. In the Great War, the cigarette proved to be a valuable piece of military equipment because it is a far more effective means of disciplining a modern army than alcoholic spirits. More portable, more rational and more flexible, the individual soldier can carry a personal supply for use as necessary to relieve either boredom or panic. No wonder their popularity in trench warfare.

In the early part of the twentieth century, smoking was quite definitely a male and not a female behaviour. Among ordinary women smoking was stigmatised and those who took up the habit may have done so as part of a challenge to conventional ideas of femininity. We have already seen that the increasing consumption of cigarettes went hand in hand with the decline in drinking. One socially legitimate drug associated with manhood was substituted for another with probably some immediate social benefit. In effect the war hastened the sort of social changes which the Temperance Movement struggled to bring about. Drink was an acknowledged social evil. It divided families, lowered their living standards, and led to conflict and violence. The cigarette also represented a drain on household resources but at least it did less overt damage to relationships between husbands and wives or fathers and children. The role of the cigarette in 'taming' the British working man, in tempting him out of the pub and into the parlour is, as yet, an unexplored terrain of sociology and social history.

The foregoing goes some way towards explaining why smoking became more prevalent among the cohorts of British men born in the decades around the turn of the century. These were the same cohorts who registered the largest sex mortality differential in Britain. The war provided a positive sanction for male smoking while making the same habit in women look unnatural and unfeminine. Equally the war experience itself taught young men the value of nicotine as a means of stress relief. Here we see both a cultural and a materialist explanation for the spread of smoking in Britain in the first half of the twentieth century. In becoming a symbol of the brave soldier, the cigarette was incorporated as part of the insignia of manhood in the inter-war years. Smoking was already more prevalent among men; the war strengthened this differential and invested it with new cultural significance. Does this mean that the attachment of British men to the cigarette is explicable solely in terms of cultural norms? Could it be merely a reflection of the structure of gender differences in the twentieth century?

The alternative explanation is to see the cigarette performing a material role as an agent of stress relief. We should be in no doubt of the capacity of tobacco to perform this role; it has proved its worth in two World Wars. But to attribute the sex differential to this function implies that men are exposed to greater stress in their daily lives than women. What grounds are there for such an assumption?

The materialist question can be extended to alcohol as well as tobacco. In short, should the partiality of men to both these drugs be taken as an indicator of greater physiological need? An affirmative answer to this question suggests that household management was less onerous than wage employment in the decades around the turn of the century when the high-risk cohorts came of age. It is hard to imagine oral historians accepting this assumption. Their accounts of working class family life in those days are redolent with memories of women depriving themselves in order to feed and to clothe their families (see for example Roberts, 1984). On the other hand, as the size of families shrank, the pressures of managing a household on a small budget may also have been reduced. As we saw in Figures 6.4 and 6.5, the cohorts which recorded the peak of sex inequality in life chances were also those where the rate of fertility was at an all-time low. These cohorts also registered the lowest female labour force participation rates in Britain. Born too late to fill the vacant jobs of soldiers at the front, these women found themselves competing with war veterans in the 1920s and facing the slump of the 1930s. Their life careers spanned a particularly unfavourable period for mounting a challenge on the bastions of male privilege in the workplace.

The low participation rates of these female cohorts must also be seen in the context of a major social transformation which emerged after 1860. This was the rise of the *male breadwinner*. In the earlier part of the century, the sex and age structure of the industrial labour force was quite diverse in the growing industrial regions of Britain. Men, women and children worked side by side in workshops, factories and even coal mines. Emile Zola's *Germinal* reveals the same reality in France. By the end of the century, women and children had retired from wage employment. Encouraged by factory legislation and compulsory education, most families in Britain came to depend for their subsistence upon the wage of the male household head. This process laid the foundations of the main axis of gender differentiation in the twentieth century. With the sanction of law, men came to monopolise opportunities for wage employment, while women were increasingly confined to domestic life; they became full-time housewives. This process happened more quickly in Britain than in France. The survival of a large number of peasant proprietors in the French countryside sustained high levels of female participation in agricultural work until well into the twentieth century even though wage employment there, as in Britain, was increasingly monopolised by men (see Tilly and Scott, 1978). We should not overlook the fact that, even in the heyday of the male breadwinner, many families continued to depend in some degree on the casual earnings of housewives generated from cleaning, washing or lodgers. However, the sexual division of labour which characterised the experience of the turn-of-the-century cohorts in both countries must surely have exposed men to industrial accidents and diseases from which women were largely protected. It seems indisputable that some part of the growing divergence in life chances between the sexes must be explained by this change.

It is difficult to determine precisely the contribution of industrial hazards to the sex mortality differential in the closing decades of the nineteenth century. The mines and factories of that period were not healthy; workplace conditions were far harsher than they are today. The working day was more than 12 hours long with no weekend break for leisure or rest. Even so, one source of evidence suggests that the overall contribution of gender differences in employment could not have been very great. In some parts of Britain, notably the textile areas, levels of female participation in work remained quite high. By comparing the mortality rates of female industrial workers we can get some idea of the additional risks faced by men in their breadwinning role. Johannsen (1977) has carried out just such a comparison. She found that the mortality rates of female factory workers were below those of the general population of women at every age. If women in factory work had better life chances than their household sisters, it seems unlikely that the excess mortality of men in the same period could be entirely attributed to industrial risks. One other aspect of the gendered structure of wage employment in the early part of the century, however, suggests a more fertile area for explanatory insight and one moreover linked closely to the sex differences in the consumption of alcohol and tobacco.

In the early decades of the twentieth century, the housewife in Britain had an economically vulnerable status. She lived off the earnings of her husband with help from older employed children still living at home. In law, the economic resources generated by households belonged to the male household head. There is plenty of evidence that housekeeping expenses were managed by women. Men either kept or were allocated some portion of their earnings as pocket money, leaving women in charge of weekly household budgeting. As keepers of the family purse they were acutely aware of the cost of living and the sacrifices required to make ends meet (see Roberts, 1984). Documentary and early social survey evidence makes it clear that in the distribution of food, the male breadwinner enjoyed the lion's share and that wives and, secondarily, children went hungry or badly clothed when resources were scarce. Indeed, there is some evidence that it was female rather than male children who were discriminated against (Wall, 1981). The male breadwinner enjoyed privileged access to the economic resources of the household. Economists use the term 'personal expenditure' in an undifferentiated way to refer to the purchasing decisions of individuals. If we take the term literally we would have to conclude that personal spending power was a male prerogative in the decades which spanned the end of the nineteenth and the beginning of the twentieth century.

The period in question was a time of relative prosperity for working class households. In part this may reflect smaller family size, but of equal importance was a growing trend in security of employment. Work was becoming less casual and household income and expenditure more stable and predictable. There is evidence that some proportion of the rising living standards recorded at the turn of the century was diverted into male leisure activities (see Dingle, 1972; Marrus, 1974). As the length of the working day was reduced and as wages rose, more resources became available for male sociability. Alcohol and tobacco were the typical breadwinner's indulgences and the pub in England and the café in France became places where men relaxed in each other's company. Sex segregation at work was mirrored in sex segregation at leisure. The possible health consequences of this particular gender division are obvious.

It is important to place these developments in their correct historical context. The widening sex mortality gradient is associated with declining mortality which is itself the product of improved living standards. Before 1870, scarcity of household resources combined with large families offered little scope for an expansion of female life chances. As living standards rose, the material circumstances of the sexes changed in different ways. Both sexes must have benefited from better nutrition, but in men such improvements were partly offset by excessive consumption of alcohol, increasingly substituted after 1900 in Britain, though not in France, by cigarettes. Underlying these tendencies, are gender differences in employment and the power and dependency relationships which flow from them. We have already remarked that the high-risk cohorts included the generations of women who recorded the lowest levels of both fertility and labour force participation. They were women most distanced from processes of both production and reproduction and their sense of economic dependency on, and subordination to, their husbands may have been correspondingly heightened. As a result, their capacity to strike a favourable bargain over the division of household income and thereby to exert some control over the spending patterns of their menfolk may have been reduced.

Among later generations, improvements in living standards were increasingly channelled into expenditure on the home. This shift may itself reflect a change in the balance of power between the sexes. The home was the province of the female and as it became a principal object for the investment of surplus income, we may infer that a redefinition of family relationships and of gender differences within them, was taking place. Sociologists have referred to this process as the emergence of the privatised home-centred worker, more interested in home and family than in work or workmates. The whole process was clearly aided by the entry of married women into paid employment after the Second World War but, in its infancy, we might infer that, in an ironic way, the cigarette also played its part in encouraging the same developments. As British men shifted their personal expenditure from alcohol to cigarettes, the pub came to play an increasingly minor part in their leisure time.

Could these trends help us to understand the reasons why men born in the first decade of the twentieth century recorded the highest level of excess male mortality in Britain? Was the lifespan of this cohort the heyday of male drug consumption; a period of small families and of increased household income where financial surpluses were channelled into male leisure rather than family living standards? The drugs in question are on the proscribed list. They were and are freely available over the counter to any adult who could afford to pay. Is it precisely because men and not women could afford to pay that they turned out to be at much greater risk to the long-term lethal effects of alcohol and tobacco? This would fit with our knowledge of the greater consumption of psychotropic drugs by women. In Britain many more medical prescriptions for these drugs are issued for women. They are obtained on the National Health Service at a highly subsidised price but their use implies a clear medical definition of depression. Is this an example of a gender division in the social construction of stress?

Men deal with stress through the purchase of alcohol and cigarettes. It is a natural feature of their lives. In women, on the other hand, stress appears pathological. Because of cultural and financial barriers, women have not used the cigarette for stress relief to anything like the extent that men have. Instead they have resorted to medical advice and consequently record much higher rates of depressive illness and of tranquilliser use. In other words, female stress has been medicalised. In keeping with their dependent economic status, housewives have less scope to be active themselves in the treatment of stress; they have become the clients of doctors, the passive consumers of medical not market drugs.

This explanation suggests that it is not the level of stress which varies between the sexes but rather the method of response. It also implies that, with the exception of tea consumption, the stresses of domestic life went unrelieved in the decades before health care and tranquilliser use became citizenship rights in Britain. The unwaged housewives born in the closing decades of the nineteenth century often lacked sufficient means to provide even basic subsistence and having little control over the generation of income, probably never knew the luxury of personal spending power and never even entertained the thought that they might try a cigarette. Never at least until they joined the workforce themselves. The entry of women to paid employment in post-war Britain has been accompanied by a growing consumption of cigarettes. The correlation between trends in employment and smoking is probably as universal as the sex mortality differential itself. As women gained access to the means of generating their own income, they chose to spend some part of it on the typical male indulgences. When men began the dangerous habit more than a century ago, the health risks of smoking were virtually unknown. The new smoker today embraces the cigarette with no illusions. The consequences for the gap in life chances look predictable. As women claim the right to be treated on equal terms with men in the worlds of work and consumption, they too may pay the price by forfeiting their distinctive advantage in longevity. The signs that this process may already be underway can be witnessed in the rising incidence of lung cancer in Britain and in the downturn in the sex mortality differential among British cohorts born since the mid-1920s. We must wait to see if trends in the other European countries follow suit in the coming decade.

Acknowledgements
The author records her gratitude to the trustees of the Fuller Bequest at the University of Essex for financial support in carrying out the analysis in the paper. Acknowledgement is also made to the Office of Population Censuses and Surveys for their permission to use their data. *Please note that this data is subject to Crown copyright.*

References
Alderson, M. (1981), *International Mortality Statistics*, London: Macmillan.
Corti, C. (1931), *A History of Smoking*, London: Harrap.
Dinkel, R.H. (1985), 'The seeming paradox of increasing mortality in a highly industrialised nation: the example of the Soviet Union', *Population Studies*, 39, pp. 87–97.
Dingle, A.E. (1972), 'Drink and working class living standards in Britain 1870–1914', *Economic History Review*, pp. 608–22.
Durkheim, E. (1897), *Suicide: A Study in Sociology*. Routledge Paul and Kegan, 1970.
Enterline, P.E. (1961), 'Causes of death responsible for recent increases in sex mortality differentials in the USA', *Millbank Memorial Fund Quarterly*, 39, pp. 312–28.

Gove, W.R. (1973), 'Sex, marital status and mortality', *American Journal of Sociology*, 79, pp. 45–67.

Hamilton, J.B. (1948), 'The role of testicular secretions as indicated by the effects of castration in man and by studies of pathological conditions and short lifespan associated with maleness', *Recent Progress in Hormone Research*, 3, pp. 257–324.

Hart, N. (1976), *When Marriage Ends: A Study in Status Passage*, London: Tavistock.

Hart, N. (forthcoming), *Life Chances; Health, Vitality and Citizenship*, London: Macmillan.

Institut National D'Etudes Demographiques: INSEE (1985).

Johannsen, S.R. (1977), 'Sex and Death in Victorian England: An examination of age and sex specific death rates, 1840–1910' in Vicinus, M. (ed.), *A Widening Sphere: Changing Roles of Victorian Women*, Methuen, pp. 163–81.

Keegan, J. (1976), *The Face of Battle*, Harmondsworth: Penguin.

Kynch, J. (1985), 'How many women are enough? Sex ratios and the right to life', *Third World Affairs*, London: Third World Foundation, pp. 156–72.

Lee, P.J. (1978), *International Trends in Cigarette Consumption*, Tobacco Research Council.

McKeown, T. (1976), *The Modern Rise of Population*, Edward Arnold.

Madigan, F.C. (1957), 'Are sex mortality differentials biologically caused?', *Millbank Memorial Fund Quarterly*, 25, pp. 202–23.

Marrus, M.R. (1974), 'Social Drinking in the Belle Epoque', *Journal of Social History*, pp. 115–41.

Martin, W.J. (1956), 'A study of sex, age and regional differences in the advantage of rural over urban mortality', *British Journal of Preventive and Social Medicine*, 10, pp. 88–91.

OPCS (1978), *Decennial Supplement of Occupational Mortality 1970–2*, HMSO.

OPCS (1979), *Variant Population Projections*, HMSO.

OPCS (1980), *Trends in Mortality*, HMSO.

OPCS (1985), *Mortality Statistics 1841–1980*, HMSO.

OPCS (1986), *Decennial Supplement of Occupational Mortality 1979–80, 1982–3*, HMSO.

Preston, S. (1976), *Older Male Mortality and Cigarette Smoking: A Demographic Analysis*, Population Monograph Series no. 7, Berkeley: University of California.

Retherford, R.D. (1972), 'Tobacco Smoking and the Sex Mortality Differential', *Demography*, 9, pp. 203–16.

Roberts, E. (1984), *A Woman's Place: An Oral History of Working Class Women*, Oxford: Blackwell.

Royal College of Physicians (1986), *Our Favourite Drug*, London: Tavistock.

Sen, A.K. (1981), *Poverty and Famines: An essay on entitlements and deprivation*, Oxford University Press.

Stolnitz, G.J. (1956), 'A century of international mortality trends: II', *Population Studies*, 10, pp. 17–42.

Sobel, R. (1978), *They Satisfy: The Cigarette in American Life*, Anchor.

Tilly, L.A. and Scott, J.W. (1978), *Women, Work and the Family*, Holt, Reinhart and Winston.

Valkonen, T. (1985), *The Mystery of the Premature Mortality of Finnish Men*, Reprint no. 128, Department of Sociology, University of Helsinki.

Wall, R. (1981), 'Inferring differential neglect of females from mortality data', *Annales de Demographie Historique*, pp. 119–40.

WHO (1980), *Annual Review of Statistics*.

Winter, J.M. (1982), 'The decline of mortality in Britain 1870–1950' in Barker, T. and Drake, M. (eds), *Population and Society in Britain 1850–1980* London: Batsford Academic.

Winter, J.M. (1986), *The Great War and the British People*, Macmillan.

Zola, E. (1933), *Germinal*, London: Everyman's Library.

7 Adult mortality and level of education: a comparison of six countries
Tapani Valkonen

Studies on socio-economic differentials in adult mortality have shown that the mortality of upper classes is lower than that of lower classes in most causes of death (e.g. Kitagawa and Hauser, 1973, Fox and Goldblatt, 1982, Valkonen, 1983). From the point of view of social and health policy it would be useful to know to what extent this 'inequality in the face of death' varies from country to country. Because of differences in the methods and variables it is, however, difficult to draw any conclusions about the relative sizes of socio-economic mortality differentials on the basis of these studies. This study is an attempt to compare differentials in total mortality and in mortality by cause of death in six countries by using the same variables and methods in all of them. The six countries for which data are available are Denmark, England and Wales, Finland, Hungary, Norway and Sweden. The study also describes changes in the sizes of the differentials in five of these countries during the 1970s. There is so far very little reliable information about the trends of mortality according to socio-economic variables.

Several different socio-economic indicators have been used in studies on differential mortality, such as occupation, income, and housing tenure. In this study, the level of education is used. Level of education is preferable to occupation-based indicators because it applies with equal validity to retired and working men, and to all women including housewives. Furthermore, weakening health tends to have a negative effect on a person's occupational status and income whereas the achieved level of education remains unaffected. This is important when we wish to study how socio-economic status influences health, not the contribution of health to one's socio-economic status (cf. Kitagawa and Hauser, 1973, p. 73).

For comparative purposes education has an additional advantage: if educational attainment is measured by a classification based on the number of years of education, it is more useful in international comparisons than occupation-based classifications, which are difficult to compare because of differences in the occupational structures of countries. The most obvious weakness of level of education in mortality research is its skewed distribution: in many countries the majority of the population has only the basic compulsory education.

Data

Special tabulations for this study were made from data files for Denmark, England and Wales, Finland, Hungary and Norway. In addition an unpublished table on mortality by level of education but without causes of death was obtained for Sweden (see Acknowledgements at the end of the chapter).

The methods of data collection, ways of structuring the data, age-groups covered, and the completeness of the information vary from country to country. To achieve maximum comparability without losing too much information this study concentrates on the 35–54 year-old populations.

The following is a short summary of the data:

Denmark, Norway and Sweden: The death records from 1971 to 1980 were linked with the 1970 Census records. Data on total mortality only are available for Sweden. Two periods are distinguished, 1971–75 and 1976–80. The age-variable refers to age at the beginning of each of the two periods. The deaths are counted cohort-wise for the 5-year cohorts which were 35–49 years old in 1970 and in 1975, respectively. Figure 7.1 shows the structure of the data in the form of a Lexis diagram.

Finland is similar to the above-mentioned countries except that the data for the period 1976–80 are based on linkage of the death records with the 1975 Census records on education.

England and Wales: A representative sample of about 500,000 persons was drawn from the 1971 Census and the deaths occurring in this sample were recorded in the periods 1971–75 and 1975–81 (April). The age-variable refers to age at the time of death. To make the age-range comparable to that used in the cohort-based Nordic data, the age-group 35–54 was used. For simplicity 'England' will be used instead of 'England and Wales' in this chapter.

Hungary: The data are not based on linked records. The death records cover the period 1978–81. The information on the level of education in the population-at-risk was obtained from the 1980 Census whereas the deceased person's level of education was derived from the death certificate. The data are thus not quite comparable with the other data sets. The age variable refers to age at death. Similarly to England and Wales, the analysis covers the age-group 35–54 years.

The educational systems, the codes used in the censuses and the

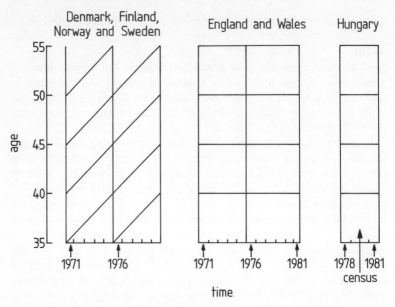

Figure 7.1   The structure of the data sets

completeness of information differ from country to country. It is therefore not possible to use the same classification of the level of education in all countries. Table 7.1 presents the classifications as they are used in this study. The original classifications have been modified by combining small educational categories.

The basic variable underlying 'level of education' is years of school education, when both general and vocational education are taken into account. The Finnish, Norwegian and Hungarian classifications are explicitly based on this variable, whereas this is not the case in the other countries. For Denmark the classification used here was specifically constructed by cross-classifying the information on general education and vocational education.

Table 7.1 gives the percentage distribution of person-years by level of education as well as the total number of deaths in each category covered by this study. The first column shows the average number of school years for each educational category. These numbers are partly estimates by the author and they may be incorrect. The estimates are needed to make the comparison of the otherwise incomparable classifications possible. In estimating the years of education for the educational categories in the British data, an unpublished table on the distribution of years of education by educational category prepared by Mildred Blaxter (see Acknowledgements) was used.

Table 7.1 Educational classifications used in the study, estimated average numbers of years of education, percentage distributions of person-years, and numbers of deaths by country and sex in the material of the study (age-group 35–54)

Educational category	Estimated years of education	Person-years % Males	Person-years % Females	Deaths Males	Deaths Females
Denmark					
1 9 years or less of school educ.	8	27.8	44.5	5464	5548
2 10–12 years of school or voc. educ.	11	40.2	30.3	6318	3160
3 Niveau 5 of vocational educ. (13–14 y.)	13.5	6.2	3.6	791	350
4 Niveau 6 and 7 of vocational educ. (15+ y.)	16	6.4	0.9	699	96
5 Vocational educ., level unknown	11.5	6.9	5.0	776	538
6 No information	9	12.5	15.8	3468	2700
All		100.0	100.0	17516	12392
Finland					
1 Basic education (9 years or less)	8	71.7	74.4	21346	7543
2 Lower secondary educ. (10–11 y.)	10.5	12.4	13.6	2505	961
3 Upper secondary educ. (12 y.)	12	7.9	5.4	1432	382
4 Lower level of higher educ. (13–15 y.)	14	4.3	5.0	605	316
5 Graduate level of higher educ. (16+ y.)	17	3.7	1.6	477	102
All		100.0	100.0	26365	9304
England and Wales					
1 No higher qualifications	10	81.0	86.2	2290	1457
2 A-levels or non-degree, higher qualifications	12	11.6	9.7	235	112
3 Degree or equivalent	17	4.9	1.5	76	16*
4 Not stated	10	2.4	2.7	64	73
All		100.0	100.0	2665	1658

*Combined with category 2 when death rates are computed. The estimated number of years of education for the combined category is 12.5.

(Table 7.1 cont.)

Educational category	Estimated years of education	Person-years % Males	Females	Deaths Males	Females
Hungary					
1 0–7 years	6	25.4	33.9	16307	9495
2 8–11 years	9.5	49.0	45.6	19329	8631
3 12 years	12	15.2	15.1	4067	2335
4 13+ years	14	10.4	5.3	2830	974
All		100.0	100.0	42533	21435
Norway					
1 Primary school, lower stage (less than 9 y.), not reported	7.5	38.9	43.2	6104	3138
2 Second level, first stage (9 y.)	9	20.8	29.7	2250	1486
3 Second level, second stage I–III (10–12 y.)	11	27.6	21.2	3000	1113
4 Third level, first stage I–II (13–15 y.)	14	8.2	5.4	575	223
5 Third level, second stage I–II (16+ y.)	17	4.4	0.5	290	34*
All		100.0	100.0	12219	5994
Sweden					
1 Primary school	8	57.3	67.5	16356	10449
2 Secondary education	11	29.7	22.1	6410	2854
3 Higher education	15	9.7	8.1	1475	781
4 Not reported	9	3.4	2.3	2397	718
All		100.0	100.0	26638	14802

*Combined with category 4 when death rates are computed; the estimated number of years of education for the combined category is 14.5

Results
Total mortality by level of education

Figures 7.2 and 7.3 are based on the age-standardised death rates for the educational categories during the whole period covered by the data. In age-standardisation the direct method was used with equal weights for the three 5-year cohorts in the four Nordic countries. To correct for the difference in the structure of the data the age-groups 40–44 and 45–49 had equal weight and the age-groups 35–39 and 50–54 half of this weight in England and in Hungary. The x-coordinate in Figures 7.2 and 7.3 is the number of years of education.

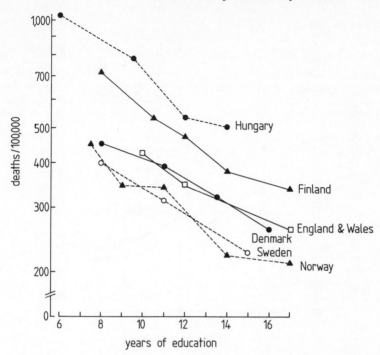

*Figure 7.2   Age – standardised mortality (per 100,000) from all causes of
death by years of education and country, males aged 35–54,
log scale.*

There are great differences in the levels of the lines in both Figures
7.2 and 7.3. These differences are due to intercountry differences in
mortality, which are also known on the basis of comparisons using
standard mortality statistics. For example, both male and female
mortality is much higher in Hungary than in the other countries. The
Finnish male mortality is quite high, but female mortality in Finland
is clearly lower than that of Denmark and England.

The main observation from Figure 7.2 is that all the lines are
approximately parallel: male mortality declines in all of the countries
with increasing education and the relative differences between countries are almost the same at all educational levels. The death rates in
the categories with longest education are 40–60 per cent lower than
the death rates in the lowest educational categories.

In five of the countries male mortality declines monotonously with
the rise of the years of education. In Norway the decline is stepwise,
the first step being between those with primary education and those

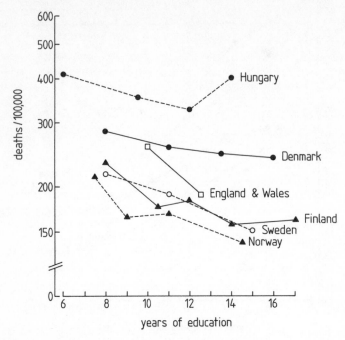

Figure 7.3   Age-standardised mortality (per 100,000) from all causes of death by years of education and country, females aged 35–54, log scale

with 1–4 years of secondary education and the second step between secondary and higher education.

The general relationship between level of education and mortality is the same among women as among men: mortality diminishes with increasing years of education. The slopes of the lines vary, however, more among women than among men, and exceptions from the pattern of monotonous decline are more common. In Norway, the same stepwise pattern as was observed for men can be seen: a clear decline from the primary to the secondary level of education and another decline from the secondary to the tertiary level of education. In two of the countries – Finland and Hungary – mortality is higher in the highest educational category than in the second highest category.

Differences in inequality in total mortality
There are several ways of measuring the size of differences or inequalities in mortality (see e.g. Preston *et al.*, 1981, pp. 247–51 and Hansluwka, 1984). In this study, a measure based on the slope of regression of the logarithm of the death rates on the years of education

is used. This measure, which will be called the 'inequality coefficient', is formed to indicate the estimated relative reduction in mortality (in per cent) per an increase of one year in the level of education. For example the value 6.0 of the inequality coefficient means that the mortality of those with, for example, ten years of education is six per cent lower than the mortality of those with nine years of education. The higher the inequality coefficient, the greater are the differences between educational categories and the steeper is the decline of the regression line. A negative coefficient shows that mortality is higher in the high than in the low educational categories. The effects of age and period are adjusted when calculating the coefficients.

The inequality coefficients were obtained by fitting a log-linear regression model by means of the GLIM program package (Baker and Nelder, 1978) to the data for each country. The method of computing the inequality coefficients is presented in more detail in Appendix 7A.

The inequality coefficients for total male mortality vary between 7.4 (England) and 9.2 (Finland) (see Table 7.2). The differences are thus relatively small, which means that the influence of educational level on total mortality is rather similar in these countries. The parallelism of the lines observed in Figure 7.2 have already indicated such a result.

The inequality coefficient for England is somewhat lower than those for the other countries. This may reflect the real situation, but it is also possible that the result is due to the weaknesses in the measurement of educational level in England (see Fox and Goldblatt, 1982).

The inequality coefficients are smaller among women than among men in all countries but England, as can be expected on the basis of Figure 7.3. There is also more variation in the coefficients for women than for men. Hungary, with its low coefficient, differs clearly from the rest of the countries. The low inequality coefficient is due to the high mortality of the highest educational category. Although the mortality of Danish women declines almost linearly with increasing education, the inequality coefficient is low, since the relative differences are considerably smaller than in the rest of the countries.

As shown in Table 7.1, one of the original educational categories for Denmark, Sweden and England is 'education not reported'. In addition, there is a category with missing information on the length of vocational education in Denmark. Assumptions about the average years of education for these categories were used when computing the inequality coefficients and are presented in Table 7.1. To check how sensitive the results are for changes in the treatment of the 'not reported' cases, the coefficients for total mortality were recomputed after the exclusion of the 'not reported' categories. The results show

Table 7.2   Inequality coefficients (relative reduction of mortality per an
increase of one year of education in per cent) by sex, country
and cause of death ('education not reported' classified as in
Table 7.1)

	Denmark	Finland	England & Wales	Hungary	Norway	Sweden
Males						
Neoplasms	5.1	5.1	3.2	3.2	3.9	—
Circulatory diseases	8.7	9.3	9.2	5.1	8.0	—
Other diseases	12.9	9.1	11.0	12.8	12.1	—
Accidents etc.	7.7	11.1	6.8	14.2	11.5	—
'Avoidable causes'	—	13.2	(28.3)	34.3	—	—
All causes	8.1	9.2	7.4	8.2	8.6	8.0
All causes, not reported excl.	5.8	—	7.4	—	—	7.7
Females						
Neoplasms	3.0	1.1	5.4	−5.3	2.0	—
Circulatory diseases	13.4	14.0	19.3	6.1	16.9	—
Other diseases	7.1	11.9	11.4	8.9	10.6	—
Accidents etc.	−5.2	1.2	−8.4	1.6	−1.8	—
'Avoidable causes'	—	14.3	(21.0)	7.5	—	—
All causes	3.8	6.1	7.8	2.2	5.8	4.8
All causes, not reported excl.	2.9	—	7.2	—	—	4.7

that in England and Sweden the coefficients computed in these two
ways differ very little. For Denmark the original coefficients are
greater due to the fact that the share of the 'not reported' is largest
there. It is possible that the inequality coefficients computed for
Denmark including the 'not reported' cases are somewhat too high.

Inequality by cause of death
Table 7.2 shows the inequality coefficients for the four main groups of
causes of death. All of the coefficients for men are positive, which
indicates that mortality declines with increasing level of education in
all of the four cause-of-death groups in all countries. It is likely that a
more detailed classification of causes of death would reveal specific
causes (e.g. cancers of the rectum and prostate) for which male
mortality increases with rising level of education.

There are systematic differences among the four cause-of-death
categories in the level of coefficients. These differences are known
already from earlier studies on socio-economic mortality. For example
the coefficients are smallest for neoplasms and highest for 'other

diseases' and accidents etc. Coefficients for circulatory diseases are intermediate and close to the coefficients for total mortality. An exception is Hungary, where mortality differentials for circulatory diseases are relatively small.

The differences in mortality from other diseases than neoplasms and circulatory diseases can be considered most interesting from the perspective of inequality in health. Mortality from neoplasms and circulatory diseases is influenced strongly by the social distribution of specific risk factors such as smoking and diet. 'Other diseases' is a heterogenous group in which general living conditions and the utilisation and quality of health services can be assumed to be relatively more important determinants of mortality than specific risk factors. Among men the inequality coefficients in mortality from 'other diseases' are highest in Denmark and Hungary and lowest in Finland. The order of the countries is thus quite different from that for total mortality.

In accidental deaths the coefficient is particularly high in Hungary and low in England.

The cause-specific inequality coefficients vary more among women than among men. The small coefficient for total mortality in Hungary is due to the increase of mortality from neoplasms with increasing level of education. In the other countries the coefficients for neoplasms are, similarly to men, low but positive. In all countries educational differences in mortality from circulatory diseases are greater among women than among men. For example, in Norway the death rate for those with 12 years of education is 64 per cent lower than that for those with eight or fewer years of education. The relationship between level of education and mortality from circulatory diseases is not linear, since most of the difference is due to the difference between those with less than 12 years and at least 12 years of education. Additional years of education after 12 seem to contribute little to the prevention of premature circulatory deaths among women in Hungary, Finland and Norway.

In female mortality from accidental and violent causes the signs of coefficients vary. The negative inequality coefficients for England, Denmark and Norway are due to high mortality in the highest educational category.

Besides the main categories of causes of death, Table 7.2 also includes inequality coefficients for 'avoidable' causes of death (see Rutstein *et al.*, 1976 and Charlton *et al.*, 1983) for three countries for which the data were available. Tuberculosis, chronic rheumatic heart disease, hypertensive disease and certain respiratory diseases are the most important of the avoidable causes of death. The coefficient for men in Hungary is very high indicating large differences. For

England, the coefficient is similarly quite high, but it is based on 108 cases of death, only 10 of which are other than the first educational category. In Finland the coefficient for avoidable causes of death is only slightly higher than that for all causes of death. In Finland the coefficient for women is about the same as for men, whereas in Hungary the female coefficient is surprisingly low compared to the male coefficient.

The absolute number of avoidable deaths in the higher educational categories is low, particularly in England, and the results are influenced by random variation. It seems, however, that mortality from avoidable deaths is worthy of further study as an indicator of social inequalities in health.

Changes in inequality

Changes in the educational inequalities in total mortality can be studied in four of the countries and in cause-specific mortality in three of them. Figure 7.4 shows the relative change in the total age-standardised mortality from the period 1971–75 to the period 1976–80 in each educational category. A horizontal line indicates that the relative change has been equally great in all educational categories and the educational inequalities have not changed. A declining line indicates an increase in inequality.

Among men, the differences between educational categories have clearly increased in England. In the category with no higher educational qualifications there has been no change in mortality, whereas a decline of 10–20 per cent has taken place in the other educational categories. In Sweden and Norway a slight increase of differences can also be observed. In Denmark an increase of mortality in the highest educational group confuses the picture which otherwise shows an increase in inequality. In Finland mortality has declined in all educational groups, but there is hardly any systematic change in the size of the differentials.

Among women, there seems to be no systematic widening or narrowing of the differences in total mortality in the four Nordic countries. On the other hand there is a very large increase of the differences between the two educational categories in England. This is due to a more than 40 per cent decline in mortality in the higher educational category. Educational inequality in mortality, both among men and women, has thus increased considerably in England and Wales in the 1970s. It must be noted, however, that the number of deaths in the high education category in the British female sample is low: 80 deaths in 1971–75 and 48 deaths in 1976–80. The result for English women may thus be influenced by random error.

To make it possible to decide more objectively whether the changes

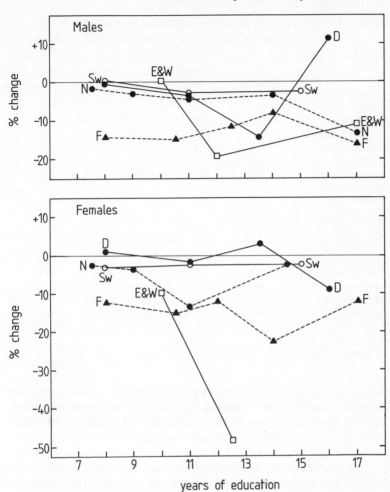

Figure 7.4   Percentage change in age-adjusted mortality from 1971–75 to 1976–80 by years of education, country and sex, all causes of death

in the educational gradients described in Figure 7.4 are real or within the range of random variation, the changes in the values of the inequality coefficients from the period 1971–75 to the period 1976–80 were calculated and the statistical significance of these changes tested. The results are presented in Table 7.3. The method of calculating the changes and their significance by means of the GLIM package is presented in Appendix 7A.

Table 7.3 shows to what extent the educational mortality differen-

Table 7.3   Change in the inequality coefficient from the period 1971–75 to the period 1976–80 by sex, country and cause of death

	Denmark	England & Wales	Finland	Norway	Sweden
Males					
Neoplasms	1.5	−0.4	−1.4	0.1	—
Circulatory diseases	1.5	8.9*	−0.2	1.7	—
Other diseases	−1.6	4.4	−0.3	0.9	—
Accidents etc.	−1.7	−2.3	−0.3	−1.0	—
All causes	0.2	4.0	−0.5	0.7	0.7
All causes, not reported excl.	0.2	4.0	—	—	0.6
Females					
Neoplasms	0.6	—	3.2	2.0	—
Circulatory diseases	0.8	—	−0.7	3.3	—
Other diseases	−2.5	—	−1.5	−5.5	—
Accidents etc.	1.8	—	3.4	2.5	—
All causes	0.2	20.9***	1.1	0.4	0.0
All causes, not reported excl.	0.4	21.5***	—	—	−0.2

* = p < 0.05
*** = p < 0.001

tials have widened or narrowed. A positive number indicates that the inequality coefficient has risen and the differences widened, whereas a negative figure indicates a decrease in the size of the differentials. For example, the coefficient for total male mortality in Finland was 9.4 in 1971–75 and 8.9 in 1976–80. This means that mortality diminished by 9.4 per cent per year of education in the data covering the years 1971–75 and by 8.9 per cent in the data for 1976–80. The change is -0.5 per cent units, which implies a slight reduction in inequality. According to the statistical test this reduction is not statistically significant.

The upper part of Table 7.3 shows that all the other changes in the coefficients for total male mortality but those for Finnish men are positive. This indicates that the tendency towards widening differences is more common than the tendency towards narrowing. None of the changes is, however, statistically significant.

Table 7.3 also shows the changes in the inequality coefficients for the main groups of *causes of death*. 'Avoidable' deaths are omitted because their numbers are too small. In Finland all of the cause-specific changes for men are negative indicating diminishing educational differentials, but none of them is statistically significant. In

Denmark, England and Norway the male cause-specific changes show increasing inequality in mortality from circulatory diseases. In England the change is statistically significant. The male inequality coefficient for circulatory diseases in England was 4.8 in 1971–75 and 13.7 in 1976–80. This change is due to the fact that there was some increase in circulatory mortality in the lowest educational category whereas there was a decline of 20–40 per cent in the other educational categories. In England there was also a considerable increase in inequality in male mortality from 'other' diseases, but this increase is compensated for by a decrease in inequality in mortality from accidents and neoplasms.

The lower part of Table 7.3 shows that the increase of inequality in total mortality among women in England is statistically significant despite the low number of female deaths. The cause-specific changes for women in England are not presented because the small number of deaths makes them very unreliable. In countries other than England, the changes in inequality in women's total mortality are small and statistically not significant.

Some of the changes in cause-specific female mortality differentials are considerably larger than those in total mortality. For example, inequality in mortality from 'other' diseases has diminished considerably, but this narrowing of differences is more than balanced by the widening of differentials in neoplasms and circulatory as well as violent causes of death.

The changes in inequality coefficients have also been calculated excluding the persons for whom the educational category was not reported. It can be seen that the results are almost the same as those for the whole sample.

According to Table 7.3, England is the only country in which there have been some statistically significant changes in inequality. In order to confirm this result, Table 7.4 was calculated using data for the age groups 35–64. The results for this wider age-group are not quite comparable to the results for other countries, but are useful to describe the trends in England. The table includes the inequality coefficients for both periods and the change from the period 1971–75 to the period 1976–81.

Table 7.4 confirms that the all-cause mortality gap between the educational categories has widened considerably during the 1970s. The change in the inequality coefficient for total mortality is statistically significant for both men and women. Among men, the change is due to increases in inequality in mortality from circulatory diseases and from 'other diseases'. There was almost no change in mortality from these groups of causes in the lowest educational category but a clear decline in the other categories.

Table 7.4　Inequality coefficients for England 1971–75 and 1976–81 by sex and cause of death, ages 35–64

	1971–75	1976–81	Change
Men			
Neoplasms	9.3	8.7	−0.6
Circulatory diseases	3.3	10.2	6.9**
Other diseases	1.4	12.4	11.0*
Accidents etc.	8.1	9.5	1.4
All causes	4.7	9.9	5.2**
Women			
All causes	3.8	13.1	9.3*

* p < 0.05
** p < 0.01

Among women, the increase in inequality in the 35–64 age-group is not as great as that observed in Table 7.3 for the 35–54 age-group. According to age-specific data not presented here, the increase of educational inequality has been clearly greater in the ages below 60 years than in the age-groups 60–64 and 65–69 years. However, the small numbers of deaths make this result uncertain.

Discussion

On the basis of earlier research it is not surprising that there are considerable differences between educational categories in mortality among both men and women in all of the countries. Many of the cause-specific findings, such as the relatively small differences in mortality from neoplasms and larger differences in the heterogeneous 'other diseases' group and in accidental mortality, are also familiar from earlier studies. The purpose of this study was, however, not to confirm these earlier results with new variables and data, but to make possible the comparison of inequalities across countries and between two periods.

The pooled data for the two periods showed that, despite considerable differences in the socio-economic conditions and in the levels of mortality, the relationship between years of education and total mortality for men was surprisingly similar in all the six countries.

The uniformity of the male inequality coefficients might be interpreted to show that there is a general 'law of male educational mortality gradient', according to which mortality among middle-aged men diminishes by about eight per cent with an increase of one year in educational attainment. The results presented by Kitagawa and

Hauser (1973) for the USA and by Desplanques (1984, pp. 76–85) for France are not comparable to the results of this study, but they may well follow approximately the same 'law'.

There are, however, at least two reasons not to take the 'law of male mortality gradient' too seriously. First, there is more variation between countries in the cause-specific inequality coefficients than in the coefficients for total mortality. For example, mortality from circulatory diseases and neoplasms is less closely connected with the level of education in Hungary than in the other countries, but this is balanced by the high inequality coefficients for other diseases and accidental deaths. On the other hand, accidental deaths are less closely associated with low educational attainment in Denmark and England than in the other countries. The similarity of the coefficients for total mortality which is the weighted sum of the cause-specific coefficients may be more a coincidence than a general law.

The second and more important finding indicating that the uniformity of the coefficients for total male mortality in Table 7.2 cannot be taken as a general rule is the change of the coefficient for England from 5.3 in 1971–75 to 9.3 in 1976–81 in age-group 35–54 (and from 4.7 to 9.9 in age-group 35–64). During the first period, educational inequality was thus smaller in England than in the other countries, but during the second period it was greater. Only the average for the two periods is close to the other countries. It is also important that, despite this rapid increase in inequality in total mortality, no increase in inequality took place in mortality from neoplasms and from accidents and violence.

The results for men discussed above show that there is more variation between the countries and more differences between the periods when cause-specific mortality is examined instead of total mortality, even when only a crude classification of causes of death is used. For women, the variation of inequality according to cause of death is even clearer, since the sizes and even the signs of the cause-specific inequality coefficients vary strongly both within and between countries. The variation in the coefficients for total mortality is also much greater for women than for men and no generalisation about the female gradients analogous to the 'law of male mortality gradient' can be made.

The observed inequalities in total mortality and their changes, particularly in England, pose an important challenge to health and social policy. It would, however, be too simple-minded to draw immediate strong conclusions about weaknesses in health services or social policy in individual countries on the basis of these results. In order to understand the causes of the inequalities and their changes, and to make practical conclusions for policy, a much more detailed country- and cause-specific analysis is needed. It is, for example, important to find out whether small educational inequality is due to exceptionally high mortality in the high socio-economic positions (as is the case in female cancer mortality in Hungary) or to exceptionally low mortality in the low socio-economic position (as is the case in male accidental mortality in England).

This study is restricted to a rather narrow age-group of population (35–54 year-olds). This restriction was done partly because of the limitations of data for Denmark and Sweden, but also because it was practical in reducing the complications caused by the variation of inequalities by age. This variation may be different in different countries depending on the life-histories of cohorts. A more thorough analysis of the influence of age would be necessary for the explanation and interpretation of the results. This should also include an analysis of the changes in the school systems and methods of recruiting students to higher education.

The level of education has been used here as a socio-economic indicator. The purpose has not been to analyse specifically the causal effect of education on mortality. This would have required a multivariate analysis in which other socio-economic variables, such as occupation and income, should also be included. The study has been based on the assumption that, on average, general socio-economic conditions improve with rising levels of education. The correlation of the level of education with other socio-economic indicators may vary from country to country. The use of another socio-economic indicator, such as occupational class or income, might have given somewhat different results on the degree of inequality in the countries studied. The results on the changes in mortality differentials are likely to depend less on the socio-economic indicator chosen.

Marmot and McDowall (1986) have shown that the mortality difference between the manual- and non-manual occupational classes widened in Great Britain from 1970–72 to 1979–83. This result was based on the comparison of the *Decennial Supplements on Occupational Mortality* published by the Office of Population Censuses and Surveys. The results presented here are based on a different set of data, on a different socio-economic indicator and cover a partly different period and area. They are, however, in agreement with the results presented by Marmot and McDowall and confirm the increase in social inequality in mortality in the 1970s.

Both the study by Marmot and McDowall and this study show that the widening of the gap is mainly due to the development of mortality from cardiovascular diseases. In the four Nordic countries the changes in inequality in cardiovascular mortality were small and also the changes in inequalities in, all cause, mortality were small compared to England and Wales.

Acknowledgements

I am indebted to the following persons and organisations for preparing and giving the permission to use special tabulations for this study:

Otto Andersen (Statistics Denmark),
John Fox and Peter Goldblatt (Office of Population Censuses and Surveys and Social Statistics Research Unit, The City University, London),
Gerd Skoe Lettenstrom and Lars B. Kristofersen (Central Bureau of Statistics of Norway), and
Peter Jozan (Hungarian Central Statistical Office)

I am also indebted to Lars-Gunnar Horte (Central Bureau of Statistics of Sweden) for sending me unpublished tabulations for Sweden, and to the Central Statistical Office of Finland for the permission to use the data files prepared for the occupational mortality study. The data files were compiled by Hannele Sauli and Ritva Marin.

I am also grateful to Tuija Martelin and Seppo Koskinen for their help and their comments on an earlier version of this paper and to Mildred Blaxter for survey data on years of education in Great Britain.

References

Baker, R. J. and Nelder, J. A. (1978), *The Glim System, Release 3, Generalised Linear Interactive Modelling Manual*, Numerical Algorithms group.

Charlton, J. R. H., Hartley, R. M., Silver, R. and Holland, W. W. (1983), 'Geographical variation in mortality from conditions amenable to medical intervention in England and Wales', *Lancet*, 1, pp. 691–6.

Desplanques, G. (1984), 'La mortalite selon le milieu social en France', *Socio-Economic Differential Mortality in Industrialized Societies*, 3, pp. 69–101.

Fox, A. J., Goldblatt, P. O. (1982), *Longitudinal Study 1971–1975, Socio-Demographic Mortality Differentials'*. Office of Population Censuses and Surveys, Series LS no. 1, London: HMSO.

Hansluwka, H. (1984), 'A note on social inequality of death in more developed countries', *Socio-economic Differential Mortality in Industrialized Societies*, **3**, pp. 345–61.

Kitagawa, E. M. and Hauser, P. M. (1973), *Differential Mortality in the United States*, Cambridge, Mass: Harvard University Press.

Marmot, M. G. and McDowall, M.E. (1986), 'Mortality decline and widening social inequalities', *Lancet*, pp. 274–6.

Preston, S. H., Haines, M. R. and Pamuk, E. (1981), 'Effects of industrialization and urbanization on mortality in developed countries', International Population Conference, Manila 1981, part 2, Liege: IUSSP, pp. 233–54.

Rutstein, D. D., Berenberg, W., Chalmers, T., Child, C. G., Fishman, A. P. and Perrin, E. B. (1976), 'Measuring the quality of medical care: a clinical method', *New England Journal of Medicine*, **294**, pp. 582–8.

Valkonen, T. (1983), 'Socioeconomic Mortality Differentials in Finland', in M. Lagergren (ed.), *Halsa for alla i Norden ar 2000*, The Nordic School of Public Health, Rapport NHW, 1, pp. 81–95.

Appendix 7A: The calculation of the values of inequality coefficients and their changes

The inequality coefficient for a specific country, sex and cause-of-death is based on the slope of regression of the logarithm of the death rate on the years of education when the effects of age and period are adjusted for. To obtain an inequality coefficient, a statistical model was first fitted by means of the GLIM programme package (Baker and Nelder, 1978). The dependent variable was the number of deaths for each age, period and level-of-education combination. The continuous variable 'level of education' and the categorical variables age and period plus their interaction were independent variables. The logarithmic link function was used and the number of person-years was taken into account by an OFFSET-directive.

The following model was used:

$$\log E\ (Y_{ijk}) = \log (N_{ijk}) + \text{constant} + \alpha_{ij} + \beta E_k$$

where

$E(Y_{ijk})$	=	the expected number of deaths for age-group i, period j and educational level k
N	=	person years
α_{ij}	=	the effect parameter for the combination of age-group i and period j (marginal effects and interaction)
β	=	the effect parameter for years of education
E_k	=	average years of education for educational category k

After fitting the model the parameter describing the effect of education was modified to indicate the fitted percentage of reduction in mortality per an increase of one year in the level of education by calculating the inequality coefficient $I = 100\ (1-\exp\ (\beta))$.

For the comparison of the two periods, a new model was fitted, which included the interaction between level of education and period in addition to the terms of the original model. Separate slopes of regression of mortality on the level of education and the corresponding inequality coefficients were computed for the two periods on the basis of this model. The statistical significance of the difference of the slopes was tested by observing whether the fit of the model with separate slopes was significantly better than the fit of the original model with the common slope. The test was based on the difference of the scaled deviances for the two models. The difference is distributed approximately as Chi-Squared (Baker and Nelder, 1978, p. 3).

References
Baker, R.J. and Nelder, J.A. (1978), *The Glim System, Release 3, Generalised Linear Interactive Modelling Manual*, Numerical Algorithms Group.

8 Mortality: a comparison of within-country differentials based on selected occupational groups reported in a variety of countries

Elsebeth Lynge, Otto Andersen and Lars-Gunnar Horte

Introduction

To identify occupational risks, it seems sensible to compare the mortality of equivalent occupational groups within different countries. In this way, mortality data are obtained for persons who carry out the same functions in different societies. The method is widely used in cancer epidemiology. The International Agency for Research on Cancer's (IARC) evaluation of evidence for carcinogenicity in humans from arsenic is based, for instance, on studies of copper smelter workers from both the United States and Sweden and from studies of vineyard workers from the Federal Republic of Germany and France (International Agency for Research on Cancer, 1970).

We report here mortality data for selected occupational groups in the Nordic countries in the period 1970–80. The selected groups represent quantitatively important occupations in the Nordic societies, and the purpose is to compare the relative position of these groups within the individual countries as well as to compare the absolute mortality level across countries. It has previously been demonstrated that observed differentials in mortality may depend on the nature of the data source. Thus the social class gradient in overall mortality for UK males was steeper in the unlinked 1970–72 occupational mortality study, than in the linked 1971–75 longitudinal study (Fox, 1980). We have limited the analysis of selected occupational groups to the Nordic countries because it is possible from these countries to obtain mortality figures derived from structurally similar data sources, i.e. census-based linkage studies.

Material and methods

The mortality figures presented here from Norway, Sweden, Finland and Denmark are all derived from linkage studies, where individual records from the 1970 Census have been linked with individual records for deaths and emigrations during the 10-year period 1971–80.

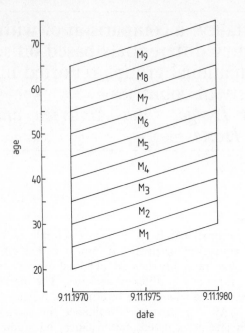

Figure 8.1 Lexis diagram. Principles for calculation of age-specific death rates in the Nordic linked mortality studies 1970—80.

Note: dates refer to dates in the Danish study.

The general design is a cohort study of the cross-sectionally registered census population. Persons aged 20–64 on the census dates are included in the study and followed up from the census date until death, emigration or end of follow-up at 31 December 1980 (for Denmark – 9, November 1980). A person is assigned to the age and occupational group he belonged to at the time of the census, and death rates have been tabulated for 5-year age groups and 10-year calendar periods as illustrated in Figure 8.1.

The Nordic occupational classification (NYK) (Department of Employment, 1969) which follows the same structure as the International Standard Classification of Occupation (ISCO), 1958, was used in the 1970 Censuses in Norway, Sweden and Finland. However, national specifications have been added, and the classifications are only equivalent across countries on the 2-digit level. A special Danish code, developed for earlier censuses, was used in the 1970 Census in Denmark, and it is necessary to take both the detailed Danish codes for occupation and industry into consideration in order to specify Danish occupational groups equivalent to those specified by the

NYK-code on the 2-digit level from the other Nordic countries. These classification problems are reported in detail elsewhere (Andersen, 1988).

There are slight differences between the Nordic countries in the definitions of persons considered economically active in the 1970 Census. The definitions are given below as the differences may be of importance for the interpretation of the mortality data.

Norway: Persons included as economically active are those who had at least 500 hours with income-giving work or work without fixed wages in a family enterprise during the last 12 months prior to the census date (Borgan *et al.*, 1985).

Sweden: Considered economically active are those persons who had at least one hour income-giving work or work without fixed wage in a family enterprise during the census week. Persons who were temporarily absent from the labour market for a maximum of four months before the census date are considered economically active (Statistika Centralbyrån, 1974).

Finland: Considered economically active are those persons with income-giving work on the census date for at least half of the industries' normal working hours. Unemployed and conscripted persons are considered as economically active (Tilastokeskus, 1973).

Denmark: Considered economically active are those persons who were or normally would be economically active on the census date. Persons temporarily absent from work are considered as economically active (Andersen, 1985).

Results

Although the Nordic countries all belong to the prosperous part of the world, mortality differences nevertheless exist within the region. The highest mortality is found among Finnish males: for the age groups relevant in the present study the expected years of life between age 22.5 and 72.5 is 42.90, i.e. on average 7.1 years of the possible 50 years of life in this age span are lost for a Finnish male. The Norwegian females are the most advantaged within the Nordic countries with 47.54 expected years of life between age 22.5 and 72.5 (Table 8.1).

The proportion of the population who passed the threshold to economic activity in 1970 varies between the Nordic countries. The highest proportion is found for Danish males where 92 per cent of males aged 20–64 were economically active, and the lowest proportion

Table 8.1   Expected years of life between age 22.5 and 72.5 in the Nordic countries 1971–80, all persons

	Norway	Sweden	Finland	Denmark
Males	45.11	45.22	42.90	44.77
Females	47.54	47.34	47.07	46.70

Table 8.2   Proportion of population aged 20–64 economically active at the 1970 Census in the Nordic countries

	Norway %	Sweden %	Finland %	Denmark %
Males	90	86	87	92
Females	41	54	60	52

is found for Norwegian females where the percentage is only 41 per cent (Table 8.2).

As a consequence of the differences in the overall national mortality and in the selection of persons into the group of economically active, the mortality rates for economically active persons, vary between the countries (Figure 8.2). These rates have been used as standard rates in calculation of national Standardised Mortality Ratios (SMR) values, and the base level to which the individual social and occupational groups are compared is consequently different from one country to another.

Table 8.3 shows the SMRs for the selected occupational groups from the four countries. Males in pedagogical work have a mortality considerably below the average for economically active males in all the Nordic countries, and males in restaurant work have an excess mortality in all countries. The mortality for males in clerical work and in printing work is close to the average in all countries. Differences between the countries are found in the relative national position for males in agricultural work; the SMR is close to 100 in Finland but considerably below 100 in Denmark.

Persons in pedagogical work are also generally advantaged among females, whereas the SMRs for females in administrative and clerical

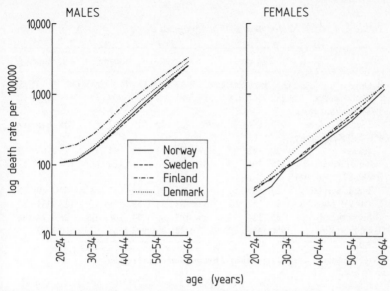

Figure 8.2 Age-specific death rates for all economically active persons in the Nordic linked mortality studies 1970–80.

Note: age refers to lower limit of 5-year age group at time of the 1970 census.

Table 8.3 SMR[1] for persons in selected occupational groups at the 1970 Census in the Nordic countries

	Norway	Sweden	Finland	Denmark
Males				
– Pedagogical work	72	75	62	75
– Clerical work	100	106	91	108
– Agricultural work	80	82	94	71
– Printing work	107	114	97	115
– Restaurant work	143	159	144	171
Females				
– Pedagogical work	84	81	78	87
– Administrative and clerical work	103	102	102	98
– Textile work	98	103	99	107
– Restaurant work	112	100	107	110

Note: 1 National standard populations: All economically active persons.

Table 8.4   SMR¹ for males in pedagogical work

	Norway			Sweden			Finland			Denmark		
ICD-8	O	E	SMR	O	E	SMR	O	E	SMR	O	E	SMR
140–209 Cancer	280	361	78	575	681	84	206	309	67	427	594	72
390–458 Circulatory diseases	519	656	79	965	1226	79	519	742	70	705	845	83
460–519 Respiratory diseases	20	42	48	57	78	73	12	44	28	43	81	53
Other diseases	139	201	69	167	279	60	81	123	66	144	246	59
E 800–827, 940, 941 Traffic accidents	23	39	59	59	88	67	33	61	54	47	69	68
E 950–959 Suicides	32	52	62	135	183	74	58	118	49	132	151	87
Other accidents	35	114	31	96	198	49	54	168	32	26	73	36
Total mortality	1050	1466	72	2054	2732	75	963	1565	62	1560	2092	75

Note: 1   National standard populations: All economically active persons.

work, females in textile work and females in restaurant work are close to the average for economically active females in all the four countries.

Table 8.4 shows the national SMRs for main causes of death for males in pedagogical work. The deficit in mortality is seen for all main causes of death. Low relative risks are found for respiratory diseases and for violent deaths, except for suicides in Denmark.

As the SMR values are weighted by the mortality level of the national populations, nationally advantaged groups may not turn out to keep the same position when the mortality rates are compared across the countries. Figure 8.3 shows the age specific death rates for males in pedagogical work in the Nordic countries. The diagram shows Finnish male teachers to have the highest mortality despite the fact that they have the lowest national SMR value. The national differences in overall mortality are even more outspoken for males in agricultural work where Finnish farmers have mortality rates considerably above those of farmers in the other countries, a reflection of the general high mortality in Finland combined with the fact that Finnish farmers have a national SMR of 94. Table 8.5 shows that age-standardised mortality rates for males in pedagogical work and in agricultural work for the main causes of death. The small excess in overall mortality for Finnish teachers compared with Swedish teachers is seen to be due almost entirely to circulatory diseases, whereas the considerable excess in overall mortality for Finnish farmers compared with Swedish farmers is seen to be due to an excess in mortality from all main causes of death.

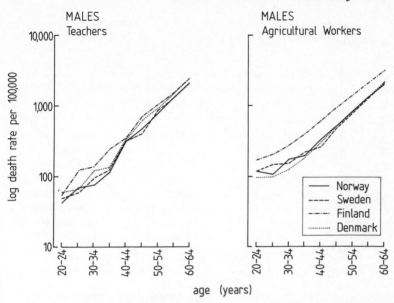

Figure 8.3 Age-specific death rates for male teachers and agricultural workers in the Nordic linked mortality studies 1970–80.

Note: age refers to lower limit of 5-year age group at time of the 1970 census.

Table 8.5 Age-standardised rates per 10,000 in the population[1] for males

ICD-8	Pedagogical Work				Agricultural Work			
	Norway	Sweden	Finland	Denmark	Norway	Sweden	Finland	Denmark
140–209 Cancer	13.0	13.9	13.9	16.1	12.6	12.9	19.3	15.2
390–458 Circulatory diseases	25.2	24.3	36.4	27.3	23.7	24.7	47.8	22.9
460–519 Respiratory diseases	1.0	1.4	0.8	1.6	1.3	1.6	3.4	2.7
Other diseases	6.3	3.7	4.6	5.1	7.8	4.4	5.6	5.0
E800–827, 940, 941 Traffic accidents	0.9	1.2	1.6	1.6	2.2	1.7	2.9	2.1
E 950–959 Suicides	1.2	2.6	2.1	3.6	2.5	4.0	5.6	3.5
Other accidents	1.4	2.0	2.4	0.8	3.3	3.2	5.4	1.5
Total mortality	49.0	49.0	61.8	57.3	53.4	52.5	89.9	53.1

Note: 1 Age distribution as of the total Nordic male 1970 Census population (excl. Iceland).

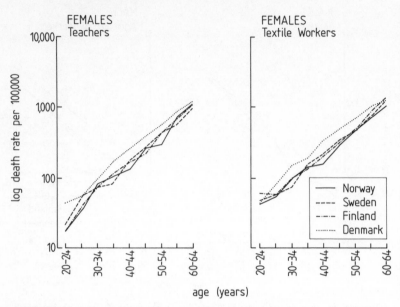

Figure 8.4   Age-specific death rates for female teachers and textile workers in the Nordic linked mortality studies 1970–80.

Note: age refers to lower limit of 5-year age group at time of the 1970 census.

As seen from Fig. 8.4, Danish females in both pedagogical work and in textile work have an overall mortality above that of equivalent occupational groups in the other Nordic countries. Table 8.6 shows the pattern of causes of death for females in these occupational groups, and the high mortality rates for Danish females are seen to be due primarily to an excess cancer mortality.

Discussion
In the age-span we are studying here Finnish males have the highest mortality among Nordic males and Swedish and Norwegian males have the lowest. The present analysis indicates that these differences are not only due to differences in the social structure of the societies, but that the same pattern is seen when mortality rates for specific occupational groups are compared across the Nordic countries. The differences may, however, be more or less obvious. Thus male Finnish teachers only have a small excess mortality in comparison to male teachers in the other countries, and this difference seems to be due almost entirely to circulatory diseases. The mortality differences between male farmers are, on the other hand, considerably more acute, and Finnish farmers seem to have an excess mortality from all

Table 8.6   *Age-standardised rates per 10,000 in the population[1] for females*

ICD-8	Pedagogical Work				Textile Work			
	Norway	Sweden	Finland	Denmark	Norway	Sweden	Finland	Denmark
140–209 Cancer	12.8	12.5	10.5	18.3	12.8	14.1	11.9	18.8
390–458 Circulatory diseases	6.1	5.0	8.1	6.1	7.8	8.5	11.3	10.3
460–519 Respiratory diseases	0.6	0.5	0.6	0.8	0.4	0.7	0.7	1.4
Other diseases	2.2	2.3	2.2	2.7	3.7	2.5	3.4	4.7
E 800–827, 940, 941 Traffic accidents	0.4	0.6	1.1	0.9	0.8	1.0	1.0	0.8
E 950–959 Suicides	0.6	1.6	0.7	2.3	0.6	1.3	1.0	2.0
Other accidents	0.5	0.8	0.8	0.6	0.3	0.7	1.1	0.7
Total mortality	23.1	23.2	24.0	32.0	26.3	28.8	30.4	38.8

Note: 1   Age distribution as of the total Nordic female 1970 Census population (excl. Iceland).

main causes of death compared with farmers in the other Nordic countries. It is interesting that the mortality of Norwegian, Swedish and Danish farmers seems to be fairly equal despite the obvious differences in climatic conditions for agriculture in these countries.

The mortality is highest for females in Denmark in the economically active age groups studied here. The mortality differences between occupational groups are generally smaller among females than among males, but, among the groups selected for tabulation in the present study, female teachers were shown to be a low-risk group in all of the four countries. The excess mortality among Danish females is seen both in the low-risk group of teachers and in females in textile work, and is primarily due to cancer in both groups.

Acknowledgements

The data presented here were collected as part of an inter-Nordic project on socio-economic differentials in mortality 1970–80. We are indebted to Lars Kristofersen, Statistisk Sentralbyrå, Norway and Hannele Sauli, Tilastokeskus, Finland, for assistance with the data collection. The study was supported by the Nordic Council (170.21–0.37).

References

Andersen, O. (1985), 'Occupational mortality in Denmark 1970–80' (In Danish) *Statistisice Undersøgelser* (41), København: Danmarks Statistik.
Borgan, J–K., Kristofersen, L. (1985), 'Occupational Mortality 1970–80 Documenation' (in Norwegian). *Interne notater*, Oslo: Statistisk Sentralbyrå.

Department of Employment (1969), *Classification of Occupation* (in Danish), København.

Fox, A.J. (1980), 'Prospects for change in differential mortality' in WHO (ed.) *Proceedings of the Meeting on Socio-Economic Determinants and Consequences of Mortality*, New York, Geneva.

International Agency for Research on Cancer (1970), 'Monographs on the evaluation of the carcinogenic risk of chemicals to humans', *Some Metals and Metallic Compounds*, 23, Lyon: IARC.

Nordisk Statistisk Sekretariat (1988), *Occupational Mortality in the Nordic Countries 1971–80*, Statistical Reports of the Nordic Countries, No. 49, Kebeuhaun.

Statistiska Centralbyrån (1974), '1970-Census Documentation' (in Swedish), *Sveriges Officiella Statistik. Folk-och bostadlds-rakningen 1970*, Del 12, Stockholm.

Tilastokeskus (1973), '1970-Census: Industry and occupation' (in Finnish), *Fos VI C: 104*, Del II B, Helsinki.

9 A compilation of some aspects of area mortality differentials in some European countries
Peter Jozan

This paper is a compilation of the main features of scientific material dealing with area mortality differentials in some European countries.

The material can be divided into three parts:

- data series
- papers describing area mortality differentials;
- papers trying to explain, at least to a certain degree, area mortality differentials by applying independent variables (socio-economic, cultural, environment etc. factors) and studying their relationship with the dependent variable: the area mortality differential.

The available material by no means covers the whole of Europe since there is no information on some very important European countries. In certain cases they exist, but for one reason or another they cannot be reached. In other cases there is an uncertainty regarding even the existence of relevant data.

Usable material is available on area mortality differentials in the following countries.

Austria
Regionale Unterschiede in der Sterblichkeit in Österreich 1969–1973; 1976
Österreichischen Statistischen Zentralamt (OSZ)

A short description of findings in German. Number of deaths by sex, age (5-year age-groups), area (9 Bundeslandern) and causes of death (29 categories).
Age-specific death rates (100,000 population). Breakdown as above.
Age-specific death rates (7 age groups – 100,000 population) by sex, administrative areas, size of settlements (population of people in agriculture) and causes of death (29 categories).

Belgium
'Regional Mortality for Adult Ages in Belgium' in Espace Populations Sociétés La Mortalité Adulte dans les Pays Industrialises; 1984
R. André

Université de Lille I, Université Libre de Bruxelles, Université Catholique de Louvain etc.

This article is based on studies carried out by the Centre de Demographie de l'Université Libre de Bruxelles, that have resulted in the calculations of regional tables 1969–72 with all causes put together and according to various causes. The regions have defined the crude death rates 1968–73 from 2,379 communities which formed the administrative groundwork of Belgium in 1970.

R. André uses as basis for this analysis of adult mortality the values of life expectancies at 15, 35 and 60 years of age as well as the quinquennial quotient from 45 to 69 years of age. Concerning men, a low-mortality for the Flemish and natives of Brussels appears to contrast with an excess mortality for Walloons; concerning women, regional differences are less marked. However, a slight excess mortality can be found for Walloons. The article ends with the presentation of regional variations of mortality for diseases of the circulatory system and neoplasms. To measure the effects of these causes, the author uses life tables.

Le cancer en Belgique et en Europe: Mortalité et Morbidité.
Josianne Duchene, Michele Van Houte-Minet, Christine Leton. Centre d'Etude de la Population et de la Famille 1983 Dossiers du Departement de Demographie, Université Catholique de Louvain.

Mortality of neoplasms in Belgium: the history of registration and the description of present and past characteristics. Neoplasms, their position among other causes of death. The development of crude and standardised death rates; the ageing of the population. The risk of dying of cancer and its development when it is considered as an independent cause of death. The distribution of neoplasms by sex, age and localisation. The effects of analysis by calendar year or by cohort. Mortality of neoplasms in Europe between 1955–75. The presentation of findings. The selection of countries and period of observation. Crude cause-specific mortality rates. Refined measures analysing the development of cancer mortality. Analysis of mortality by localisation of neoplasms. The morbidity of malignant tumours in Belgium and in Europe. The registration of new cases in Belgium. The incidence of cancer in Belgium and certain European countries. Morbidity rates of new cases by sex and age in Belgium and Europe. The distribution of new cases by localisation of neoplasms in Belgium and in Europe.

Conclusion: the study, conducted for both sexes, has shown, in the 16 countries, similar developments towards increase or decrease: the general decrease of mortality of cancers in the digestive system and the increase in lung cancer mortality and in the mortality of neoplasms of lymphatic and haematopoietic tissues. A decrease of malignant neoplasms of the breast and other female genital organs also can be observed. An attempt was made to classify the European countries by frequency of neoplasms. In the case of neoplasms of the respiratory and digestive system the Nordic countries have a lower mortality rate than the European average. For each site of cancer, developments have been related to several possible causes in the environment, lifestyle, nutritional habits and to particular age cohorts.

Denmark
Regionale Dodeligheds forskelle I Danmark 1971–79; 1983
Danmarks Statistik

A short description of findings in Danish in 25 tables on number of deaths and death rates by sex, age, area and causes of death.

Dodelighedsindeks for kommuner of amted 1971–80; 1984
Dansk Institut for Klinisk Epidemiologi

English summary of scope, methods and findings. Head and lateral text of tables also in English. The study is descriptive in character.

England and Wales
Mortality Statistics Area; microfiche Series DH 5 no. 10
Office of Population Censuses and Surveys

Review of the Registrar General on deaths by area of usual residence in England and Wales 1983.

Death rates per 1,000 population: sex and age-group, 1983 – England and Wales, England, Wales standard regions, Greater London, metropolitan and non-metropolitan countries. Regional health authorities.

Standardized Mortality Ratios: Cause, 1983 – as above.

Microfiche: deaths: cause, sex and age-group, 1983. England and Wales, England, Wales standard regions, Greater London, City of London, London boroughs metropolitan and non-metropolitan counties and districts. Outside England and Wales. Regional and district health authorities.

Atlas of Cancer Mortality in England and Wales 1968–1978; 1983
John Wiley and Sons

This book records, in atlas form, deaths from cancer which occurred in England and Wales during the years 1968–78. Death rates from cancers of selected sites of the body are shown on maps on two different scales. The numerically more important cancers are depicted on a small area basis using local authority area boundaries, with the remaining sites being on a county level.

Atlas of Mortality from Selected Diseases in England and Wales 1968–1978; 1984
John Wiley and Sons

This atlas is based on deaths which occurred in England and Wales during the years 1968–78. It maps the geographical distribution of mortality from selected individual causes of death other than cancer. It is divided into two sections which reflect the two different scales used to depict the death rates: the first section shows the numerically more important causes of death on a small area basis (using local authority area boundaries) and the second section shows the remaining diseases on a county level.

'Approaches to studying the effect of socio-economic circumstances on geographic differences in mortality in England and Wales'
A. J. Fox, D. R. Jones, P. O. Goldblatt
Social Statistics Research Unit, The City University, London and Medical Statistics Division, Office of Population Censuses and Surveys, London

British Medical Bulletin, Vol. 40, No. 4, 1984, pp. 309–14

Characteristics of geographic areas must be considered as distinct from those of individuals living in these areas. Geographic correlation studies provide a weak basis for making inferences about the relationships between the health of individuals and their lifestyle, socio-economic circumstances and their personal exposure to environmental hazards, at least when the units of area used are large. Difficulties arise because in more affluent areas there are poor people and in less affluent areas there are people who are welloff, etc. This type of difficulty is often termed the ecological fallacy. Since data are available on 'usual residence at the time death' and about the last occupation of the deceased, analyses can be performed by social class within each area to measure the degree to which geographic differences reflect the socio-economic variation between areas. The OPCS *Longitudinal Study* (LS) described mortality differences in 1971–75 between administrative areas – such as regions. This paper presents some early results of a project using the full decade of deaths between the 1971 and 1981 Censuses to investigate geographic mortality differentials further. Differences in mortality between areas of the country are defined in terms of the socio-demographic characteristics of people living in them. For four selected socio-demographic areas, the authors look at the degree to which differences in mortality between the areas are explained by the housing tenure, social class and the economic position of the individual people living in those areas. Social classes are grouped on the basis of occupations as follows: professional, administrative, junior non-manual, skilled manual, semi-skilled manual, and unskilled manual occupations. A preliminary investigation has been made on the extent to which differences in socio-economic characteristics explain differences in mortality by housing tenure, social class, etc. This paper uses area of usual residence, economic position (i.e. whether or not the sample member was working the week before the census), social class and housing tenure.

Mortality is compared in 36 geographic clusters derived by grouping census wards on the basis of 40 census variables. The 36 geographic clusters are grouped into seven families:

Family 1: Areas of young and growing population
Family 2: Areas of older settlement
Family 3: Rural areas
Family 4: Urban council estates
Family 5: Areas in Scotland suffering from acute social disadvantage
Family 6: Areas of multi-occupancy – students and immigrants
Family 7: Areas of established high status and resorts.

Male mortality in four clusters is analysed in this paper. The object of these initial analyses is to obtain an indication of the extent to which the socio-economic characteristics explain the cluster differences or the cluster differences explain the socio-economic differences.

The cluster with the most significantly raised SMR is inner areas with low quality older housing. Other clusters with significantly raised SMRs include overspill estates, urban local authority estates with good job opportunities, mining areas, inner-city council estates and multi-occupied and immigrant inner areas. The clusters with significantly lowered SMRs include modern high-status areas, established high-status suburban areas, residential retirement areas, rural established high-status areas, very high-status areas, modern high-status housing, young families and high-status rooming-house areas. These areas are found with a high proportion of two-car households, professional people and owner-occupiers with large accommodation.

Four clusters are analysed in detail. They are: residential retirement areas (35), new towns (1), older industrial settlements with less stress (9). These have mortality near to average. Cluster 11 (inner areas with low-quality older housing) has high mortality.

Cluster differences persist within tenure groups. Furthermore, tenure might explain some, but not all, of the geographic cluster differences. Tenure differences, within geographic clusters show that owner-occupiers have substantially lower SMRs than local authority tenants. Men in privately rented accommodation in Clusters 35, 9 and 11 have similar mortality rates to local authority tenants. Within each cluster category the relationship with the tenure is similar and within each tenure category the relationship with the cluster is similar.

The analysis of mortality by social class within geographic clusters indicates that both social class and cluster contributes to observed differences. There is an area component which is independent of the social classes of the men in these types of area. Also within each geographic cluster, men in Social Classes I and II had lower mortality than men in Social Classes IV and V, with those in Social Class III in between.

Differences in SMRs by housing tenure within geographic clusters are wider than those by social class within clusters.

Within each geographic cluster the employed have low mortality and the retired have higher mortality.

Marked differences between clusters were found; high-status areas having low mortality and those identified as low-status areas having high mortality. In most instances, only a part of the geographic cluster differences could be explained by differences in the distribution of people by socio-economic characteristics. Within each geographic cluster, socio-economic differences in mortality were found by housing tenure, by social class and by economic position.

France

Statistique des causes medicales de deces, tôme II, Année 1978 Resultats par région; 1982
INSERM – Institut National de la Sante et de la Recherche Medicale

Number of deaths, crude death rates (per 1,000 population) by regions and départements. Number of deaths by sex, age-group (11 age-groups) and by regions, *départements* and agglomerations, by types of settlements, causes of death (74 causes – 8th Revision), deaths by sex, age, region, *département*, agglomeration and by size and type of settlements.

Données de démographie régionale – 1975; 1981
Michel de Saboulin
INSEE – Institut National de la Statistique et des Etudes Economiques

Main characteristics of mortality: number of deaths, crude death rates, standardised mortality rates (SMRs), infant mortality rates, life expectancies at birth and at age one for males, females and both sexes by regions and *départements*, settlements: cities and towns and agglomerations, by types of communities. Age-specific mortality rates (5-year age-groups), by regions and *départements*, settlements: cities and towns and agglomerations, by types of communities – for males and females separately. Life table indices: probabilities of dying between different ages and number of survivals at different ages for males and females separately by regions etc. (see above). The publication is the result of a combination of the data of the 1975 Census with mortality statistics for 1974, 1975 and 1976. (Other vital statistical events are also tabulated.)

'Cancer and food. The case of cancer of the intestine and cancer of the rectum'
France Mesle, INED
Population, no. 4–5, 1983, pp: 733–62

Cancers of the intestine and rectum are the second most important cause of death from malignant tumours in France. The development of mortality of cancer of the colon since 1950 has been completely different for the two sexes: mortality of women from this cause has fallen, that of men has risen. In 1973 mortality was higher for men; this development was recent for cancer of the colon, but excess mortality of men from cancer of the rectum goes back a long time.

Regional differences in mortality are marked. In the Mediterranean Littoral these two malignant tumours are less frequent. The North, Britanny and Aquitaine are among the most affected regions. A comparison of mortality and dietary habits leads us to suspect a link with the intake of certain foods: animal fats, beer and potatoes.

The mortality rates from cancer of the intestine and the rectum in 29 developed countries are widely divergent. In the Anglo-Saxon countries, mortality from cancer of the intestine is very high as is mortality from cancer of the rectum in German-speaking countries. An examination of dietary patterns brings out the relationship between intestinal cancer and consumption of meat, fats and sugar, and between rectal cancer and the consumption of beer, fats and potatoes.

'Causes of mortality in France III. An interpretation of geographical differences for the period 1974–76'
Graziella Caselli, INED – University of Rome
Population, no. 6, 1984, pp. 1011–44

In this paper, variations in cause and geographical distribution of mortality are confronted by a group of economical, social, environmental and cultural variables. This involves the use of Vallin and Nizard dual etiological and anatomical classification and the Department mortality data for 1974–76.

A large portion of the geographical variations is due to differences in incidence of alcoholism. But for men, this did not prevent other etiological processes, less linked to individual behaviour, also playing a significant role. Thus, for example, several etiological processes concern the respiratory apparatus (whether tumours, infection or degeneration) which are the sum of the negative effects of smoking, poor working and economic conditions and an unhealthy climate. In the case of degeneration of the circulatory system, very wide differences are seen between diseases affecting the heart and non-cerebral blood vessels and cerebro-vascular degeneration. For the former, the most important external factors are the same as those which affect diseases of the respiratory apparatus (smoking, working conditions), whilst the latter are more related to problems inherent in the physical and sanitary conditions of the population and its level of economic development.

Finland
Kuolleisuuss-ja elvonjaamisolukuja 1983, Life tables 1983
Central Statistical Office of Finland, 1985

Expectation of life at birth by sex and province between 1966–83. Differences between the life expectancies of females and males as absolute figure ($e_o^F - e_o^M$) and as percentage of the quantity e_o^{MS}.

Influence of Socio-economic and Other Factors on the Geographic Variation of Mortality in Finland, Sweden and Norway
Tapani Valkonen and Veijo Notkola
Publication no. 105 of the Department of Sociology, University of Helsinki. Reprint from the *Yearbook of Population Research in Finland*, XV, 1977

There is high mortality in Finland as compared to that of the other Scandinavian countries. Clear and systematic geographic differences exist within countries. Factors which can be responsible for geographic mortality differences: geographic and historical factors; those living conditions which have a direct effect on the biological health of the population; variables indicating the level of health or risk of becoming ill among the population. Furthermore, general level of living, especially when the cohorts now dying were young; the impact of urbanisation and industrialisation is ambiguous. The mechanisms through which urbanisation is linked with higher mortality are not known. Mortality in urbanised areas is not high among all groups. The quality of health care and the climatic factors can be assumed to be more important when the level of living is low and when outdoor work is common. The influence of dietary and smoking habits on mortality has not been analysed in this study. When the influence of the groups of factors mentioned above has been taken into account, some systematic regional variation is likely to remain. To explain this remainder, the genetic composition of the population and various cultural factors associated with, for example, level of social integration may be relevant.

The Development of Male Mortality by County and Cause of Death in Finland in 1961–75
Tapani Valkonen and Marja-Liisa Niemi
Working paper no. 12. Department of Sociology, University of Helsinki, 1980

This research report is part of a larger study on regional mortality differences and their development in Finland. The report contains results on the development of age-standardised male mortality in Finland as a whole, in urban and rural areas and by county. There are twelve counties in Finland. The data on total mortality cover the period 1961–77 and the data on cause-specific mortality the period 1961–75. Death rates are presented on the following groups of causes of death: diseases of the circulatory system, ischaemic heart disease, cerebrovascular disease, neoplasms, malignant neoplasms of the trachea, bronchus and lung, other diseases and accidents, poisonings and violence. Age-standardised death rates were computed separately for the 35–64 year-old males, the 65–74 year-old males and the 35–74 year-old males. Mortality from circulatory diseases rose in Finland in the 1960s. The increase was greater, and also lasted longer, in rural than in urban areas. In urban areas, mortality from circulatory diseases started to decline after 1967; in rural areas at the beginning of the 1970s. The main trend in mortality from other than circulatory diseases has been declining, whereas mortality from accidents, poisonings and violence has increased. The analysis of cardiovascular mortality by county reveals two distinct regions: a southern and western region characterised by low mortality and an eastern region characterised by high mortality. In both of these regions mortality from cardiovascular diseases increased in the 1960s. The decline started in the southern and western counties at the end of the decade. In eastern Finland the outset of the decline was later – the beginning of the 1970s. The differences among counties in the development of mortality from other causes than cardiovascular diseases are mostly small and unsystematic. The role of the change in the consumption of animal fats (especially butter fat), smoking habits and medical care as causes of the observed changes in cardiovascular mortality is discussed in the last part of the report. It seems that changes in the consumption of butter fat correlates better with changes in cardiovascular mortality than changes in smoking habits. The improvement of medical care may have contributed to the decline in the 1970s.

The High Ischaemic Heart Disease Mortality in Finland. International Comparisons, Regional Differences, Trends and Possible Cause
Kalevi Pyorala and Tapani Valkonen, Skandia International Symposia, 1980

In both sexes (for men aged 35–64 and women 35–74 by counties in Finland in 1969–72) there is a clear pattern of increased IHD mortality from the south-west to north-east. The most eastern county, North Karelia, shows the highest IHD mortality rates. The IHD mortality rate in the Aland islands is much lower than in other parts of Finland. The excessively high mortality of east Finns is almost entirely caused by their high mortality from cardiovascular diseases, particularly from IHD. Possible cause: dietary fats and serum cholesterol, high blood pressure, smoking, genetic factors, environmental factors (e.g. mineral and trace element content of the soil and water), socio-economic factors (the lower socio-economic groups show the highest IHD incidence rates), lifestyle, health care.

The Development of Cardiovascular Mortality in Finland from 1951 to 1978
Tapani Valkonen and Marja-Liisa Niemi
Reprint no 120, Department of Sociology, University of Helsinki
Reprinted from *Yearbook of Population Research in Finland*, XX, 1982

The rural-urban mortality differentials have generally been considerable for men but very small for women. Since cardiovascular mortality in urban areas started to decline much earlier than in rural areas the former excess mortality regarding cardiovascular diseases has disappeared in urban areas. In mortality from other than cardiovascular diseases the urban excess mortality has remained approximately the same as in the 1950s. The general pattern of regional differences in male cardiovascular mortality has remained the same during the whole period covered by the study. In almost all provinces, an increase and a later decline in mortality can be observed. The maximum mortality was, in general, reached earlier in the western and southern provinces (which otherwise have had, by national standards, the lowest mortality). In most of the eastern high-mortality provinces the rise continued longer and the decline started at the beginning of the 1970s. The regional differences in the timing of the rise and decline of mortality are not independent from the rural–urban difference. The western and southern provinces are more urbanised and economically more developed than the eastern provinces: the maximum mortality was reached in the more urban and industrialised areas in the latter part of the 1960s and somewhat later, around the year 1970, in the rural and more agricultural areas. Several factors influencing death rates may have changed simultaneously: improvements in the medical prevention and care of cardiovascular diseases (increase in antihypertensive treatment and in the proportion of diagnosed hypertensive subjects receiving treatment), improvements in the social security system, which have made early retirement easier. No hypotheses connecting changes in mortality with changes in the economic situation are plausible. Animal fat is considered to be a major factor influencing the incidence of coronary heart disease. The changes in male, cardiovascular mortality correlate closely with changes in the consumption of milk fat. Therefore this might explain the trend in cardiovascular mortality. Changes in mortality have followed changes in the consumption of milk fat with a three-year lag.

'Psychosocial stress and sociodemographic differentials, in mortality from ischaemic heart disease in Finland
Tapani Valkonen
Reprint no.121, Department of Sociology, University of Helsinki
Acta Med Scand (suppl) 660, 1982, pp. 152–64

This report describes differences in mortality from ischaemic heart disease (IHD) and other selected causes of death according to region, marital status, language group (Finnish or Swedish), social group and rural–urban divisions in Finland. The data include all deaths in Finland during 1971–75 in the cohorts of men aged 35–64 and women aged 35–74 on 1 January 1971. IHD mortality was found to be higher than average in Eastern Finland in the Finnish-speaking population and in lower social groups. The findings are discussed in the light of differences in stress-related mortality.

Regional Differences in Mortality from Cardiovascular Diseases and Other Causes of Death in 1971–75
Seppo Koskinen, Tapani Valkonen, Hanna Kulokari, Marja-Liisa Niemi, Ja Hannele Sauli
Research Report no. 220, 1983
Department of Sociology, University of Helsinki

The study describes regional mortality differentials in Finland by cause of death in several sub-groups of population and explores regional correlations between various causes of death. Attention is directed primarily to cardiovascular diseases; other causes of death are mainly considered for comparative purposes.

The data were originally compiled in the Central Statistical Office by linking death certificate records covering all deaths in the period 1971–75 with the 1970 Census by means of the personal identification code. This study is limited to those who were 35–74 years old on 1 January 1971. The population at risk is classified in sub-groups according to age, sex, degree of urbanisation and education. Finland is divided into 40 areas, and cause of death is grouped in eight classes. Regional mortality rates are calculated using the indirect method of age-standardisation.

Mortality from cardiovascular diseases is lowest on the west and south-west coast and highest in East Finland and, particularly among men, in North Finland. There is a relatively sharp division, following a line from Porvoo to Pietarsaari, between the high-mortality and low-mortality regions. Among middle-aged men crossing the above-mentioned division, mortality rate from ischaemic heart disease is 36 per cent higher, which constitutes more than half of the difference between areas of the lowest mortality on the south-west coast and the high-mortality region in far north-east Finland. Regional variation in mortality from ischaemic heart disease is almost uniform in sub-groups of the population. Among the middle-aged, mortality from ischaemic disease and cerebrovascular diseases varies similarly by region. The correlation between lung cancer and ischaemic heart disease is positive and fairly high among men but negative among women. Cancer among women and ischaemic heart disease for both sexes show a strong negative correlation.

The results suggest that regional differences in mortality from cardiovascular diseases are largely due to factors which exert a similar effect on different groups of population. Moreover, crossing the Porvoo–Pietarsaari line from south-west to north-east greatly strengthens this effect. The determinates of observed regional variation in mortality remain unknown, but especially genetic factors and/or some features in the natural environment might be essential.

'Transition of mortality in Finland and Sweden'
Tapani Valkonen
Beitrage zur Demographie, (*Demographic Transition*) no. 7,
Humboldt-Universität zu Berlin, 1983, pp. 185–208

The chapter of the paper 'Regional and socio-economic differences' deals partly with area mortality in Sweden. Fridlizius states that decline occurred in the course of a marked regional conformity for all the mortality series and the relationship between different regions remained unaltered. According to Norberg, Norman and Akerman there were marked discrepancies in the changes of mortality during the second half of the nineteenth century. The two statements are the result of different approaches, (investigation of different areas, using different mortality data). In Finland, Turpeinen and Strommer studied the decline in area mortality rates. Before the transition, mortality was higher in the southern and south-western regions where the death rates declined faster than average. As a consequence, death rates were lower than average in these regions already at the turn of the century. This reversal of the regional differences in mortality is analogous to the reversal of the urban–rural differences, which took place at about the same time.

'Trends in coronary heart disease, mortality, morbidity and related factors in Finland, 1985'

Kalevi *Pyorala, Jukka T. Salonen, Tapani Valkonen
Department of Medicine and Research Institute of Public Health and
Department of Community Health, University of Kuopio and
Department of Sociology University of Helsinki – published in
Cardiology, 72, 1985, pp. 35–51

A marked increase in the coronary heart disease (CHD) mortality of
working-age men and women occurred in Finland from the 1950s
until the 1960s. Around the year 1970, CHD mortality started to
decline and this decline still continues. In the age-group 35–64 years,
the average annual decline of CHD mortality in the 1970s was 1.8 per
cent for men and 3.4 per cent for women. Limited data available on
trends in CHD morbidity show that the decline in CHD mortality is
accompanied by a decline in the incidence of non-fatal myocardial
infarction.

CHD mortality and incidence are higher in East Finland than in
West Finland and this east–west difference has so far persisted during
the declining trend. The decline in CHD mortality and incidence in
the 1970s had been preceded and paralleled by changes into a
favourable direction in dietary fat consumption and population mean
levels for serum cholesterol, prevalence of smoking among adult
Finnish men, control of hypertension by antihypertensive drug
therapy, and management of patients with symptomatic CHD. Both
the changes in lifestyles and CHD risk factor levels, as well as changes
in the management of patients with CHD, appear to have been
contributing to the decline in CHD mortality and incidence in
Finland.

Federal Republic of Germany (Bundesforschungsanstalt für Ländeskunde und Raumordnung)
*Regional Unterschiede der Sterblichkeit Untersuchung am Beispiel der
Länder Nordrhein–Westfälen und Rheinland–Pfalz*

Frank Heins,
Gerhard Stiens

Regional mortality differentials. A study on the Länder Nordrhein-
-Westfalen and Rheinland–Pfalz life expectancy at birth, sex-specific
differentials, age-specific mortality for males and females separately.
Standardised mortality indices. Cause-specific mortality differentials:
standardised indices for males and females separately. Cause-specific
life table indices. Malignant neoplasms of the respiratory system.
Alcohol-psychosis, alcohol dependence and cirrhosis of the liver.
Ischaemic heart disease. Diseases of the respiratory system (without
infections and neoplasms) motor vehicle traffic accidents. Interpre-

tation of findings. The risk factor concept. Socio-economic, environmental factors, types of settlement mortality differentials.

'Regional Mortalitätsunterschiede in der Bundesrepublik Deutschland', *Daten und Hypothesen*, pp. 37–63
Hans-Peter Gatzweiler and Gerhard Stiens
Source: Jahrbuch für Regionalwissenschaft Gesellschaft Für Regionalforschunge, 3, 1982
Göttingen, Vandenhoeck and Ruprecht

(Regional differences in mortality in the Federal Republic of Germany.) This article is concerned with major regional differences in mortality and life expectancy in the Federal Republic of Germany. Death rates remarkably above the average are found predominantly in two different types of areas – the densely populated centres of large agglomerations dating back to early industrialisation (like the Ruhr area) on the one hand and, on the other hand the sparsely populated peripheral rural areas (e.g. regions near the eastern Bavarian border or in central parts of the Eifel mountains) where the social and economic structures are rather underdeveloped. Both types of areas offer living conditions far below the average quality of the country. However, the reasons for the inferiority of the living conditions in different areas are not identical. This becomes obvious when the patterns of death causes are examined, which turn out to be not identical either. The centres of early industrialisation, in contrast to the rural areas concerned, have a significantly higher mortality from cancer (especially cancer of the respiratory organs), diseases of the digestive organs, bronchitis, and cirrhosis of the liver. In the rural areas, on the other hand, a significantly higher incidence of death caused by specific chronic heart diseases, by cerebrovascular diseases, and by traffic accidents has been observed. On the basis of these empirical data, the authors discuss hypothetical correlations between the different patterns of death causes and the probability of different pathogenous influences from the ecologic, social environment and housing. Conclusions are drawn with further investigations in view and with regard to certain specific consequences in the range of regional policy.

Hungary
An Ecological Approach in Revealing Socio-economic Differentials in Mortality: Some Preliminary Results of the Budapest Mortality Study
Peter Jozan
Hungarian Central Statistical Office
Presented in the Seminar on Social and Biological Correlates of Mortality Organised by the National Institute for Research Advancement of Japan and the IUSSP in Tokyo in 1984

The Budapest Mortality Study is part of a research programme started by the Central Statistical Office in 1983 in order to reveal mortality differentials in the early 1980s in Hungary. This study was initiated in 1984 and will be finished in 1986. It has to be emphasised that only some preliminary results are currently available. Since mortality differentials are more substantial among males than among females, in this paper only some data of the male sub-population, already available, are analysed. When the study is completed, the data on mortality differentials in the female sub-population will also be discussed. Likewise some of the independent and dependent variables are omitted here from analysis. They will be dealt with in detail in the final paper of this study.

Budapest has 22 districts. Each of the districts represents a particular entity. Their populations are by no means homogeneous, yet there are socio-economic and other variables relevant in mortality differentials which can be found in substantially different frequencies in the 22 municipalities. This variation makes Budapest a suitable laboratory for the ecological approach of socio-economic differentials in mortality.

The following independent variables are used in order to describe the socio-economic characteristics of the population:

1. Education

(a) The proportion of 25 year-old and older males who had completed less than eight grades (including those who never attended school);

(b) The proportion of 25 year-old and older males who completed eight grades (usually it means the completion of primary school including those who have had some years in secondary school without finishing it);

(c) The proportion of 25 year-old and older males who had completed some types of secondary school (in most cases it means 12 grades, including those who have had some college education without finishing it);

(d) The proportion of 25 year-old and older males who had completed college education;

(e) The proportion of males, aged 40–59, who had completed less than eight grades (including those who had never attended school);

(f) The proportion of males, aged 40–59 years, who had completed eight grades (usually it means the completion of primary school, including those who have had some years in secondary school without finishing it);

(g) The proportion of males, aged 40–59 years, who completed some types of secondary school (in most cases it means 12 grades; including those who have had some years in college education without finishing it);

(h)   The proportion of males, aged 40–59 years, who completed college education;

(i)   The proportion of males, aged 40–44 years, who completed less than eight grades (including those who never attended school);

(j)   The proportion of males, aged 40–44 years, who completed eight grades (usually it means the completion of primary school; including those who have had some years in secondary school without finishing it);

(k)   The proportion of males aged 40–44 years, who completed some types of secondary schooling (in most cases it means 12 grades, including those who have had some years in college education without finishing it);

(l)   The proportion of males, aged 40–44 years, who had completed college education;

(m)   The average number of completed grades by males;

2. Occupation

(a)   The proportion of male manual workers among active male breadwinners;

(b)   The proportion of male non-manual workers among active male breadwinners;

(c)   The proportion of skilled and semi-skilled male workers among active male breadwinners;

(d)   The proportion of unskilled male workers among active male breadwinners;

(e)   The proportion of males in managerial positions among active male breadwinners;

3. Housing

(a)   The number of people per 100 rooms in occupied dwelling units;

(b)   The proportion of flats with bathroom or with wash-basin among the occupied dwelling units;

(c)   The proportion of one-room dwelling units among the occupied dwelling units;

(d)   The proportion of dwelling units with four and more rooms among the occupied dwelling units;

4. Health Provision

(a)   The number of general practitioners per 10,000 population.

In the study of socio-economic differentials in mortality in Budapest the residential population of the capital at the 1980 Census has been used as the denominator population. Deaths which occurred to the population at risk in the period 1980–83 have been used as the nominator. Abridged life tables have been constructed separately for each of the male and female sub-populations of the 22 districts in order to decribe general mortality.

Standardised mortality ratios (SMRs) of the most important groups of diseases and of the relevant nosological entities have been calculated in order to present cause-specific mortality for the whole male and female sub-populations and for certain, bigger age-groups having particular importance.

The following dependent variables are used in order to discover mortality differentials among the 22 districts:

A.   expectation of life at birth;
B.   expectation of life at age 30;
C.   probability of dying between age 40–45.
D.   SMR[1]: age 1-x, I[2]. Infectious and parasitic diseases;
E.   SMR: age 1-x, II. Neoplasms;
F.   SMR: age 1-x, VII. Diseases of the circulatory system;
G.   SMR: age 1-x, VIII. Diseases of the respiratory system;
H.   SMR: age 1-x, IX. Diseases of the digestive system;
I.   SMR, age 1-x, External causes of injury and poisoning;
J.   SMR, age 1-x, Malignant neoplasms of lip, oral cavity, pharynx and oesophagus (140–150),
K.   SMR, age 1-x, Malignant neoplasm of stomach (161);
L.   SMR, age 1-x, Malignant neoplasms of trachea, bronchus and lung (162);
M.   SMR, age 1-x, Ischaemic heart disease (410–414);
N.   SMR, age 1-x, Acute myocardial infarction (410);
O.   SMR, age 1-x, Cerebrovascular disease (430–438);
P.   SMR, age 1-x, Intracerebral haemorrhage (431);
Q.   SMR, age 1-x, Pneumonia and influenza (480–487);
R.   Chronic obstructive pulmonary diseases and allied conditions (490–496);
S.   SMR, age 1-x, Chronic liver disease and cirrhosis (alcoholic) (571, 0–571, 3);
T.   SMR, age 1-x, Motor vehicle traffic accidents (E810–E819);
U.   SMR, age 1-x, Suicide and self-inflicted injury (E950–959).

SMRs of the same causes of death are also calculated for the age-

---

[1]SMR: Standardised Mortality Ratio. Budapest as a whole equals 100 per cent.
[2]The Roman numbers show the main groups of diseases; the Arabic numbers indicate the three- and four-digit categories of the 9th Revision of the ICD.

groups 15–44, 45–64 and 40–59 years. Here only SMRs for the age-groups 1–x, and 40–59 years are used.

Substantial mortality differentials can be found among the 22 districts. The expectation of life at birth for males is 69.73 years in district II and it was only 64.22 years in district VII in the early 1980s. The second district is one of the most fashionable residential areas in the green belt and district VII is one of the depressed neighbourhoods in downtown with many economic and social problems. Those males who live in district II enjoy a life expectancy of about four years longer than the national average and 5.5 years longer than those who live in district VII. The differences between the highest and the lowest values of the expectations of life at age 30 and at age 40 are relatively even bigger: 4.9 and 4.5 years respectively. In the critical age-group, in which the biggest increase can be observed in age-specific mortality rates in the country as a whole, namely in the age-group 40–45, the probability of dying is 3.3 times as high in the 'worst' than in the 'best' district.

Without exception, the districts with the most favourable mortality record are those which are situated on the west side of the Danube, in the green belt and in the old, historical quarter of the city. They are the neighbouring districts I, II and XII. The districts with the most unfavourable mortality records can be found exclusively on the east side of the Danube: either in the deteriorating areas of downtown (districts VI, VII, VIII), or in the outer parts of the capital where presumably considerable immigration from the countryside has substantially increased the proportion of males with low educational attainment (districts XVII, XX).

The differences among SMRs are less remarkable regarding the whole male sub-population (except those under age one) than in the age-group 40–59. They are most striking for alcoholic cirrhosis of the liver, suicide and malignant neoplasm of the stomach. In these cases the ranges can be found between 15–179, 70–149, 51–129 per cent respectively when SMRs were calculated for the whole population. In the age-group 40–59 the ranges of the three SMRs are even bigger: alcoholic cirrhosis of the liver: 50–196, suicide: 52–198, and malignant neoplasms of the stomach: 47–159 per cent. The green belt districts in the above-mentioned three categories, have the lowest extreme values and some deteriorating downtown districts and districts in the industrial belt have the highest extreme values.

The differences among SMRs are also rather conspicuous for intracerebral haemorrhage, cerebrovascular disease and external causes of injury and poisoning. The differences among SMRs for lung cancer, acute myocardial infarction and ischaemic heart disease are less remarkable.

Some Features in Area Mortality Differentials in Hungary in the Early 1980s; p. 22
Peter Jozan
Hungarian Central Statistical Office
Presented at the Ninth International Conference on The Social Sciences and Medicine in Korpilampi in 1985

A Project of Mortality Differentials has been carried out. It was initiated in 1983 by the Hungarian Central Statistical Office, with the assistance of the United Nations Fund for Population Activities (UNFPA) and in technical cooperation with the WHO Regional Office for Europe, in order to reveal the causes of the rising secular trend in, and the high level of, mortality differentials. Life tables and standardised mortality ratios (SMRs) by causes of death have been applied in order to explore the mortality differentials:

– between urban and rural populations;
– among the nineteen counties;
– by population size of settlements and;
– between urban and rural populations in each county separately.

The period of observation is 1970–82. Some time series start in 1970. In these cases each year is covered separately. However, most of the data originate from the years around the 1980 Census.

In the early 1980s (average for the years 1980–82) the expectation of life at birth for males was 66.0 years in the country as a whole. Life expectancies at birth for males in urban areas were almost equal in the capital (66.7 years) and in other cities (66.8 years), whilst the expectation of life at birth in rural areas developed less favourably (65.2 years).

Looking at the development of life expectancies at birth in the 19 counties it is not justified to say, that substantial mortality differentials exist among the six regions of the country. Yet it can be stated that, in the early 1980s probabilities of survival were greater in the north-western, western, south-eastern and eastern counties respectively than in counties situated in the middle of the country. The expectation of life at birth was between 67.2 – 67.5 years in the counties of Györ-Sopron, Vas, Békés and Csongrád, whilst it was only 64.2 – 64.4 years in Bács-Kiskun and Pest counties.

Recently the life expectancy at the age of 30 has acquired particular importance in Hungary since the increase in the probability of dying occurred in the age-groups over this age (except in the age-groups of 85-x). Life expectancy for males at the age of 30 was 39.0 years in the early 1980s in Hungary; in Budapest it was 39.6 years, in all other cities and towns it was 39.4 years and much less in rural areas: 38.4 years.

Expectation of life at age 30 is the longest in Békés county and the shortest in Bács-Kiskun county. The difference is 2.9 years. The differences in the probabilities of dying increase substantially over the age of 30.

The prospects of survival by the population size of settlements was as follows: expectation of life at birth is the longest in the cities with 30–50 thousand inhabitants (66.8 years), there is a direct ratio between the decrease in population size of settlements and the decrease in life expectancy at birth in the case of cities, towns and villages with a population less than 30,000. In villages with a population less than 1,000, the expectation of life at birth is only 64.0 years. In contrast with this the differences in terms of expectation of life at birth are negligible among the settlements in the three upper ranges: Budapest, cities with more than 100,000 and cities with 50,000 – 100,000 inhabitants on the one hand, and cities with 30,000 – 50,000 inhabitants on the other at the expense of the three former. The low life expectancy at birth in the smallest villages can be partly attributed to the impact of emigration: healthy people leave these settlements and the less healthy ones remain there. However, it cannot be excluded that the quality of life, especially the standard of health provision, is worse in the smallest villages than in the more populous settlements.

In general, mortality differentials are much smaller among female sub-populations than among the male ones. It might be supposed that those elements of lifestyle which are relevant to health do not differ too much among females living in towns, cities or villages. The longest life expectancy at birth can be found in the western and north-western counties: Vas, Gyor-Sopron. Also, the prospect of survival is rather good in Csongrád and Nograd counties. In these four counties the values of expectation of life at birth are between 74.7 – 74.0 years. Life expectations at birth are shortest in the south, south-western part of the country: in the Somogy and Baranya counties. The differences between the longest (Vas) and shortest (Somogy) expectation of life at birth is 2.1 years.

At the age 30 life expectancies are about the same by types of settlements: it is 45.5 years in the country as a whole, 45.3 years in Budapest, 45.6 years in towns and cities and 45.5 years in villages. In the county of Vas, in which it is the longest, it is 46.4 and in the county of Komárom, where it is the shortest, it is 44.8 years.

Expectation of life at birth for females by the population size of settlements show similar features to those for males. Yet the differences are smaller and less consistent. More health-conscious behaviour can help a lot to decrease the disadvantages regarding health provision which can be found in villages.

Standardised Mortality Ratios have been applied in order to reveal cause-specific mortality differentials. In this approach the cause-specific morality rate of the country as a whole equals 100 per cent.

SMRs have been used deliberately to explore mortality differentials by types of settlements and by counties. They have been calculated for:

- all causes of death;[*]
- all natural causes of death (without violent causes);
- II Neoplasms;
- VII Diseases of the circulatory system;
- VIII Diseases of the respiratory system;
- IX Diseases of the digestive system;
- External causes (Icode)
- all other causes together and
- those three-and-four-digit categories separately which have a high frequency as cause of death.

In this preliminary report, only the SMRs of four causes of death (groups of causes of death) are evaluated. They are those which either have the highest frequency or they are relevant in revealing harmful health practices (e.g. excessive alcohol consumption) or in exploring the standard of health care, especially primary health care indirectly regarding some chronic diseases (e.g. hypertensive disease).

Italy

La Mortalita per causa nelle regioni Italiane
Tavole per contemporanei 1965–66 e per generazioni 1790–1964
(Mortality by causes in the Italian regions Momentum life tables 1965–66 and cohort life tables 1790–1964, 1973
Marcello Natale, Amadeo Bernassola
Instituto di Demografia Facolta di Scienze Statistiche Demografiche ed Attuariali Universita di Roma

Results of the research on male excess mortality in the Italian regions. Life tables by sex, regions and principal causes of death, cohort life tables for the whole of Italy. In the mid-1960s, male excess mortality was the highest in those regions and in those causes for which the levels of age-specific mortality rates were the highest. The development and possible explanation of male excess mortality 1790–1964 are given. However, there are still significant differences among the various regions – in fact the range between the largest and the smallest regional value is about 4 years – for both males and females. Infant mortality, which is closely associated with socio-economic develop-

[*]According to the 9th Revision of ICD.

ment, is higher in the southern regions than elsewhere in the country. Against this, people, especially males, live longer in the less developed southern regions than in the more developed northern regions. This particular feature of regional mortality differentials has not changed since 1950–52.

Tavole di mortalita ridotte per le regioni e le ripartizioni Italiane 1951–1961–1971
(*Abridged Life Tables for the Italian Regions and Divisions*), 1977
Antonio Golini, Lamberto Soliani, Giovanni Giavelli, Romano Zanni

The volume contains abridged life tables by five-year age groups covering the periods 1950–52, 1960–62, and 1970–72. These tables have been constructed for single Italian regions as well as for divisions and, in general, for all those regional aggregations on which the analysis of the Italian population is usually centred. These results show how the Italian population, with an expectation of life at birth of 69 years for males and 75 years for females, achieved one of the lowest mortalities in the world in the years 1970–72.

Le differenze Territorialy di mortalita in Italia: Tavole di mortalita provinciali (1971–72); (Geographical Differences in Mortality in Italy Life Tables by Provinces 1971–72), 1980
Graziella Caselli, Viviana Egidi

The volume analyses rates and structural characteristics of mortality in relation to place of residence and contains provincial life tables. In the first part, mortality levels in the Italian provinces are examined using indices such as average life expectancies and probabilities of dying for broad and fairly homogeneous age-groups which make it possible to describe the main characteristics of mortality at different ages. For males, an area for excess mortality was identified which includes the provinces of Northern Italy to the north of the Po river and a small area in the south covering Naples and Caserta. Among females the high-mortality area is geographically smaller in the North and broader in the south. Analysis of mortality by age also shows that geographical differences are, for the most part, related to differences in risk of dying in the middle age-groups. Among males especially, a ranking order among the various provinces begins to emerge as early as from the age of 15 and remains the same, with few exceptions, for subsequent age-groups. In general, male mortality is higher in the northern and central provinces. The second part presents abridged provincial life tables for males and females separately for the years 1971–72 with reference to resident populations.

Norway
Dodsarsaker Causes of Death, 1980, 1981
Statistisk Sentralbyra

Number of deaths by sex, cause and counties (A-list)
Number of deaths by sex, age and cause in Oslo and in Bergen (A-list)

Regional Dodelighet–Oversikt og Opplegg til behandling i Befolkningsframskrivingene (regional mortality – Overview and design for handling of population prognoses), 1979
Knut O. Sorensen

Sex- and age-specific mortality indexes of counties 1971–75. (7 age-groups, 18 counties); life expectancies at birth for males/females by counties. Truncated SMRs between 1929–32 – 1971–75. Standardised mortality by types of communities. Prognosis of regional mortality by counties up to 2010.

Statistisk Sentralb yras Befolknings-prognosemodell: regionale forskjeller i dodelighet (The CBS's Model for population prognosis: regional differences in mortality), 1982.
Dag Helge Tronnes
Statistisk Sentralbyra

Causes of variations in mortality. Data and methods mortality index. The variables results by counties and regions, types of communities and regions and by age-groups.

Regional Dodelighet 1976–1980, (Regional Mortality 1976–1980), 1982
Statistisk Sentralbyra
Central Bureau of Statistics of Norway

Some main results:
   In the period 1976–80, the lowest mortality was observed for males in Son og Fjordane and for females in More og Romsdale. The highest mortality was observed in Finmark for both males and females.
   The mortality observed was much higher for males than for females in all counties. More than half of all deaths were caused by cardiovascular diseases, and particularly from these causes, the excess mortality for males was high.
   The standardised death rates for the various types of municipalities showed that in the period 1976–80 the total death rate for males was lowest in agricultural municipalities while central service and industrial municipalities, and fishing municipalities had the highest death rate. For females, the highest death rate was found in central service and industrial municipalities.

Regional Variations in Mortality in Norway
Central Bureau of Statistics of Norway
Paper presented at the third meeting of UN/WHO/CICRED Network
and Socio-Economic Differential Mortality in the Industrialised
Societies in Rome in 1983

Studies on mortality by region in Norway have been made for several
periods. They show that there is a high regional differentiation in
mortality, in particular in male mortality. This mortality pattern has
remained nearly unchanged over time. In all counties, male mortality
exceeds female mortality, and the male excess mortality has shown an
increasing tendency.

Corresponding calculations for municipalities grouped by type may
give an impression of the influence exerted by population density,
centralisation and industrialisation on morbidity and mortality.

The standardised rates clearly show that the most central and
industrialised municipalities, together with fishing municipalities, are
in the least favourable position when mortality is looked at. Agricultural municipalities have the lowest rates for both sexes. Compared to
male mortality regional differences in female mortality are smaller.

Nearly the same pattern is found for the two most frequent groups
of causes, malignant neoplasms and heart diseases.

An indication of the possible connection between mortality differentials found for types of municipalities and for counties can be traced
from the distribution of deaths by municipal types within regions.

For North Norway, including Nordland, Troms and Finnmark
counties, more than 60 per cent of all deaths occurred in types of
municipalities having high mortality rates. More than half of all
deaths in fishing municipalities were related to North Norway. In
Finnmark county, 74 per cent of the population lived in fishing ang
and mixed service and manufacturing municipalities.

In East Norway, more than 40 per cent of the deaths were assigned
to especially central, mixed service and manufacturing municipalities,
a type having high mortality rates. In this group, Oslo plays a
dominating role.

For West Norway, including Hordaland, Sogn of Fjordane and
More og Romsdal, all counties on a low mortality level, nearly 30 per
cent of the deaths referred to agricultural and mixed agricultural and
manufacturing municipalities. In Sogn og Fjordane, 54 per cent of the
population lived in such municipalities.

Editor's footnote
Unfortunately Dr Jozan was unable to complete this review. As geographic
comparisons probably offer the most realistic opportunity for a systematic
analysis of within country variation in mortality it was decided to include the
chapter in its incomplete state.

PART III
DIFFERENCES IN
MORBIDITY

10 A comparison of measures of inequality in morbidity
Mildred Blaxter

Introduction: morbidity and mortality

Most nations confess to a lack of information about social differences in morbidity, compared with statistics of mortality. Frequently there are pleas for better morbidity statistics (for example, WHO, 1980), and it can be noted that none is disseminated by WHO except for notifiable infectious diseases and cancer registrations (and neither of these by any social variables). Life expectancy, or overall or disease-specific mortality rates, are the most unambiguous and easily available statistics. Most nations record them, with greater or lesser sophistication, and they are used because they are there.

It could, however, be argued that morbidity or general health status are increasingly more important indicators of inequality (in developed countries) than mortality. As mortality rates level off, and degenerative or multi-caused disease becomes prominent, the usefulness of death rates decreases. All men must die, and though premature death is certainly a part of inequality in health, it may be that the lifelong experience of health and illness most clearly demonstrates the difference between social groups.

A simple preliminary point which can be made is that indicators of morbidity may show quite different patterns to rates of mortality. The comparisons of mortality and morbidity shown in Figures 10.1 and 10.2 and in Table 10.1 are not unproblematic, even though examples have been chosen which derive from the same study or statistical sets. However, some generalisations are illustrated. Figure 10.1 shows that the ranking of countries in the incidence of a specific disease, and ranking in the rates of those who die from it, do not necessarily match exactly (for obvious reasons which include health-service provision); the same could be shown to be true of the ranking of social groups.

Figure 10.2 is a very simple demonstration of typical trends in British data. Chronic disease and disability commonly show much steeper social gradients than mortality, and gender differences are almost always reversed (with women always showing more morbidity than men but lower mortality rates, and often showing steeper social gradients in morbidity). That women live longer than men, but appear to experience proportionately more illness, demonstrates that

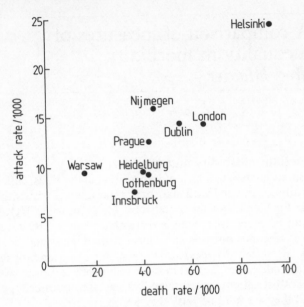

Figure 10.1   Correlation between attack rate of AMI and death rate, age 55–64 years, selected centres in the WHO Cardiovascular Disease Programme in Europe

Source: *Public health in Europe*, **15**, WHO, 1981.

two quite different aspects of health are concerned. Lastly, Table 10.1 is an example of the way in which areas may be ranked differently for mortality, and for various morbidity measures.

What do we mean by morbidity?

The title allocated to this chapter specifies measures of morbidity, and this clearly reflects the common emphasis upon measuring ill-health rather than health. A simple but fundamental first point which would probably receive agreement is that 'health' is a continuum, with no simple cut-off point or division into those who are healthy and those who are not. Health surveys or statistics almost always describe ill-health, and are confined to arbitrary 'lower' sections of the continuum. Accepting this for the moment, five other general conceptual points seem important.

1. Health and ill-health are not unitary concepts, and the notion of a continuum is in a sense misleading. The possibility of disease without illness, and of illness without disease, is a commonplace observation, defining these terms in the usual vocabulary of medical sociology. Disability is not the same as disease, and

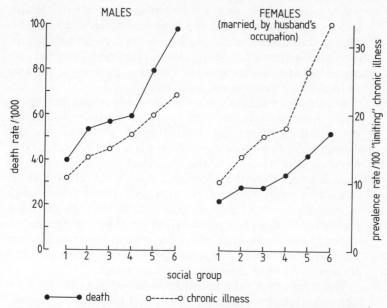

Figure 10.2 *Trends by socio-economic group in Britain, comparing mortality rate (1970–72) and rates of 'limiting chronic illness'*

Source: *General Household Survey*, 1982.

Table 10.1 *Ranking on various health measures compared, in four centres in the WHO Collaborative Study (all rates standardised)*

	Mortality/ 1000		Healthy persons/ 1000		Restricted activity days in 2 weeks/ 1000		Persons with bed days in 2 weeks/ 1000	
	Rate	Rank	Rate	Rank	Rate	Rank	Rate	Rank
Liverpool	8.3	3	147	1	599	3	104	1
Helsinki	8.2	2	120	4	181	1	175	2
Lodz	7.9	1	124	3	722	4	176	3
Banat	9.1	4	137	2	494	2	176	3

Source: Kohn and White, 1976.

psychosocial malaise may not be the same as illness. Health surveys very properly tend to use several different measures – perhaps the existence of chronic diseases, rates of 'illness', rates of functional restriction, the incidence of symptoms – but the conceptual status of each is not always clear, nor the ways in which they are being or can be compared.

2. Confusion also commonly arises because indicators of temporary health states (at a given moment of time, is this individual or this group suffering from any sort of health problem?) are not distinguished from indicators of long-term health status (at a given moment of time, is this individual or this group to be identified as basically healthy or unhealthy?). Either may of course be a useful concept: for one purpose, rates of sickness-days (a measure of state) may be required, and for another, the prevalence of abnormal physiological conditions (a measure of status). They are likely to bear some relationship to each other, but our conceptual models seem inadequate, at present, for any attempt to combine them into a unitary measure.

This is important because there is some evidence that they have differing relevance for health inequalities. In Figure 10.3, derived from the British *General Household Survey, (GHS)*, the trends by socio-economic group shown by a measure of health state and the trends shown by a measure of health status overlap, as would be expected. If they are combined, the differences (especially for men) between socio- economic groups are small. The proportions of those with no health problems at all are very similar. Nor are there conspicuous differences between social groups in the experience of acute illness. However, the measure of health status – chronic illness – shows considerable socio-economic variation.

3. It should be also noted that the nature of the problems which go to make up temporary ill-health or permanently disadvantaged health status will differ. For instance, in the CREDOC review in France (Lecomte, 1984), a measure of status (existence of disease) distinguishes 'dental conditions' as the most common category, while a measure of state (illness experienced during 14 days) places 'ear, nose and throat conditions' first. It should be clear that the distinction is not entirely the one, adopted from medicine, between the chronic and the acute (though these are, indeed, the terms used in the *GHS* example of Figure 10.3). An attempt to force all ill-health into one of these categories complicates many surveys. Chronic disease results in, or is accompanied by, varying degrees of acute illness at any particular time, and it is possible to be a chronic sufferer from conditions medically defined as acute: both these situations contribute to the overlap in

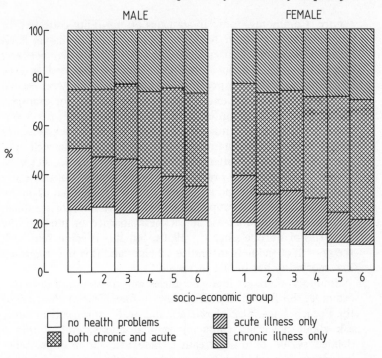

MALE   FEMALE

socio-economic group

☐ no health problems   ▨ acute illness only
▨ both chronic and acute   ▨ chronic illness only

Figure 10.3 Proportions of the population with acute and/or chronic health problems, by socio-economic group, Great Britain
Source: *General Household Survey*, 1977.

Figure 10.3. Nor, of course, is the distinction identical with prevalence/incidence. Incidence produces changes in state, but (depending on the nature of the condition) sometimes also in status.

4. The nature of enquiries about health (at all levels from clinical screening to simple self-reports) means that cross-sectional health is almost inevitably taken as a surrogate for health status. However, patterns of inequality demonstrated by cross-sectional data may not be representative of eventual outcomes. It is possible that short-term illness may be adaptive or preventive, postponing or avoiding more serious consequences (WHO, 1975). It is also possible that prognosis may differ by social variables. Many questions in this area remain to be answered by longitudinal studies, but meanwhile the analysis of cross-sectional findings must bear them in mind.

5. Especially in countries with national health services, there may be good information about the use of various components of the

service. Commonly, 'official' statistics of morbidity collected for administrative or public health purposes are also available. Such statistics have obvious uses (depending on their completeness and reliability) within nations, but none can be regarded as true morbidity statistics, especially for comparison between social groups or between nations. Formal registration as, for example, absent from work, or suffering from a specific disease, is system-dependent. Rates of contact with health services are a product of supply of services and admission or referral policies, as well as of perception of need. Differential rates of, for example, sickness, absence from work or premature retirement may depend more upon unemployment and social security structures than upon the actual health of the groups concerned. There has, for instance, been a consistent increase in sickness absence in most of the countries of Europe since the 1950s, but this is coincident with the growth of sickness insurance schemes and it is not suggested that morbidity has in fact increased.

Similarly, there are many enquiries into consultation rates (for example, the British *Morbidity Surveys from General Practice*, or the French *Enquête de Morbidité*), and health surveys commonly ask about physician contacts, hospitalisations, etc., within a defined period of time, treating these rates as in some sense indicators of morbidity. Consulation statistics often show interesting differences between social groups by type of condition, but on the whole say more about inequality in rates of, and differences in the nature of service-use, or about the effect of different types of service-provision, than they do about inequalities in morbidity (Blaxter, 1984). For these reasons, none of these official statistics or utilisation statistics will be discussed further here.

Measures of morbidity

The examination of measures of morbidity – viewed generally, rather than in an epidemiological or disease-specific way – has been approached in this chapter by a 'survey of surveys'. The conceptual basis of the measures commonly used in a wide range of European countries was considered. The conclusion was that a basic division into three different models might be appropriate: a biological or medical model, defining ill-health in terms of pathology or deviation from physiological (or psychiatric) norms; a social interactional or functional model, defining ill-health as a lack of ability to perform 'normal' tasks or roles; and a subjective model, defining ill-health in terms of the individual's perception. Although these were derived empirically from the analysis of survey questions or measures, in fact

Table 10.2 Measures of health which are commonly used in mortality surveys

(1) Medical or physiological/ psychiatric model	(2) Social – interactional or functional model	(3) Subjective or 'illness' model
Clinical examination, physiological/psychiatric screening for abnormality	Tests of physical or psychological disability	Self-assessment of health
and/or	and/or	and/or
Medical diagnosis of physical or psychiatric disease	Ascertainment of functional status associated with ill-health (e.g. bedridden not working)	Reported experience of physical symptoms of ill-health
and/or	and/or	and/or
Self-reports of the existence of medically defined disease or abnormality	Inability to perform 'normal' tasks because of disease, impairment or illness	Reported experience of psychosocial malaise

they represent no more than the conventional distinction which is commonly made between disease, sickness and illness. The types of measure used for each are shown in Table 10.2, and they will be discussed in turn.

1. Medical model
Clinical or physiological screening
For obvious reasons, actual large-scale screening or testing of populations is rare. Such screening programmes are usually orientated towards specific disease processes and do not always document the social variables essential for the study of inequalities. The great majority of large-scale programmes have investigated hypertension or other coronary risk factors. Blood pressure is, of course, relatively easy to measure on a large scale. The marked emphasis on cardiovascular disease does seem, however, to be an example of the priority of mortality over (perhaps less dramatic) measures of morbidity. Indeed, in claiming that the MONICA (Multinational Monitoring of Trends and Determinants in Cardiovascular Diseases) project is 'the first model for monitoring morbidity in non-communicable disease', WHO has specifically noted that 'the stimulus . . . was given by mortality statistics' (WHO, 1982).

Examples of studies which have investigated social variables include the prospective study of coronary risk factors in middle-aged blue-collar workers in the Federal Republic of Germany (Siegrist, Chapter 17 in this volume), the prospective study of different grades of occupation in the British Civil Service (Marmot *et al.*, 1978), an area study in France of coronary risk factors including overweight and hypertension (ALPHA, 1979), a study of the relationship of physical activity to coronary risk by the Irish Heart Foundation, measuring blood pressure, cholesterol and weight (Hickey *et al.*, 1975), and the large-scale multiphasic screening programme, including blood pressure, in Finland 1966–72 (Aromaa, 1983).

The international MONICA project of WHO (1983) calls, in its recommended core study, for the measurement, in samples of the population, of blood pressure, cholesterol, weight and height as a basic minimum. To these electrocardiograms and other biochemical tests on blood and urine may be added. In certain of the centres it is anticipated that socio-economic factors will be studied in great detail, including migration, occupation and work characteristics. National projects are, of course, being conducted in a large number of centres, including (in Europe) Britain, the Federal Republic of Germany, Hungary, Italy, Finland, Belgium, the Netherlands, Spain, Czechoslovakia, Yugoslavia and the German Democratic Republic.

One other example of a large-scale population sample survey which includes some physiological measures in addition to blood pressure is the British Health and Lifestyle Survey (Cox *et al.*, 1987). One example of the very regular gradients by social class which have been found for every measure of physiological fitness investigated is shown later in Figure 10.8, p. 225.

Screening for specific physiological dysfunction can also be performed, in population studies, by questionnaire methods rather than actual measurements. Certain standard sets of questions are available, including, for instance, the British Medical Research Council's (1966) questionnaire on bronchitis and emphysema, or questions for the identification of ischaemic heart disease (Rose, 1962), or arthritis (Ropes *et al.*, 1957). Such instruments are intended for cross-national use, and there is some literature on the reliability and validity of questionnaire screening for specific dysfunctions (for example, Milne *et al.*, 1970). There have, however, been few social variables available in reports of studies using these methods.

Survey ascertainment of disease
A common factor of most health surveys is an attempt to ascertain the prevalence of disease, variously defined as chronic conditions, long-standing illness, lasting complaints, health problems, etc. Typical

forms of the question are: 'Do you have any long-standing health problem or chronic illness?' (WHO International Collaborative Study); 'Do you have any serious and/or chronic diseases nowadays?' (Zala County Survey, Hungary); 'Do you have any long-standing illness, disability or infirmity? That is, anything that has troubled you over a period of time or is likely to affect you over a period of time?' (British General Household Survey); 'Do you suffer from a physical infirmity, handicap or chronic illness which will continue to affect you in the future?' (CREDOC Survey, France).

Simple as it is, this type of question appears to tap a response with face validity and comparability. Of course, only known disease is reported, and it is possible that there are social inequalities in 'silent' disease. The acceptance of self-reports may be thought problematic, but in fact, where comparisons have been made, the agreement with doctors' assessments or medical records has been high (for example about 80 per cent in a small study; Blaxter, 1985).

Most of the conditions declared in answer to such questions will be medically diagnosed. Some will not, but it could be argued that a true record of morbidity ought indeed to include those conditions which respondents suffer from, can identify in broad clinical terms, but never consult about; common examples include chronic headache, complaints in the general class of rheumatism/arthritis, and disorders of menstruation. The British Health and Lifestyle Survey asked, for all the most common conditions, whether they had been medically diagnosed, and at least 73 per cent of the conditions offered were, it is claimed, named by doctors. The most common self-diagnosed conditions declared (over 50 per cent of each) were, in order, varicose veins, migraine, and haemorrhoids.

A more serious problem is to know what the respondent 'counts' as a disease worthy of mention. There is no doubt that both the level and kind of disease which is spontaneously reported differs by social groups. The forms of question quoted above attempt to solve this by stressing chronicity. An earlier form of the British General Household Survey question specifically referred to '. . . any health problem that keeps recurring or which you have all or most of the time'.

An alternative method is to offer a check-list of diseases or syndromes, to provide respondents which an appropriate vocabulary and indicate to them the level of ill-health which is being sought. There is no doubt that such a check-list stimulates reporting, sometimes to a degree which is not very useful: it seems that, faced with a list of health problems, most people in most populations can identify themselves. In the British General Household Survey before 1977, about one-quarter to one-third of the population declared chronic illness, but in the 1977 edition when a check-list was introduced, 56 per cent of men and 70 per cent of women claimed to suffer from one or more of the conditions offered.

It is common to analyse disease conditions by broad ICD categories. It may, of course, be useful to know that the predominant disease of one group of the population is in the class of gastro-intestinal, and of another the respiratory system. On the whole, however, the shortcomings, for descriptions of morbidity, of a system which places both upper respiratory infection and chronic emphysema in the same broad category of diseases of the respiratory system, are obvious. A new classification oriented to illness as well as disease, and particularly that illness which does not often lead to death, is badly needed. If ICD categories are not used, each health survey tends at present to use its own *ad hoc* classification.

In all surveys, this measure of long-standing illness, or chronic disease, demonstrates great inequality between social classes. Figure 10.4 offers some examples. In these different surveys, the definition of 'chronic illness' may not be the same, nor may the social groups be entirely comparable. The intention is not therefore to draw attention to the actual rates, but simply to indicate the similarity of trends. In general, inequality in chronic illness is especially notable in middle age, when rates are quite uniformly 40–50 per cent higher in the lowest social groups – however defined – than in the highest. Disease inevitably rises with age, but the timing of the rise may be an important indicator of unequal chances.

2. Functional model

In many surveys, the medical model is combined with the functional by eliciting, exclusively or additionally, that disease which has an effect upon the subject's daily life. Thus, disease may be 'counted' only if it has some functional consequences, or a second category of 'limiting' disease may be formed. Examples include the General Household Survey in Britain, which asks, of any disease declared, 'does this limit your activities in any way'? or the WHO Collaborative Study which asked 'Does this [condition] affect your ability to do your usual work'?, in order to form a category of 'activity-limiting impairment or chronic illness'.

Disease which is 'limiting' commonly shows even steeper gradients among social groups – again, especially in middle and older age (Figure 10.5). There may be some effect of differential reporting or identification: that is, there is some evidence that those in the more disadvantaged circumstances may be less likely to mention disease which has no functional effect. Also, the extent to which a given condition limits activities depends to some extent upon the nature of

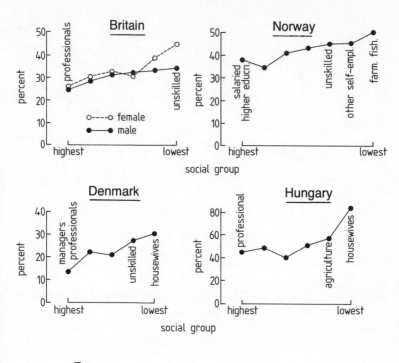

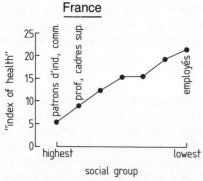

Figure 10.4   Some examples of social trends in chronic illness

Sources: Britain – *General Household Survey*, 1983.
   Norway – *Level of Living Survey*, 1980.
   Denmark – National Institute of Social Medicine, 1979.
   Hungary – *Zala County Survey*, 1979.
   France – *Boulogne – Billarcourt Survey*, 1972.

those activities, especially the nature of work. However, it appears to
remain true, despite these questions of interpretation, that this is the

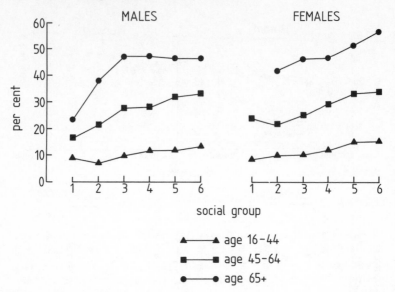

Figure 10.5   Proportion of the populaton with 'limiting chronic illness' by socio-economic group, Great Britain

Source: *General Household Survey*, 1983.

greatest mark of inequality in health between social groups. Those who are socially disadvantaged are not only more likely to experience chronic disease before old age, but their disease is also more likely to be more functionally incapacitating.

Specific functional measures
It is also a common practice to 'measure' specific loss of function, however caused, by eliciting the number of 'sick days', 'days lost from work', etc., over a defined period. There are obvious attractions in defining ill-health solely by its effects, which are easier to define and elicit than either pathologies or feelings. Advantages of this approach are that it encompasses a wider view of health, and persons can be characterised by degree of incapacity rather than simply the absence or presence of disease.

'Bed-days' describes the most serious loss of social function, with 'restricted activity days' or 'absence from work days' as additional measures. Fourteen days (usually considered to be maximum recall period) is a standard period used in most surveys. 'Bed-days' (including days hospitalised) plus 'restricted activity days' are often combined into a concept called 'sick days'. Occasionally, 'days with symptoms' are also included, though this is perhaps to be deprecated as confusing quite different models of ill-health: the concept of 'sickness' is essentially a functional one.

Although 'bed-days' is an easily defined measure, the concept of 'restricted activity days' is not without problems. At its broadest, it can be defined, as in the British GHS, by such a question as 'Did you have to cut down on any of the things you usually do (about the house or at work or in your free time) because of illness or injury?' Similarly, the Norwegian Health Survey 1975 defined sick days as days with activity reduced from the normal, the WHO Collaborative Study asked 'Were there any days . . . when you were not able to do your usual activities because you were not feeling well?', and the Finnish Survey (Purola *et al.*, 1974) enquired about days absent from work or 'failed to attend to normal duties' (though in this case over a longer time period).

From these, various measures can be derived: persons reporting/not sick days within the period, mean number of sick days/year for a group, bed-days/year, etc. Obviously, these may not vary together, for the incidence of illness and duration of episodes may vary differentially by social characteristics (and, of course, by conditions).

Though defining illness in this way may seem more objective, in fact the comparison of these measures is not easy. 'Normal' activity remains a subjective judgement, and social groups may vary in the extent to which any given level of ill-health has functional consequences. There are always problems about applying the concept of 'restricted activity days' to the elderly. In fact, rates of 'sick days' or of social dysfunction tend to vary more widely, if different surveys or societies are compared, than do mortality rates or rates of disease. They may also show little difference between social groups, as illustrated in the British or Spanish figures of Figure 10.6. Women in general, and housewives in particular, generally record higher rates: part of this excess would seem (from declarations of symptom experience) to be the effect of higher rates of illness, but obviously the definition of 'restricted activity' is relevant. For some occupational groups, there is little middle ground between being able to work and being totally incapacitated. For others, including housewives, there is more flexibility and freedom to perform 'restricted' activities.

The measures of the incidence of illness days, and the mean numbers of illness days, may show different trends because of greater severity or slower recovery in lower social groups. This is again demonstrated in the British figures. Number of illness days is probably the more satisfactory measure. Bed-days may show different trends again, and indeed may be as high in the most advantaged classes as in the least (as illustrated from Norway and Spain); obviously, there is an area of voluntary choice, or an effect of what is

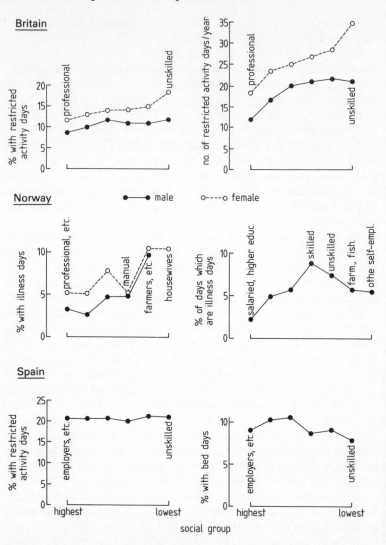

Figure 10.6   Some examples of social trends in illness defined in functional categories

Sources: Britain – *General Household Survey*, 1983.
Norway – *Level of Living Survey*, 1980.
Spain – *Barcelona Survey*, 1983.

practicable in different social circumstances, in determining what level of illness necessitates the complete giving up of normal functioning.

Disability and handicap

Ill-health defined as 'inability to function normally' shades into the concept of disability or handicap. There is, however, a distinction between surveys which include 'functioning' as part of health, and surveys which seek to select out groups specifically defined as 'the disabled'. The measures of function discussed above are measures of health state (in a given period). Disability is usually meant to refer to (permanent or long-term) health status.

The social and economic problems caused by disability mean that such surveys are very common, because the information is often required for administrative or service provision purposes. Examples have been conducted, for instance, in Poland, Denmark, the Netherlands, the Federal Republic of Germany and Britain. The underlying purpose of the British national survey (Harris, 1971, a survey which is currently being repeated) was the assessment of numbers and needs for a particular social security provision. It subsequently became a legislative requirement that local authorities should also conduct enquiries (see Knight and Warren, 1975 for a summary of these), as a basis for the provision of a wider range of services.

Disability surveys have the advantage that, since the WHO classification (1975), there are at least common and clearly defined concepts available. It is now generally agreed that impairment should be defined as any loss or abnormality of psychological, physiological or anatomical structure or function; disability as any restriction or lack of ability (resulting from impairment) to perform an activity in the manner or within the range considered normal; and handicap as the disadvantage resulting from impairment or disability. Disability surveys also have the advantage that measurement may be easier, and can use well tried and validated instruments – for instance, Activities of Daily Living scales based on the ability to perform 'normal' activities unaided (for example, Garrad and Bennett, 1971).

Fundamental problems remain, however, about indicators of disability. Comparison of rates is complicated by whether institutionalised persons are included, and if they are not, by particular patterns of institutional provision. The WHO definition of impairment logically includes all chronic illness. Surveys (such as the British Survey of the Handicapped and Impaired) have been found to identify the mobility-disabled or those needing practical help with much greater certainty than those suffering the functional consequences of chronic illness. There are problems in distinguishing short-term and long-term disability: how permanent does an impairment have to be before it is counted? Also, the capacity to perform tasks, and the actual performance of the tasks, may not be the same thing. Performance, or the extent to which disabilities are actually handicapping, depends on personal factors and variables of the social environment: the 'normal' activities of the WHO definition of disability are obviously relative. 'Inability to work' is one of the most obvious and frequently used categories. The meaning of this category, however, depends on social, economic and industrial structures and regulations, as well as on systems of social security. As has been pointed out in connection with a large disability survey in Poland (Niklas, 1978), such surveys are difficult to interpret both in terms of true morbidity and in terms of social inequality in morbidity.

Their principal value is probably in demonstrating, rather, the way in which disadvantaged health *causes* social inequalities. 'The disabled', however defined, are commonly shown to be among the poorest groups of a nation. The consequences of disability are also unequal, varying by social circumstances, clinical conditions, and geographical areas. The inequality of the disabled, and inequalities among the disabled, are important topics in their own right.

3. Subjective model

The most usual way to measure self-perceived illness, whether or not it is associated with known clinical disease, is by means of symptom lists. Commonly, these are elicited during a recall period (often 14 days) and the lists provided may attempt to be exhaustive, covering all possible manifestations of health disturbance (for example, Hannay, 1978) or may simply include a convenient number of the most common symptoms. Differential recall, and the possibility that different social groups may place varying emphasis upon different kinds of symptom, complicate analysis: there has been a considerable amount of work asking who, under what circumstances, is likely to report what symptoms (Aiach *et al.*, 1981). An alternative method, though it may be practised only on a smaller scale, is the use of health diaries, and again there have been several studies comparing these with recall methods. In general, a symptom list appears to result in the reporting of a larger number of symptoms (Aiach and Cèbe, 1983).

The justification of including the declaration of symptoms as a measure of morbidity lies in the demonstration of how different service-identified and experienced morbidity are, especially at the less serious end of the spectrum. Diary methods, in particular, have shown how small a proportion of self-perceived illness is ever taken for medical diagnosis or treatment, and how frequent 'illness' is. Typical rates are a mean 4.3 symptoms in 14 days (Hannay, 1978), or 6.2 symptom episodes in four weeks (Banks *et al.*, 1975, women aged 20–44), or 53 per cent (M) and 58 per cent (F) reporting at least one symptom in 14 days (*General Household Survey*, 1977). In the British Health and Lifestyle Survey, 28 per cent of females and 16 per cent of males reported three or more different symptoms within the last month. In a French study (Aiach and Cèbe, 1983) the ratio of symptoms/consultations ranged from 0.1 (circulatory problems, insommnia, migraine) to 1.3 (respiratory problems). A British six-week diary study (Scambler *et al.*, 1981) found ratios of consultations to symptoms ranging from 1 to 9 for 'sore throat' to 1 to 60 for 'headache', with an overall ratio of 1 consultation to 18 symptom episodes.

Rates of illness, defined as the number or frequency of symptoms an individual declares, have been found to be a useful measure inasmuch as they do distinguish different social groups, or different life situations quite clearly (though not necessarily in the same way as disease prevalence, or measures of functioning). It may be noted, as a universal finding, that rates of symptoms tend to be much higher at all ages among women than among men. The analysis of the way in which these patterns vary by social position is complicated by the problems of categorising women, but 'housewives not occupied outside the home' are often a group with particularly high rates. The degree to which this represents selection depends, of course, on the economic activity rates which are normal for the woman of any given society. The general 'inequality' in morbidity between the sexes is perhaps not susceptible to precise interpretation. It seems that women do experience more illness symptoms, but factors of perception and what Aiach *et al.*, (1981) calls 'une relation tout à fait privilegée entre la sexe feminine à tout ce qui touche à la maladie et à la santé' are also involved.

One problem which remains is the measurement of degrees of illness: symptoms such as headache or gastric pain may be of very different degrees of (perceived) severity, and this is rarely taken into account (except for the effect upon function). Pain, distress and worry are dimensions of physical illness which are neglected in morbidity measures. The WHO Collaborative Study made one brave attempt to categorise severity of illness by asking, after eliciting each type of illness, 'At its worst, did this bother you/hurt or pain you/were you worried or concerned about this, (a great deal/somewhat/etc)'. In fact, this bother–pain–worry index did not substantially alter the patterns of declared illness, which it was suggested lent some credibility to the validity of self-perceived illness as a concept.

Psychosocial illness

Questions on pain or worry are more usually included in instruments specifically designed to measure psychosocial ill-health. The common inclusion among symptom lists of items which are more properly called 'malaise' (depression, nerves, sleep and appetite disturbance, worry, social isolation, etc.) is a recognition that total health involves more than physical symptoms, but it is not always clear what status is being assigned to such 'symptoms' – whether, for instance, they are being seen as illness *per se*, or as the cause or consequence of any association found with subjective physical symptoms.

The distribution in populations of psychosocial ill-health, or mild psychiatric morbidity, is of course interesting in itself, and indicators for its measurement range from elaborate, validated instruments (in Britain, three which are frequently used are the General Health Questionnaire, Rutter's Malaise Inventory, and the Nottingham Health Profile) to simple questions about the most common 'symptoms'. The Norwegian Level of Living Survey, 1980, for instance, based an index of 'nervous conditions' on being often troubled by three conditions: palpitations without prior effort; nervous anxiety or restlessness; and depression (identifying 5 per cent of the population).

Concepts of the nature of nervous illness or psychological malaise, and the kinds of lay vocabulary available for discussing them, probably differ more among nations than do concepts of physical illness. For this reason, comparability between societies is difficult. This is, however, an area where the development of simple instruments for comparative purposes has been neglected. The WHO Collaborative Study used questions from the Cornell Medical Index to measure anxiety, but found difficulty in interpreting the very wide variation in results across the study areas (approximately fourfold, compared with twofold at most for specific physical dysfunctions).

Positive health and self-assessments of health

As already noted, nowhere as yet has there been much attempt to measure total health, including the more positive aspects. As ill-health has several dimensions, so positive health – as in the WHO definition – can be conceived in different ways. The equivalent positive measures to the measures of morbidity in Table 10.2 are perhaps those shown in Table 10.3.

In many surveys, the 'healthy' are defined simply as those who report no morbidity: no attempt is made to distinguish different levels of health and fitness in the absence of illness. This is the definition of 'the healthy' in the British General Household Survey (as in Figure 10.3), for instance, or in the Finnish Survey (Purola *et al.*, 1974). Measures of social inequalities in health at the most positive extreme remain to be developed at both the conceptual and practical levels. It is at least possible that they are more pronounced than inequalities at the lower end of the healthy–unhealthy continuum.

The nearest approach to the description of health, rather than illness, is the common request in many surveys that the respondents

Table 10.3   *'Positive' measures of health   equivalent to the morbidity measures of Table 10.2*

(1) Medical or physiological/ psychiatric model	(2) Social–interactional or functional model	(3) Subjective or 'illness' model
Tests or clinical measures of the fitness of physical or psychological systems	Tests of physiological or psychological functioning and/or Reports of activity levels, social role performance	Reports of well-being, happiness

should define their own health: 'Do you feel yourself to be healthy?' (Hungarian survey); 'Over the last 12 months, would you say that on the whole your health has been good, fairly good, or not good?' (British General Household Survey). Of course, the answers cannot be presumed to say anything about objective health. Measures of self-perceived 'healthiness' are subject to distortion because of variation of norms by education, age, family support or health experience. Nevertheless, it is common to find a remarkably steep and regular gradient by social class. Figure 10.7 shows the regular trends produced by dividing the population of the British Health and Lifestyle Survey into four income bands.

Whether or not a good measure of inequality in health, self-perceived health is an important topic in equality. Self-assessments, in combination with other data, can be used to examine the relationship of self-perceived health to other lifestyle and psychological variables, and also social variation in norms of what it is to be healthy. What affects the definition of whether one is healthy or not? Even those with serious disease have been known to claim to be in 'excellent' health. There is some evidence that positive 'fitness' is a more important component for the young, and those in higher social classes. For the old, and those in lower social classes, the functional dimension may assume greater importance, and psychosocial malaise is certainly associated with depressed self-assessment of health (Blaxter, 1985).

Social variables by which inequality is measured
Some general trends across different countries were offered in the preceding discussion of morbidity measures. A few more specific

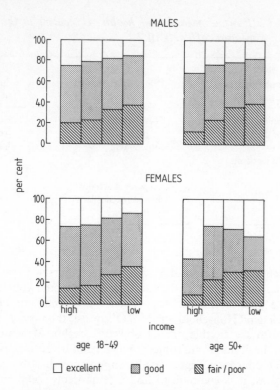

Figure 10.7   Self-definition of own health as excellent, good, or fair/poor'
'compared with someone of your own age', differences in
four bands of household income, Great Britain
Source: *Health and Lifestyle Survey*, 1986.

comparative findings will now be discussed. It must of course be
noted that the independent variables – social class, occupation,
income, education, social circumstances – by which inequality is
distinguished are as problematic as the health measures themselves.
Their comparability is not discussed, since the issue is not peculiar to
morbidity but is of equal importance for mortality. For both, it must
be borne in mind that social classes are not necessarily defined in the
same way in different countries, and the meaning of categories of
education or income depends on specific societal structures. Even the
meaning of gender, or age (as a cohort variable rather than a biological
one), may depend on specific historical processes in the society
concerned.

Unskilled labourers appear in all national statistics as a disadvantaged group. In countries which single out agricultural workers as a 'class', however, their rates of morbidity are usually the highest. There is a contrast between countries where disadvantage is still concentrated in rural areas, and industrialised nations where much smaller agricultural populations have more favourable health characteristics than urban workers. All class relationships have to be viewed in the light of specific social histories.

Also, the classification of social variables is affected by the meaning which is given to 'inequality'. Usually, what is meant, in the context of health, is unacceptable inequalities, or alternatively dysfunctional, preventable, unnecessary or unjust inequalities – the definition is ultimately an ideological one. Variation in health is part of the human condition, and the degree or nature of variation which is unacceptable has political and historical dimensions.

The interest may be in particular groups which fall below an accepted population norm. Thus, the most vulnerable groups may be selected out: the Norwegian Level of Living Survey (1980), for instance, specifically analysed six groups considered to be 'exposed' (for example, pensioners with a minimum pension, persons with a specified low wage, those unemployed over four weeks). Similarly, the INSEE–CREDOC National Survey in France (1970) selected out for special analysis those with low incomes, low education, or 'precarious' housing conditions.

Alternatively, the interest may be in an overall continuum, with an implied commitment to general social equality. It could be argued that, in this case, the good health of the privileged ought to be of as much interest as the poor health of the disadvantaged, though the focus is more usually on the lower end of the continuum.

Occupation and working conditions

Occupation *per se* and the risk of specific disease associated with industries has, of course, been an important focus of epidemiological research. This specialised area will not be discussed here. Increasingly, however, explanations for occupational–class differences in morbidity are being sought by examination of the actual content or circumstances of work, more broadly defined. The initial focus has been strongly upon coronary risk factors, with some study of mental health, and the extension of this type of investigation to other groups of diseases or to more general measures of ill-health is perhaps to be recommended.

Examples include the identification, among males 35–64 years-old in Germany surviving a first myocardial infarction, of risk factors such as stress, insecurity and night-shift work (Bolm-Audorff and Siegrist, 1983), and again in Germany, the pinpointing of economic pressure, fear of job loss, and exposure to noise as associated with the development of coronary risk factors (Siegrist *et al.*, 1986, and Chapter 17 in this volume). Similarly, Alfredson *et al.*, (1982) studied the psychosocial work environment in Sweden, and Hasan (Chapter 18 in this volume) in Finland. Within one broad occupational group – civil servants – a British study showed very regular gradients in psychosocial health from administrators through clerical and executive to manual workers, matching the gradients observed in mortality. These measures related, for instance, to reported satisfaction with work (for example, perception of fair treatment or under-use of skills), activities outside work, and social supports and contacts (Marmot *et al.*, 1978). In a more general way (but confined to younger people) the investigation in Hungary of Szalai and Antal identified an association of physically or psychologically strained working conditions with chronic ill-health.

Unemployment

Of recent years there has been much interest in the health effects of unemployment. There are well known problems associated with the separation of the effects of poverty and of lack of employment, and of disentangling cause and effect (the 'healthy worker' phenomenon). However, it should be noted that lack of occupation is consistently shown to be associated with poorer health especially in the middle years (for example, in Britain, Hill, 1973, Daniel, 1974). In the British General Household Survey (1982), for instance, 'long-standing illness' prevalence among the unemployed was only slightly elevated at ages 16–44 (males) but at ages 45–64 was 49 per cent compared with 33 per cent for the employed. Acute illness or the incidence of symptoms is often shown to be only slightly greater, however, and illness defined as 'limitation of normal activities' may actually appear to be less. In the Norwegian Level of Living Survey (1980) the unemployed, selected as an 'exposed' group, did not in fact have more 'illness days' than the population norm. In the British Health and Lifestyle Survey, 'illness', represented by a high rate of symptom experience, was no different among the employed and unemployed below the age of 40. After that age, however, the unemployed declared rates almost twice as high as the employed.

There have been several special studies in various countries of Europe of the long-term unemployed (for example, Bungener *et al.*, 1980), industrial closures etc. (for example, Iversen and Klausen, 1981). The usual findings include some increase in mental disturbance or depressed level of well-being (for example Warr, 1981), but inconclusive results with regard to other aspects of health. Comparability of studies between nations, or over time, is of course complicated by the fact that 'unemployment' has different social meanings, and selects different groups.

Income

Income is an indicator of inequality used by many nations for the analysis of morbidity, sometimes as a surrogate for social class. Obviously, poverty is relative and can be measured and defined only in relation to the standards of a given society. The political and economic structure of the society will determine patterns of distribution, which will in turn affect whether the interest is in individuals who fall to the bottom of the distribution, or in the relative position of whole communities or classes, however defined. In either case interest may focus on absolute poverty – the inability to provide for basic needs in nutrition or shelter – which may *a priori* be expected to affect health adversely. Or, interest may be in relative poverty – the inability to participate fully in the social or consumption patterns of the society – which may bear a more complex but still significant relationship to health.

In recent years there have been many attempts to apply a comparative perspective to poverty in Europe (see, for example, Townsend, 1983). Both the wealth of the society (GNP) and the patterns of distribution of income or wealth are relevant. Of course the countries of Europe are, largely, privileged in comparison to less developed countries. However, Townsend has suggested that there are growing regional inequalities within Europe as a rapidly evolving mass consumer lifestyle becomes increasingly inaccessible to those with low incomes. A complication of comparative study is that the levels of social security systems, and the extent to which welfare systems are ameliorative, are obviously relevant.

There are few direct comparisons which can be made of the association of income and health in different countries. The only (rather obvious) generalisations are that income is everywhere associated with morbidity, and that those countries with the greatest inequality of income and wealth tend to display the greatest inequalities in health. Some examples of figures are shown in Table 10.4. It can be noted that, like social class gradients, morbidity differences by income are most prominent for chronic illness and disability, and the differences are greatest in the middle years.

Education

As a variable, education is of course closely associated with social class. As a component of, or surrogate for, social class it is likely to show the same associations with morbidity: indeed, in the Norwegian Helseundersokelse; 1975, the gradients were somewhat steeper by

Table 10.4   Examples of morbidity variation by income

Finland	% with chronic illness	
	Lowest income group	*Highest income group*
Urban communes	42	18
Rural communes	49	27
	(Services Use and Health Status, 1974)	

France	% with chronic illness	
	Lowest income group	*Highest income group*
	57.2	30.5
	(INSEE – CREDOC Survey, 1970)	

Norway	% with chronic illness	
	Lowest income group	*Highest income group*
	52	39
	(Level of Living Survey, 1980)	

Hungary	% 'unhealthy', age 31–50		
	Poor	*Middle Level*	*Well-to-do*
Urban	62	54	35
Rural	89	63	
	(Zala County Survey, 1979)		

Britain	% with high rates of symptoms, age 40–59	
	Lowest income group	*Highest income group*
	M: 31.2 F: 40.3	M: 11.6 F: 24.3
	(Health and Lifestyle Survey, 1986)	

education than by occupational class, especially for 'illness days'. Similarly, in the Level of Living Survey 1980 the 'exposed' group identified as 'young people with low education' declared a high rate of illness days, and also of nervous conditions, and in the INSEE–CREDOC Survey 1970 the variable 'low education' was almost as salient as low income in increasing chronic illness or functional disability for the middle-aged (but not the elderly). In Hungary (Ferge *et al.*, 1985), the proportions of 'unhealthy' people in the lowest and the highest educational groups were again widely divergent (85 per cent with less than eight years education, 46 per cent of secondary school graduates), though in this case the income-plus-urban/rural dimension produced greater differences. Again, the middle-aged showed proportionately the greatest differences by education.

The distribution of educational standards differs, of course, from country to country, and age-group effects demonstrate that there will be a historical dimension. Education is perhaps more commonly used as a variable in small studies, or studies of health behaviour, with some tendency to regard the relationship between education and health status as essentially a direct one, through 'uneducated' and risky behaviour. The strength or otherwise of any general relationship may, however, depend largely on the extent to which education is related, in a given society, to occupation and general social advantage.

Area: Living Amenities; Housing

Area (prosperous or disadvantaged areas of a country, the urban-rural distinction, types of living environment) is another component of social class differences. In some countries the urban-rural dimension is treated almost as a class distinction of itself. Obviously, this dimension has different meanings in different societies. For example, in Eire, Greece, Finland or Hungary, the most disadvantaged health is found in rural areas. In Eire and Hungary it has been suggested that part of the explanation lies in the selective migration of the healthiest out of the rural areas. In highly industrialised countries, however, health disadvantage clusters in large cities; this is certainly true of Britain. In large part, of course, this simply indicates where poverty and poor living conditions cluster. In many countries with the greatest urban-rural differences, relevant morbidity figures are lacking, but indirect evidence is provided by extreme differences in living standards or household amenities. An example is Spain, where 72.2 per cent of the agricultural population, compared with 48.4 per cent of the non-agricultural population, lack a shower or bath in their household (INE, 1975). The physical environment *per se* (pollution, climate), types of occupation associated with areas, and the availability of medical care, are however also relevant.

The health disadvantages suffered in broad administrative areas of a country are always of continuing national interest. Closer examination of the actual living conditions within areas, and the more precise association of poor housing or lack of amenities with different aspects of the health of individuals, seem to have been neglected for some time or studied only, on a small scale. The British General Household Survey has not, for instance, used these in analyses of health since the editions of the early 1970s. At that time, however, analysis by living conditions produced some wider variations than income or social class: among those people living in households without a bath, 25.6 per cent were identified as chronically sick (compared with 15.5 per cent of those in households with the sole use of a bath), and 23.5 per cent of those with an outside WC (compared with 15.4 per cent of those with an indoor WC). Both these (overlapping) deprived groups, were, of course, relatively small. The health deficit appeared to be in this measure of chronic illness, rather than in any marked excess of acute episodes. It would thus appear that the phenomenon was one of the poorest and most deprived tending to live in the worst housing, rather than an immediately causal effect of living conditions on health.

In Britain, housing tenure has been shown (in the Longitudinal Study of Mortality) to be a useful tool for investigating a dimension of social class differences in mortality. Again, this is not a variable used in the health analysis of the General Household Survey since the early 1970s, but at that time it similarly showed a marked excess of chronic illness among the least stable tenure group – private tenants. Owner-occupiers showed particularly low rates, with public (local authority) tenants in an intermediate position.

Again in Britain, there has recently been some revival of interest in the classification of communities or areas at a relatively small level, using socio-demographic or housing variables. It has been possible in this way to identify and characterise small areas with particularly high rates of morbidity. However, the relative weights of area variables (i.e. living conditions and the physical and social environment *per se*) and the individual characteristics of the persons clustering there (i.e. the social class, poverty, education, etc. variables already discussed) remain to be studied (Morgan, 1983).

Lifestyle and health risk factors
Behaviour, or health risk factors, are not precisely a morbidity measure, but ought to be mentioned briefly, if only to note that there is more information – and more comparable information – about certain factors which may affect health than there is about health itself. Many countries have detailed and up-to-date survey material on smoking and alcohol consumption, and some on diet. It is a very general finding (for example from the Federal Republic of Germany, Switzerland, the Netherlands, Britain) that smoking is associated with lower education (and so with lower social class).

It should be noted, however, that single behaviours are never a total explanation for social inequalities in health. Figure 10.8 presents a particularly clear example. Smoking is, of course, associated with poorer lung function. Controlled for smoking, however, regular differences between non-manual and manual social groups remain.

Concepts of health
Finally, health ought to be considered in its most subjective aspect by some discussion of work on the different concepts which may be found in populations. These are not easily susceptible to measurement, nor are they morbidity measures. To the extent that the link between socio-economic circumstances and health experience is seen as a direct one, attitudes to health may not be considered relevant.

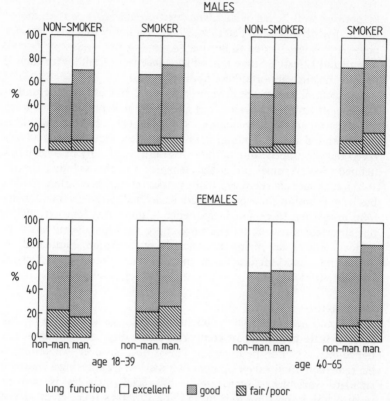

Figure 10.8   Measured lung function (achieved forced vital capacity compared with predicted value, age and height taken into account) for smokers and non-smokers in non-manual and manual socio-economic groups, Great Britain

Source: *Health and Lifetyle Survey,* 1986.

Increasingly, however, behaviour and attitudes, risk-taking and perceptions of health as a value, are being considered as possible linking variables.

There is a relatively recent, but growing, volume of work on social differentiation in the meaning of health. In general, higher social classes, younger age-groups, and the better educated are found to have more positive and self-orientated concepts of health (Calnan, 1984; Pill and Stott, 1982). Lower social classes may offer images of health which are entirely negative (simply the absence of illness) or are instrumental (health as the ability to perform social roles) (d'Houtaud and Field, 1984). The lower expectations and lack of a sense of health as positive well-being of disadvantaged groups may of itself be an 'inequality' (Blaxter and Paterson, 1982). Studies of this sort have, for obvious reasons, tended to be small-scale, but the large-scale British Health and Lifestyle Survey, in which concepts of health were elicited in some detail, supports these findings.

Concepts of health are obviously relevant, not only to the understanding of health behaviour, but also to the interpretation of survey self-assessments and responses. The role of norms of health is demonstrated by the finding, across countries, that the least advantaged tend to underestimate their ill-health, medically or objectively defined (Scott-Samuel and Szalai, Chapter 3 in this volume; Blaxter 1985). It should also be noted that a marked social class differentiation has been found in concepts of health as defined in the abstract, rather than in relation to personal experience (Calnan and Johnson, 1985). Social variables also seem to be more important when overall health or minor illnesses are being considered, but become dominated by health-experience factors when more serious illness is concerned (Wright, 1985).

Conclusion

A first (and not unexpected) conclusion of this review has to be that there is little possibility of comparing morbidity information across the countries of Europe in detail. This is not, however, something to be 'remedied' by the development of indices or by agreeing a choice of standard variables. Comparability by social variables is perhaps intrinsically impossible to achieve. The variables themselves – even those which may seem to be more objective, such as absolute poverty – have different meanings in different cultures. And if morbidity or ill-health (and still more, health in its entirety) is to be defined in any but strictly biomedical terms, then its measures – 'sick days' or 'disability', for instance – are crucially affected by social differences.

This is not to suggest that international comparisons are useless, especially when confined to one geographical area of the world. Indeed the very variety of social situations attached to such variables as gender, occupation, education, sickness absence from work, self-perception as healthy and so on, is an advantage in helping to tease out the relationships between social inequality and health.

Though individual rates of morbidity are rarely susceptible to comparison, certain generalisations accumulate. It is these general trends (or in some cases anomalies) which are important. This review has suggested that they might include, in random order:

1. *The fact that clinical measurements, or disease structures in terms of diagnostic classes, do not necessarily produce social trends which match either mortality, or ill-health more generally defined.* The latter

measures commonly produce sharper differentials. This might suggest that health must be defined in wider terms than 'disease'.

2. *The varying trends by social variables (but on the whole comparable across nations in general shape) which are produced by different sorts of indicators of ill-health.* This suggests that in measuring 'illness days', 'functional incapacity', or 'incidence of symptoms', one must be clear about what exactly is being measured. Measures of function, in particular, are partly dependent on the social categories by which they are analysed.

3. *The universal disadvantage in health, on almost all measures, of unskilled occupational groups (and in many countries, agricultural workers).* It may be simply that these groups are predominantly the poor. In all countries, income is a salient variable for distinguishing health chances.

4. *The (associated) universal disadvantage in health of populations in the most economically deprived areas of countries.* The relative weights of selection effects, and effects caused directly by poor living standards, remain to be examined.

5. *The relatively poor health of women not working outside the home.* Again, it is not clearly known how much of this is due to selection of the least-fit out of the labour market, taking societal norms and economic structures into account.

6. *The fact that it is very generally shown that social inequality in health is much greater for health status – for example the existence of chronic or handicapping ill-health – than it is for measures of 'temporary' health.* 'Random' acute illness or the experience of symptoms may show little social differentiation.

7. *The demonstration, by comparison of age-groups, that this burden of chronic ill-health appears to be clearly related to life situations.* There is usually some social differentiation at younger ages (which might be held to include the effects of poor heredity). There is also usually some social differentiation among older people, though this may be lessened by a 'healthy survivor' effect. It is in middle age, however, that health diverges most strikingly.

8. *The growing evidence that ways of conceiving of health may themselves be 'unequal'.* As Mizrahi et al. (1983) point out, 'the very concept of illness, or poor health . . . is probably different for the poor'. These issues are of importance in connection with health-orientated behaviour.

9. *The fact that indicators of morbidity may show different patterns to statistics of mortality: it is health throughout the stages of life that we must be concerned with.* One implication of this is that, ideally, longitudinal studies of lifelong health effects could eventually offer clearer explanations for social inequality in health than will

ever be possible by cross-sectional description. Examples of longitudinal or cohort studies include the British cohorts, two of which (children born in 1946 and 1958) have now reached adult years, or the Swedish study which began in 1963 of one-third of all men born in Gothenberg in 1913 (Tengwald and Faresjo, 1984).

Some of the objectives of the latter study may serve as an exemplar: to examine the dynamic relationship between the development of health problems and the development of social and economic factors, to see how different social conditions and events (especially those related to class, like unemployment, early retirement, economic problems, etc.) interrelate with health problems, and to study the varying acceleration over time of increasing health problems in different social strata.

It may seem that such cohort studies present special problems in comparability between nations, embedded as they must be in local and historical contexts. However, if – as this review has suggested – it is general trends, or considerations of broad cause and effect relationships, which offer more fruitful areas of comparison than precise statistics of morbidity, then the further development of cohort studies of all kinds may be a way forward.

References

Aiach, P. Cèbe, D. (1983), 'La perception dans les symptômes: Variations dans les declarations selon differentes procedures', *Cahiers de Sociologie et de Demographies Medicales*, **XXII**, (i), pp. 3–27.

Aiach, P., Leclerc, A. and Phillippe, A. (1981), 'Facteurs de differentation dans la déclaration de symptômes, *Revue Epidemologie et Santé Publique* **29**, pp. 27–44.

Alfredson, L., Karaskek, R. and Theorell, T. (1982), 'Myocardial infarction risk and psychosocial work environment: an analysis of the male Swedish working force', *Social Science and Medicine* **16**, p. 463.

ALPHA (1979), 'Hypertension arterielle et catégorie socioprofessionelle, rôle de la surcharge ponderale', *Revue Practicien*, **1**, pp. 99–100.

Aromaa, A. (1983), *Epidemiology and Public Health: Impact of High Blood Pressure in Finland*, Helsinki: Social Insurance Institution.

Banks, M.H *et al.* (1975), 'Factors influencing the demand for primary medical care in women aged 20–44 years', *International Journal of Epidemiology*, **4** (3), p. 189.

Bennett, A.E., Garrad, J. and Halil, T. (1970), 'Chronic disease and disability in the community: a prevalence study', *British Medical Journal*, **3**, pp. 762–4.

Blaxter, M. (1963, 1984), 'Equity and consultation rates in general practice', *British Medical Journal*, p. 288.

Blaxter, M. (1985), 'Self-definition of health status and consulting rates in primary care', *Quarterly Journal of Social Affairs* **1** (2), pp. 131–71.

Blaxter, M. and Paterson, E. (1982), *Mothers and Daughters*, Heinemann.

Bolm-Audorff, U. and Siegrist, J. (1983), 'Occupational morbidity data in myocardial infarction', *Journal of Occupational Medicine*, **25**, p. 367.

Bungener, M., Horell, E.V., Lafarge, C. and Louis, M.V. (1980), *Chomage et Santé*, CNRS.

Calnan, M. (1984), 'Patterns in preventive behaviour: a study of women in middle age', *Social Science and Medicine* **20**, pp. 263–80.

Calnan, M. and Johnson, B. (1985), 'Health, health risks and inequalities', *Sociology of*

Health and Illness, **7** (1) pp. 55–75.

Cox, B.D. *et al.* (1987), *Health and Lifestyle Survey*, Cambridge: The Health Promotion Research Trust.

CREDOC (1970), 'Survey on consumption of medical goods and services', Paris.

CREDOC (1978–79), 'Survey on situations and attitudes concerning the living conditions and quality of life of the French', Paris.

CREDOC (1982), 'Morbidité et conditions de vie', Paris.

Daniel, W.W. (1974), *A National Study of the Unemployed*, London: PEP.

d'Houtaud, A. and Field, M.G. (1984), 'The image of health: variations in perception by social class in a French population', *Sociology of Health and Illness*, **6**, pp. 30–60.

Ferge, Z., Kremer, B., Losonczi, A and Szalai, J. (1985), 'Health and Poverty: The Hungarian Case' (mimeo).

Garrad, J. and Bennett, A.E. (1971), 'A validated interview schedule for use in population surveys of chronic disability and disease', *British Journal of Preventive Social Medicine.*, **25**, pp. 97–104.

Hannay, D.R. (1978), 'Symptom prevalence in the community', *Journal of Royal College General Practitioners*, **28**, pp. 492–9.

Harris, A.I. (1971), *Handicapped and Impaired in Great Britain*, London: HMSO.

Helseundersokelse (1977), Oslo: Central Bureau of Statistics.

Hickey, N. *et al.* (1975), 'Study of coronary risk factors related to physical activity in 15,171 men', *British Medical Journal*, **3**, pp. 507–9.

Hill, M. J. *et al.* (1973), *Men out of Work*, Cambridge University Press.

INE (1975), *Encuesta de Equipiamento Y Nivel Cultural de las Familias*, Madrid.

Iversen, L. and Klausen, H. (1981), *Luknigen af Nordhavns – Vaerflet*, Copenhagen: Institute for Social Medicine, Publication 13.

Jougla, E., Maguin, P. and Hatton, F. (1984), *Morbidité ayant entrainé un recours aux soins, France 1980–1981*, Paris: INSERM., Paris.

Kalimo, E., Nyman, K., Klaukka, T., Tuomikoski, H. and Savolainen, E. (1983), *Need, Use and Expenses of Health Services in Finland 1964–76*, Helsinki: The Social Insurance Institution.

Knight, R. and Warren, M.D. (1975), *Physically Disabled People Living at Home: a study of numbers and needs*, London: HMSO.

Kohn, R. and White, K.L. (1976), *Health Care: An International Study*, Oxford University Press.

Leclerc, A., Aiach, P., Phillippe, A. and Vennin, M. (1971), 'Morbidité, mortalité et classe sociale', *Revue Epidemologie et Santé Publique* **27**, pp. 331–58.

Lecomte, T. (1984), *La morbidité declarée, description et évolution France 1970–80*, CREDOC.

Marmot, M.G., Rose, G., Shipley, M. and Hamilton, P.J.S. (1978), 'Employment grade and coronary heart disease in British Civil Servants', *Journal of Epidemology and Community Health*, **32**, pp. 244–9.

Medical Research Council (Great Britain) (1966), *Questionnaire on Bronchitis with Instructions*, London: HMSO.

Milne, J.S., Hope, K. and Williamson, J. (1970), 'Variability in replies to a questionnaire on symptoms of physical illness', *Journal of Chronic Disability*, **22**, pp. 805–10.

Minvielle, D. *et al.* (1977), 'Problèmes de santé de Inegalités Sociales. Santé Securité Sociale', *Statistiques et Commentaires* **4**, A.

Mizrahi, Andree, Mizrahi, Arie and Sermet, C. (1983), *Health Medical Care and Poverty*, Paris: CREDOC.

Morgan, M. (1983), 'Comparison of ACORN and social class classification in predicting mortality', St Thomas's Hospital, London (mimeo).

Niklas, D. (1978), 'What use to count the disabled?', *Health and Society*, Warsaw: Polish Academy of Sciences Institute of Philosophy and Sociology.

Pill, R. and Stott, N.C.H. (1982), 'Concepts of illness causation and responsibility', *Social Science and Medicine* **16**, pp. 42–51.

Purola, T., Kalimo, E. and Nyman, K. (1974), *Health Service Use and Health Status under National Sickness Insurance*, Helsinki: The Social Insurance Institution.

Ropes, M.W. et al (1957), 'Proposed diagnostic criteria for rheumatoid arthritis', *Journal of Chronic Diseases*, 5, pp. 630–5.

Rose, G.A. (1962), 'The diagnosis of ischaemic heart pain and intermittent claudication in field surveys', *WHO Bulletin*, 27, pp. 645–58.

Scambler, A., Scambler, G. and Craig, D. (1981), 'Kinship and friendship networks and women's demand for primary care', *Journal of Royal College General Practitioners*, 26, pp. 746–50.

Siegrist, J., Siegrist, K. and Weber, I. (1986), 'Sociological concepts in the etiology of chronic disease: the case of ischaemic heart disease', *Social Science and Medicine*, 22, pp. 247–53.

Subarea de Salut Publica, Ajuntament de Barcelona (1983), *Enquesta de Salut de Barcelona*.

Szalai, J. (1985), 'Inequalities in access to health care in Hungary' (mimeo).

Szalai, J. and Laslo, A. (1983), 'Social differences in the health condition of young people' (mimeo).

Tengwald, K. and Faresjo, T. (1984), 'Health and healthcare utilisation in the welfare state' (summary of a research programme), mimeo, Linkoping University.

Townsend, P. (1983), 'Understanding Poverty and Inequality in Europe' in Walker, R., Lawson, R. and Townsend, P. (eds), *Responses to Poverty: Lessons from Europe* London: Heinemann.

Warr, P.B. (1981), 'Some studies of psychological well-being and unemployment', SAPU Memo 43.

Warren, M.D. (1976), 'Interview survey of handicapped people: the accuracy of statements about the underlying medical conditions', *Rheumatism and Rehabilitation*, 15, pp. 295–302.

WHO (1975), *I.C.D. Classification of Impairments and Handicaps*, Geneva: PHN Wood.

WHO (1980), 'Information systems for health services', *Public Health in Europe* 13, Copenhagen.

WHO (1981), 'The cardiovascular disease programme of WHO in Europe' (G. Lamm), *Public Health in Europe*, 15, Copenhagen.

WHO (1982), MONICA News No. 1, Geneva.

WHO (1983), 'Proposals for the Multinational Monitoring of Trends and Determinants in Cardiovascular Disease and Protocol' (MONICA Projects), Geneva.

White, K.L. *et al.* (1977), *Health services: Concepts and Information for National Planning and Management*, Geneva: WHO.

Wright, S. (1985), 'Subjective Evaluation of Health: A Theoretical Review', *Social Indicators Research*, 16, 169–79.

11 Measuring European inequality: the use of height data
Roderick Floud

The measurement of welfare and inequality

This chapter explores a new method of measuring inequality within and between different sections of the European populations during the past 200 years. Traditionally, measures of inequality have been based on indicators of welfare, such as the mean income of selected groups, the incidence of mortality or morbidity in those groups, or by more specialised indicators such as distributions of wealth, of landed property or housing or access to various services. The particular indicator which has been chosen reflects the focus of the investigator, the availability of data and, to some degree, the fashions and preoccupations of various different disciplines within the social sciences. Thus economists and economic historians have tended to use measures of income to approach issues of inequality, while demographers have concentrated on mortality, sociologists on morbidity, housing tenure or access to social security benefits.

Faced with a plethora of such indicators, it may seem redundant or even positively unhelpful to propose another, for one of the greatest problems in the measurement of welfare or of inequality lies in aggregating, in a sensible manner, the indicators which we already possess. Thus, within economic history, a great deal of attention has been devoted to the measurement of changes in the standard of living in the past and to adjusting the primary measure, per capita real income, to take account of numerous changes affecting living standards other than income; such changes range from increasing or decreasing urban pollution to improvements in heating technology or an increase in the supply of tropical foodstuffs. In most cases, such adjustments to the primary measure, real income, have been impressionistic and unquantified; it has been argued, for example, that despite the urban pollution of the late nineteenth century, those men and women who lived in the cities improved their living standards because of their greater access to sporting or cultural facilities.

Some social scientists have, however, attempted more systematic adjustments. In particular, Usher has proposed a method by which changes in real income might be adjusted for changes in mortality. Applied to Canadian data for the period 1926–74, his 'imputation for life expectancy' raised the measured rate of economic growth 'by about one-half of one per cent per year from 2.83% without the imputation to about 3.35%, give or take 0.03%' (Usher, 1980, p. 245). The method had even more dramatic effects when applied to underdeveloped economies, where mortality rates had shown greater changes. More recently, Williamson has applied Usher's methods to the description of economic growth in nineteenth century Britain, concluding that '. . . conventional indices of real income growth may understate true living standard growth by 25% or more', with the greatest effects being seen in the second half of the nineteenth century and the first third of the twentieth. Thus British growth is seen, by these measures, to have accelerated much more sharply since the middle of the nineteenth century than is suggested by more conventional measures (Williamson, 1984). Adjustments of this kind can therefore be expected to produce radical revisions to our view of changes in welfare in the past and, by extension, to our view of differences in welfare between different groups within a society at a particular point in time.

Yet, as I have suggested elsewhere, adjustments of the kind made by Usher and Williamson are not a satisfactory solution to the problem of aggregating different aspects of welfare, (Floud, 1985). There are, for example, manifold problems of double-counting; in principle one should adjust income for changes in both morbidity and mortality, but separating these is an impossibility. In addition, as both Usher and Williamson pointed out, it is necessary to adjust only for influences on welfare which are exogenous to changes in real income; changes in welfare, for example an increase in expenditure on fuel, which are the *result* of an increase in income, must not be counted. In many important cases, in particular that of changes in morbidity, such a split between exogenous and endogenous changes may be almost impossible to determine. Last, the method does little to solve the central problem of the measurement of the welfare of groups within the population, unless it is possible to discover not only their real income (as conventionally measured) but their morbidity and mortality schedules. Both tasks are immense, as the long-standing controversy over the standard of living of the working class in England in the Industrial Revolution has shown, and to combine them seems likely to lead to despair.

The initial argument of this chapter is that it may be possible to solve some of these difficulties in the measurement of welfare and inequality by the use of an anthropometric approach and the exploitation of the millions of observations held in European archives about the physical appearance of people in the past and in the present. That such an approach is possible rests on a very large volume of work by human biologists who have demonstrated the value of anthropometric data as measures of the nutritional status of human populations. Various aspects of physical appearance are affected by nutritional status, but the focus of this discussion will be on measures of height, which is a particularly sensitive indicator.

Briefly, mean height is a direct measure of the average 'net nutritional status' of the members of a human population during their childhood and adolescence. It reflects, and sums up, the effects of multiple influences upon the human body, including inputs of energy in the form of food and warmth and outputs such as bodily activity, work and the struggle against disease. Measurement of changes in mean heights over time thus provides an index of changes in the nutritional status of a population. If measurements can be made of the mean height of sub-groups within a population, such as regional or class groups within a national population, then those mean heights will, similarly, reflect the different nutritional status of those groups. As the distinguished human biologists Eveleth and Tanner comment, the measurement of mean height thus provides:

> . . . a powerful tool with which to monitor the health of a population, or to pinpoint subgroups of a population whose share in economic and social benefits is less than it might be (Eveleth and Tanner, 1976, p. 1).

The measurement of mean height is therefore useful in understanding past changes in welfare and in delineating differences in welfare between populations and sub-groups of those populations during their formative years. In addition, however, there is increasing evidence that nutritional status during those years can significantly affect welfare, productivity and morbidity during the rest of life and even the length of life itself. Heights may therefore offer some predictive information for use in the formulation of social policy for the reduction of inequality.

Sources of data for the measurement of height

Evidence about the mean heights of populations is derived essentially from three types of sources. First, height has traditionally been one of the major criteria used to assess the health and strength of young men and thus their fitness for military service. It has therefore been common, even possibly universal, for military records compiled since the middle of the eighteenth century to contain information about the heights of recruits; sometimes information is recorded about all those who were measured, whether or not they ultimately joined the armed services, sometimes it is recorded only for those accepted for service.

Second, height has frequently been recorded to serve as a means of identification. This was probably a secondary motive behind the recording of military heights – to aid, for example, in the apprehending of deserters – but it was primary in the case of the measurement of criminals and, in the early nineteenth century, of slaves (Friedman, 1982).

Third, height has been recorded in the course of medical and social scientific investigation. In the late nineteenth century, for example, the intense popular and scientific interest in genetics and anthropometry stimulated a number of enquiries in which large numbers of people were measured. In this century, interest in human biology and the process of physical growth has stimulated many enquiries in which height has been either a primary or a secondary focus of interest; these enquiries culminated in investigations carried out as part of the International Biological Programme (Tanner, 1981; Eveleth and Tanner, 1976). There have also been a small number of studies of height carried out for commercial purposes, such as the design of clothing or furniture.

The primary source of information about the heights of large fractions of human populations remains, however, the military records and in particular the conscription records of the European nations and of the United States. Conscription has been used as the primary means of recruiting in most European countries, although only intermittently in the case of Britain and the United States and, in many cases, the results of the measurement of recruits have been published in summary form in the national statistical yearbooks which typically began to be published in the late nineteenth century. In many cases, indeed, such statistics can be found grouped with other material on the health of the populations.

This investigation is the first systematic attempt to collect and collate such measurements. Not all European countries publish such material, and there are often gaps in the data for those who do. Height data have been published in some years, but not in others, in the form of calculated means or as grouped frequency distributions, and in some cases for regions, in others only for the whole nation. It is, moreover, often very difficult to discover the exact age at measurement, since the age at which recruits were conscripted is reported only intermittently.

There are, in addition, some further difficulties in the use of military conscription data for the exploration of variation in mean heights. Such data can give only a snapshot, at one moment in time, of the complex process of human growth and moreover, of a moment at which the process of growth in those measured has largely but not entirely ceased. Ideally, one should be able to observe the whole growth process, from birth to maturity, since it is known that environmental influences affect not only the absolute height which is achieved at a given age but also the tempo of growth. It is well known, for example, that the age at menarche in girls has become earlier since the nineteenth century and the same applies to the timing of the adolescent growth spurt in boys and girls and to the age at which final height is achieved. This last point is highly relevant to conscription data; whereas in the past an 18 year-old male might well not have achieved final height at the point when he was measured for military service, today he would certainly have done so. A comparison of the mean height of a cohort of 18 year-olds today with a cohort of 18 year-olds from one century ago will therefore probably *overestimate* the change in final height; on the other hand, it may well give an *underestimate* of the impact of environment on growth, since some of the impact will have been reflected in the earlier maturity – perhaps at the same absolute height – of the modern cohort. This problem arises because, although the tempo of growth and the final height are linked, they are to some extent independent of each other; there are early maturing groups who are short, and late maturing groups who are tall (Tanner, 1982, pp. 574–5).

Military recruitment data must therefore be interpreted with great care. Nevertheless they offer by far the most consistent set of evidence available for the description of changes in mean height and by far the largest set of evidence in terms of the underlying number of measurements. They therefore form the principal source which is used in the remainder of this chapter, although they have been supplemented by other published materials.

The evidence of height data
National populations
The average height of the European adult male population has varied, during the last 200 years, between 159 and 181 cm. The shortest mean height yet recorded or computed for conscripts recruited on a national basis is that of 159.1 cm for recruits aged 18 to the Habsburg armies in the eighteenth century, (Komlos, 1985) while Kiil (1939) estimated that the height of recruits aged 18.5 to the Norwegian army in 1761 was 159.5 cm. Svimez gives 162.2 cm as the mean height of Italian recruits aged 20 in 1874–6, a figure confirmed by the *Historical Statistics of Italy 1861–1965* (1978) which shows that the mean height of 20 year-old recruits born in 1854 was 162.39 cm. Spanish recruits, as late as 1931, had a mean height of 163.6 cm (Rodriguez n.d.).

Since growth would probably have continued after the age at which these recruits were measured, it is likely that these measurements are a slight underestimate of final adult heights for those communities. On the basis of modern populations in the underdeveloped world, who have similar mean heights, it is reasonable to add an estimate of about 3 per cent for further growth after the age of 18, giving an estimated minimum mean final height for European national populations of about 165 cm.

Measurement of the upper end of the observed range can rely on modern data. Army recruits of age 17.5 in The Netherlands had a mean height of 180.7 cm in 1982 (*Statistical Yearbook of The Netherlands*, 1983). These men, the tallest in Europe, were closely followed by the Norwegians with a mean of 179.4 cm in 1983 (*Statistisk Arbok*, 1984).

The range of European final mean heights over the past two centuries has therefore been about 16 cm for national populations. This may seem small, but it can be compared with ranges in the modern world such as that shown in Figure 11.1. It can be seen that Norwegian recruits of the 1760s were as short as African bushmen, while today they are as tall as the Dinka of the Sudan. This comparison is not meant to imply that it is expected that, given adequate nutrition, bushmen will ultimately grow as tall as the Dinka – we do not know whether this would be so – but rather to emphasise, by the use of a modern analogy, how different the Norwegians of the 1760s would have looked from their descendants of today.

Moreover, most of this range has been covered within the past century. Only Great Britain among the populations of Europe had a mean height of more than 169 cm in 1880, while the majority of nations averaged less than 166 cm. Today, few have mean heights of less than 169 cm. All European countries have experienced change so rapid as to enter clearly into public consciousness and to be regarded as one of the most visible signs of economic and social development. Figures 11.2–11.7 give the course of growth in mean height (at the time of recruitment) for Denmark, The Netherlands, Belgium, Norway, Italy and Spain, countries for which series of heights have been collected, while Figures 11.8–11.9 give similar information for France and Sweden, where the data are less complete. It is likely that similar material exists for other countries, and for other periods within countries shown in the figures, but it has not yet been located.

These figures demonstrate that every European country has experienced very significant changes in mean male heights during the past century. In most cases, change seems to have been most rapid during the twentieth century, but the actual timing has varied substantially. Nor, despite the common growth overall, has the process been one of convergence to a common European mean height. While several northern European countries have exhibited very similar patterns of growth, they have, in the process, grown faster – or perhaps simply earlier than some southern countries. Table 11.1, for example, shows the differences between mean male heights in Holland, (although

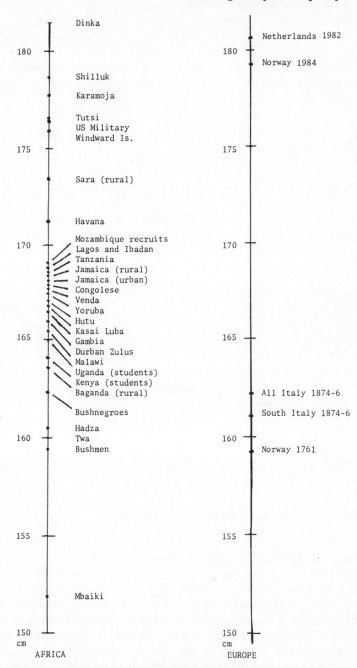

*Figure 11.1   Range of European final height over 200 years compared
with that of present day African tribesmen*

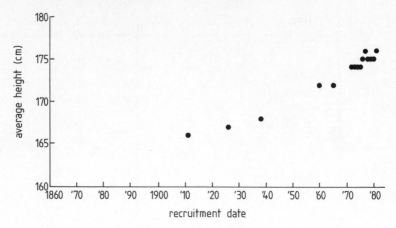

Figure 11.2   Average height of recruits: Belgium

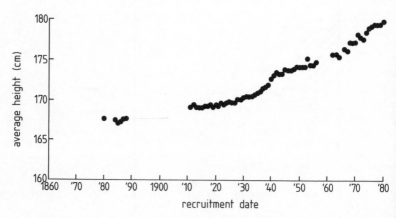

Figure 11.3   Average height of recruits: Denmark

Norway would be an almost exact substitute) and Italy.

As Table 11.1 shows, the gap in mean heights between Italian and Dutch males has grown consistently, both in absolute and in relative terms, since 1874, although the rate of increase in the gap has slowed since the 1950s. It seems likely that, as Italian prosperity increases in the 1980s, the gap will begin to narrow again; it should always be remembered that, to a considerable degree, the heights of recruits reflect the nutritional status of a population some fifteen to twenty years before the date or recruitment.

Table 11.1 Differences between the mean height of the Italian and Dutch populations, 1874–1984

Date	Italy	Holland	Diff.cm	Diff. %
1874	162.4	164.9	2.5	1.5
1894	163.4	166.7	3.3	2.0
1914	164.7	169.2	4.5	2.7
1934	166.3	171.8	5.5	3.3
1954	167.8	175	7.2	4.3
1974	171.1	179	7.9	4.6
1982	172.8	180.7	7.9	4.6

Note: It is uncertain, given the nature of the data sources, that measurements were made at exactly the same age in each country at each date.

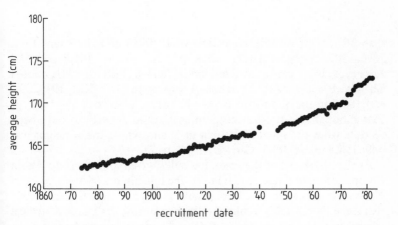

Figure 11.4 *Average height of recruits: Italy*

Just as there is substantial variation in mean final heights, between European countries, and over time, so there is considerable variation within those countries. This variation, either between those living in different geographical areas within a country or between members of different social groups, reflects the differing nutritional status of those groups and, therefore, can be a useful measure of the degree of inequality within a national society.

Areas within countries
Several European regions or provinces record mean heights of less

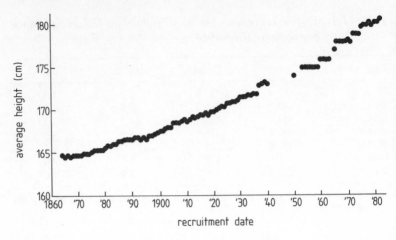

Figure 11.5   Average height of recruits: Netherlands

than 162.5 cm, including Sardinia in 1879–83 at 161.19 cm (Livi, 1896–1905, quoted Chamla, 1964, p. 228), Glaris (161.5 cm) and Appenzel (160.7 cm) in Switzerland in 1884–6 (Pittard, 1931, quoted Chamla, 1964, p. 228), Akershus in Norway in 1761 (Kiil, 1939: 39), and 160.7 in the Somme in France in 1819–26 (Aron *et al.*, 1972, p. 55), although the shortest geographical group appears to have been recruits from the town of Murcia in Spain, whose mean height was only 158.8 cm in 1895 (Carrion, 1986, p. 7).

At the upper end of the scale, the tallest geographical group within Europe recorded today appears to be the inhabitants of Aust-Agder in Norway, at 180.8 cm (*Statistisk Arbok*, 1986), although it seems likely that some Dutch areas would have higher means; the Dutch statistical yearbook unfortunately ceased to record regional height data after the Second World War.

While these observations extend the overall range of European height means, more interest resides in the extent of variation in height means within a given country, and in the change in that variation over time. Long-run published series for regional heights exist for three countries, The Netherlands, Norway and Italy, and there is a shorter series of observations in recent years for Spain; data from France exist, but only at decadal intervals. There has, unfortunately, not been time to calculate mean regional heights for The Netherlands or, for some early years, for Italy, where the published data give only height distributions; while it might appear to be a simple task to calculate means from grouped frequency distributions, the existence of truncation in the lower tail (caused by the rejection of some

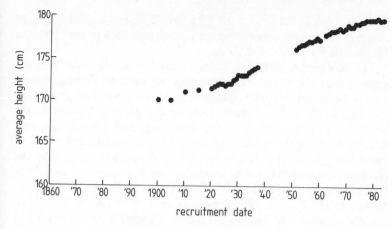

Figure 11.6   Average height of recruits: Norway

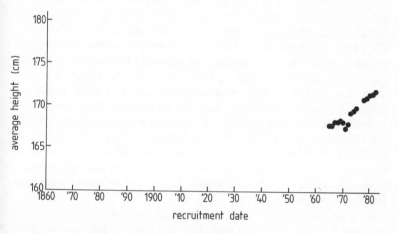

Figure 11.7   Average height of recruits: Spain

extremely short recruits) makes it necessary to employ maximum likelihood estimation.

Norway and Italy provide, however, a contrast between one of the tallest and one of the shortest peoples in Europe in recent years. The series of regional height means runs from those recruited in 1936 to 1985 in the case of Norway (although with no observations for 1938–51 and 1958–60) and from those recruited in 1949 to 1982 in the case of Italy. The mean height of Norwegians recruited in 1936 (and therefore born at the time of the First World War) was already 173.74 cm, greater than the mean height of Italians recruited in 1982 (born in 1962), who were then 172.83 cm.

The Norwegian data exhibit significantly less variation between regions than do Italian data, although the men of Finnmark have always been substantially shorter than those from other parts of Norway. In 1936, for example, with the exception of Finnmark, the shortest region in Norway, Nord-Trondelag, had a mean height of 172.83 cm, while the tallest, Vest-Agder, had a mean height only 3.33 cm greater, at 175.16 cm. At the end of the period covered by the statistics, the recruits of 1985 showed even less variation, only 2.7 cm between the shortest region, Troms, at 178.1 cm and the tallest, Aust-Agder, at 180.8. Even the exceptional area of Finnmark has drawn slightly closer to the Norwegian norm; it lagged 4.72 cm behind in 1936, but only 3.9 cm in 1985. In general, therefore, the effect has been to reduce the disparity between the southern and northern areas of the country.

The Italian pattern is somewhat more complex. The Italian anthropologist, R. Livi, studied the conscripts of 1879–83, collating information about the region of birth and occupation of 299,355 recruits. He found a difference of 4.7 cm between the tallest and shortest regions, the Veneto at a mean of 166.6 cm and Sardinia at 161.9 cm; the shortest region of mainland Italy was Basilicata at 162.6 cm. The same north–south division was observable in the earliest published official recruitment statistics, those for recruits of 1949, but the gap had widened very sharply. The recruits of 1949 exhibit a range of 8.86 cm from the men of Friuli-Venezia Giulia at 171.21 cm to those of Basilicata at 162.65 cm. By the end of the period in 1982, the range was still 6.53 cm, between the same two regions, although Sardinia is now once again the shortest region in Italy, 0.31 cm shorter than Basilicata at 169.27 cm.

In France, also, the variation in height means appears to have declined between the 1820s and 1880, and increased slightly between 1880 and 1960, although it is possible that there has been a convergence since that date. Le Roy Ladurie's work on the French conscripts of 1819–26 found that the shortest *département* was the Somme, with a mean height of 160.7 cm, while the tallest was Doubs at 168.9 cm, a difference of 8.2 cm. The work of Chamla (1964), who took samples of recruits from each French region at ten-year intervals between 1880 and 1960, shows that in 1880 the gap between the shortest *département*, the Dordogne at 163.29 cm, and the tallest, Ain at 168.07 cm, was 4.88 cm. The gap then widened, reaching 6.6 cm by 1920, before stabilising at approximately that level. By 1960, the gap was 6.35 cm, between Morbihan at 166.2 cm and Seine at 172.55

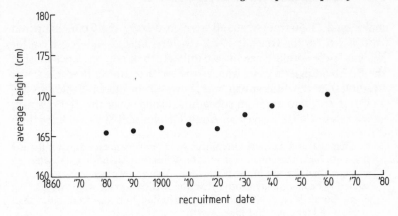

Figure 11.8   Average height of recruits: France

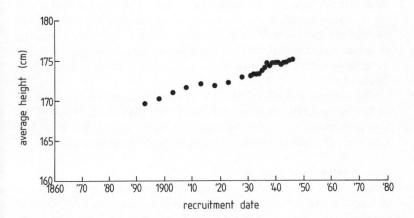

Figure 11.9   Average height of recruits: Sweden

(Chamla, 1964, p. 211–12). However, as Chamla shows, these departmental statistics conceal wider regional movements in which the northern and southern regions grew faster than the central belt of the Loire, Burgundy and Lorraine, producing an overall convergence; the fastest growth of all was to be found in the mountain areas of central, eastern and south-eastern France.

It seems likely that in Britain there has been a reduction in regional differences in height, although the lack of conscription makes the scattered evidence suspect and difficult to interpret. The British Association for the Advancement of Science found in 1883 that adult males aged 23–50 from Scotland were on average 174.6 cm, compared with 172.6 cm for Ireland, 171.2 cm for England and 169.4 cm for Wales. These absolute heights are unlikely to be correct, since most of the BAAS adult data came from Army recruits subject to severe lower height limits; the differentials may, however, be more reliable (BAAS, 1883). If so, there has been substantial change over the past century, as the recent OPCS Survey on Adult Heights and Weights finds that:

> . . . regional and national differences were not very great though it is clear that both male and female residents of Wales were significantly shorter, on average, than the rest of the population. Men and women in Scotland also tended to be marginally shorter than the British average while those living in the South West and South East (excluding London) were taller than average (Knight and Eldridge, 1984).

The range of variation was, for men, from 171.9 cm for residents of Wales and 173.0 cm for Scotland to 175.1 cm for the South-West of England; for women, the range was from 159.4 cm for Wales and 160.0 cm for Scotland and the North of England to 161.9 cm for the South-East and South-West of England. Another interesting regional variation was that both men and women residents of Greater London were shorter than residents of the surrounding areas of South-East England.

The analysis reported above is crude and preliminary, particularly in its concentration on extreme values rather than on the shape of the full distribution of heights by region in each country, but it is clear that some intriguing patterns require further investigation.

Socio-economic groups
Much less is known explicitly about variation in mean height between different social, economic or occupational groups within national populations, since the data are rarely collected or published in an appropriate form. Information is available, however, for Italy and Britain in the nineteenth century and for Britain today. In his survey of Italian recruits, Livi found very substantial differences between the mean height of students and peasants, the two most extreme groups. He arranged his data by region, but found that in all regions the gap between students and peasants was at least 1.8 cm. In the poorest regions of the south – which also had the shortest people – the gap was larger, up to 3.7 cm in Abruzzi e Molise, Basilicata and Sicilia. The student population was not of uniform height across all regions, ranging from 168.2 cm in the Veneto down to 165.9 cm in Basilicata and 164.1 cm in Sardegna, but the range in the peasant population was greater, from 166.5 cm in the Veneto to 162.2 in Basilicata and 161.9 cm in Sardegna. Finally, Livi was able to show that tempo of

growth was different between the two socio-occupational groups and between the taller and shorter regions. Since the recruits were measured both at entry and one year later, he was able to examine the change in their heights over the year. Students in the tallest region, the Veneto, grew by 3.3 per cent over the year and peasants by approximately the same amount, 3.2 per cent. By contrast, in the south the peasants grew by almost twice as much as did the students; in Basilicata, for example, students grew by 2.8 per cent and peasants by 5.0 per cent. The effect of this differential rate of growth, which implies that students were closer to their maximum height on enlistment at age 20, would of course be to diminish socio-economic differences in final height.

British recruitment data also show that there were significant differences between different occupational groups within the working class in the eighteenth and nineteenth century. Evidence collected in the early 1880s by the British Association for the Advancement of Science, largely based on recruitment records, shows that substantial differences in mean height existed between the working and 'professional' classes (BAAS, 1883). Such differences are also shown in samples of recruitment records. While the most dramatic differences were to be found in adolescence, for example between the children of Sandhurst and of the Marine Society (Floud, 1984, Table 4), Table 11.2 shows the results of the maximum likelihood estimation of occupational and regional differences in heights of recruits, almost all drawn from within the working class between 1820 and 1824.

While such differences have diminished over time, the recent Survey of Adult Heights and Weights (Knight and Eldridge, 1984) in Britain shows that they have not disappeared. As the survey states:

. . . it is clear that there is a class effect on height independent of age and sex. In almost every age group people from households headed by a manual worker were shorter, on average, than people from non-manual worker households. Overall, the average height of men was 175.5 cm (5'9") in Social Classes I and II but 172.3 cms (5'8") in Social Classes IV and V. Similarly female height in Social Classes I and II was 162.5 cms (5'4") compared with 159.6 cms (5'3") in Classes IV and V" (Knight and Eldridge, 1984).

Discussion

Over time, adult male height has varied greatly in Europe, between different geographical areas and between different segments of the European populations. While the causes and correlates of a particular measurement of height may be difficult to discern, overall the series of measurements given in earlier sections of the paper constitute, as Eveleth and Tanner suggested of height measures in general, 'a growth was different between the two socio-occupational groups and between the taller and shorter regions. Since the recruits were measured both at entry and one year later, he was able to examine the change in their heights over the year. Students in the tallest region, the Veneto, grew by 3.3 per cent over the year and peasants by approximately the same amount, 3.2 per cent. By contrast, in the south the peasants grew by almost twice as much as did the students; in Basilicata, for example, students grew by 2.8 per cent and peasants by 5.0 per cent. The effect of this differential rate of growth, which implies that students were closer to their maximum height on enlistment at age 20, would of course be to diminish socio-economic differences in final height.

British recruitment data also show that there were significant differences between different occupational groups within the working class in the eighteenth and nineteenth century. Evidence collected in the early 1880s by the British Association for the Advancement of Science, largely based on recruitment records, shows that substantial differences in mean height existed between the working and 'professional' classes (BAAS, 1883). Such differences are also shown in samples of recruitment records. While the most dramatic differences were to be found in adolescence, for example between the children of Sandhurst and of the Marine Society (Floud, 1984, Table 4), Table 11.2 shows the results of the maximum likelihood estimation of occupational and regional differences in heights of recruits, almost all drawn from within the working class between 1820 and 1824.

While such differences have diminished over time, the recent Survey of Adult Heights and Weights (Knight and Eldridge, 1984) in Britain shows that they have not disappeared. As the survey states:

. . . it is clear that there is a class effect on height independent of age and sex. In almost every age group people from households headed by a manual worker were shorter, on average, than people from non-manual worker households. Overall, the average height of men was 175.5 cm (5'9") in Social Classes I and II but 172.3 cms (5'8") in Social Classes IV and V. Similarly female height in Social Classes I and II was 162.5 cms (5'4") compared with 159.6 cms (5'3") in Classes IV and V" (Knight and Eldridge, 1984).

Discussion

Over time, adult male height has varied greatly in Europe, between different geographical areas and between different segments of the European populations. While the causes and correlates of a particular measurement of height may be difficult to discern, overall the series of measurements given in earlier sections of the paper constitute, as Eveleth and Tanner suggested of height measures in general, 'a meaning for the student of welfare, such measures must be translatable into a form which relates to personal experience. As he puts it:

> . . . statistics of economic growth may be interpreted and proposals for improvement may be judged appropriate or otherwise by means of an analogy between a country and a person: economic growth to a country is like a raise in salary to an individual . . . For without such a translation, measures of real income and economic growth are mere numbers with no apparent effect upon our lives and no status as indicators of progress towards goals that people might want the economy to achieve. Without the possibility of such a translation, the measurement of economic growth is nonsense. Why, after all, would we want to measure economic growth, why is public policy directed to the promotion of economic growth, why do economic historians and specialists in economic development search for the explanation of economic growth, if we are not better off after economic growth than we were before? (Usher, 1980, pp. 1–2).

An exactly equivalent question can be asked about height. Is there any point in measuring height, and in regarding those measurements as indicators of welfare, if we are not in some way better off for being, on average or as individuals, taller today than our ancestors were a century ago?

This question can be answered in two ways. First, height can be regarded essentially as a proxy; it represents the average nutritional status of whatever group has been measured and that average nutritional status, in turn, represents a whole complex of environmental and welfare-related influence on the individuals in that group. That is, their nutritional status embraces the food they are able to eat, the warmth they can buy in the form of fuel and clothing, the diseases they are able to combat. Thus differences in nutritional status, proxied by differences in height, reflect basic differences in welfare – more fundamental and more comprehensive than those proxied by income or wealth.

Such a justification for the measurement of height is given greater point by the increasing evidence that nutritional status in childhood and adolescence, as reflected in final height, has lifelong effects on individuals and, in fact, helps to determine how long those individuals will live. This is the clear implication of studies in Norway by Waaler and in Britain by Marmot, both of which have established that individual height (reflecting, presumably, nutritional status in childhood) has a significantly positive impact on expectation of life many years later (Waaler, 1984; Marmot *et al.*, 1984).

This evidence leads to a second way of answering the question about the translation of height to welfare. Just as the acquisition of money capital is an indication of past income levels and gives some assurance of future welfare, so the possession of height denotes past nutritional status and some assurance of future welfare. This is reinforced in societies where height is a clear signal of class differences. Such an argument helps us to understand what is, to many people, one of the most puzzling features of the measurement of height, that, like income, it seems to be regarded as desirable in itself. The work of Illsley and the OPCS study of height and weight are representative of a number of studies which have found that taller members of a group are more likely to be upwardly socially mobile than shorter members of the same group (Illsley, 1955; Knight and Eldridge, 1984).

To see the heights of European nations, set out in Figures 11.1–11.9, as indicators of welfare, is to raise a number of intriguing questions about the nature of economic development in Europe. First, it appears that most of the increase in height in Europe has taken place during the twentieth century, although in some countries there was some increase late in the nineteenth century. This suggests that the economic development of Europe in the nineteenth century did little to affect the welfare of the bulk of the European populations: although per capita real incomes were certainly growing in many countries, it would appear that either distributional shifts, or such factors as the disease environment, prevented many of the benefits of this income growth from being translated into improved nutritional status or welfare.

It seems, indeed, that there may well have been distributional shifts within the European populations. In several cases, differentials in height between the tallest and shortest areas within nations widened during the earlier period of economic development, converging again considerably later. This pattern corresponds very well with that known to economists as the Kuznets curve – the insight of Simon Kuznets, that economic development might well lead initially to increased inequality, has been widely documented in the contemporary under developed world. Recently Williamson (1985) has suggested that the same pattern can be seen in Britain during the nineteenth century. It is intriguing that the same pattern appears in height statistics, suggesting that further investigation of regional height data would be worthwhile.

This chapter has, indeed, merely touched the surface of the voluminous material available for the study of trends and variation in European heights. It has used only published abstracted data, while the European military archives – other than those in Britain and Sweden – have remained largely untouched. But what has been done suggests that further investigation will give worthwhile material for the delineation of welfare, and inequality, in Europe over the past century and further.

References

Aron, J., Dumont, P., and Le Roy Ladurie, E. (1972), *Anthropologie du conscrit français*, Paris: Mouton.

BAAS (British Association for the Advancement of Science), (1883), *Report of the Anthropometric Committee*, London: BAAS.

Carrion, J.M.M. (1986), 'Estatura, Nutricion y Nivel de Vida en Murcia, 1860–1930' *Revista de Historia Economica* **IV**, (1), pp. 67–99.

Chamla, M.C. (1964), 'L'Accroissement de la Stature en France de 1880 à 1960; Comparaison avec les Pays d'Europe Occidentale', *Bulletin de la Société Anthropologie de Paris* T.6 Xi series, pp. 201–78.

Eveleth, P.B. and Tanner, J.M. (1976), *Worldwide Variation in Human Growth*, Cambridge: Cambridge University Press.

Floud, R.C. (1985), 'Measuring the Transformation in the European Economies: Income, Health and Welfare', *Centre for Economic Policy Research Discussion Paper* 33, also published in *Historical Social Research*, 33.

Floud, R.C., Gregory, A.S. and Wachter, K.W. (1985), *The Physical State of the British Working Class, 1870–1914: Evidence from Army Recruits*, NBER working paper 1661.

Friedman, G.C. (1982), 'The Heights of Slaves in Trinidad', *Social Science History*, **6**, (4).

Historical Statistics of Italy (1978), *Sommario di statistiche storiche dell 'Italia 1861–1975*, Rome: ISTAT.

Illsley, R. (1955), 'Social Class Selection and Class Differences in Relation to Still Births and Infant Deaths', *British Medical Journal*, ii, p. 1520.

Kiil, V. (1939), 'Stature and growth of Norwegian men during the past 200 years', *Skr. norske Vidensk Akad*, **6**.

Knight, I. and Eldridge, J. (1984), (For the Office of Population Censuses and Surveys and the Department of Health and Social Security), *The Heights and Weights of Adults in Great Britain*, London: HMSO.

Komlos, J. (1985), 'Stature and Nutrition in the Habsburg Monarchy: the standard of living and economic development', *American Historical Review*, **90**, (5) pp. 1149–61.

Livi, R. (1896–1905), *Antropometria Militare*, Rome.

Marmot, M.G., Shipley, M.J. and Rose, G. (1984), 'Inequalities in Death – Specific Explanations of a General Pattern?', *The Lancet*, 5 May, p. 1003–6.

Pittard, E. and Dellenbach, M. (1931), 'L'augmentation de la stature en Suisse au cours de 25 ans', *Journal de Statistiques et Revue economique suisse* fasc. 2, pp. 308–22.

Rodriguez, M.G. (no date), 'La Estadistica de Reemplazo y Reclutamiento de los Ejercitos', Madrid.

Statistisk Arbok, Norway (Annual).

Statistical Yearbook of the Netherlands (Annual).

Tanner, J.M. (1981), *A History of the Study of Human Growth*, Cambridge: Cambridge University Press.

Tanner, J.M. (1982), 'The Potential of Auxological Data for Monitoring Economic and Social Well-Being', *Social Science History* **6**, (4).

Usher, D. (1980), *The Measurement of Economic Growth*, Oxford: Blackwell.

Waaler, T.H. (1984), *Height, Weight and Mortality: The Norwegian Experience*, Oslo: Gruppe for helsetjenesteforskning.

Williamson, J. G. (1984), 'British Mortality and the Value of Life, 1781–1931', *Population Studies*, **38**, pp. 157–72.

Williamson, J.G. (1985), *Did British Capitalism Breed Inequality?*, London: Allen and Unwin.

12 Gender and class inequalities in health: understanding the differentials
Sara Arber

The debate on inequalities in health has neglected class inequalities in health among women. Data are presented here on inequalities in health, based on the 1981 and 1982 General Household Survey. To understand the pattern of class inequalities for women, it is necessary to disaggregate women by marital status and employment status. An analysis of the similarities and differences in the pattern of health inequalities for women compared to men provides clues to an understanding of the explanations of inequality – in particular the relative importance of health selection compared to materialist explanations.

Background
This chapter addresses the question of whether or not there are less differentials in health for women than for men. Women have lower mortality rates than men, and women's mortality advantage has been increasing this century throughout Europe (Hart, Chapter 6). In all European countries women report more ill-health and use more health care services than men. This apparent paradox of men having higher mortality and women higher morbidity has been the subject of numerous studies (Nathanson, 1975, 1977; Waldron, 1976, 1983; Mechanic, 1978; Verbrugge, 1979; Gove and Hughes, 1979). However, many of these studies can be criticised for treating women as an undifferentiated category, paying little attention to differences in health between women occupying varying roles and in different types of occupation.

Women have been relatively invisible in discussions of socioeconomic inequalities in health. Awareness of social class inequalities in health in the UK increased with the publication of the *Inequalities in Health* report (DHSS, 1980). This report relied heavily on data on class inequalities in mortality of men below retirement age drawn from the *Decennial Supplement on Occupational Mortality* (Office of Population Censuses and Surveys (1978). Women are of marginal concern in the *Decennial Supplements* and in the *Inequalities in Health* report; they appear primarily as married women classified by their husband's occupation. The major published source of data on class differences in morbidity are the General Household Survey (GHS) reports which classify married women by their husband's occupation and all other women by their own occupation (OPCS, 1984).

Analyses of occupational class and health differentials need to consider the relationship between employment status and health. Unemployed men and women are either left out of analyses, treated as a separate category, or classified by their last occupation. There is a need to consider the implications of these alternative practices for the relative pattern of class inequalities for men and women. The relationship between health and unemployment has been the subject of debate over recent years (Stern, 1983a, 1983b; Hart, 1983; Moser, Fox and Jones, 1984), but women have been largely excluded from this research, perhaps reflecting an assumption that women's unemployment is less important because women can fall back on their other 'legitimate' non-active role, that of housewife. Housewives have considerably poorer health than employed women, yet there has been relatively little research to explain this association. Research in the field of mental health suggests that paid employment is conducive to better mental health because it provides a sense of self-worth and self-esteem, as well as providing social contacts, compared with the isolation, monotony and lack of prestige derived from being a housewife (Brown and Harris, 1978; Gove and Tudor, 1973; Gove, 1978; Warr and Parry, 1982). Research on the relationship between paid employment and women's physical health has highlighted the complexity of the relationship (Nathanson, 1980; Waldron, 1980), for example, demonstrating that employment may have a negative impact on health where the woman has childcare and domestic responsibilities as well as a full-time job resulting in role conflicts and role strain (Arber, Gilbert and Dale, 1985). There has been no systematic research which measures the extent of 'health selection' in women's labour force participation. This is particularly likely after a period of time spent childbearing when a woman's decision to re-enter the labour force may be influenced by the woman's health status.

Problems in analysing socio-economic inequalities for women

Analyses of socio-economic inequalities in health for women may lead to questioning of the appropriate *unit of analysis*. Should analyses of health inequalities be based on individuals, families or households? Since a man's own class and his household's class are usually treated as synonymous, it is unnecessary to debate whether the analysis should be at the individual or household level. Analyses of occupational mortality for men are predicated on the assumption that occupational mortality measures both the adverse health consequences of working conditions in specific occupations, and indicates the health effects of lifestyles and material circumstances associated with men's occupations. It is assumed that the husband's occupation determines the family's lifestyle and this is explicitly stated in the *Decennial Supplements*, prior to 1970–72. For each occupational group, the mortality of husbands and their wives are compared to separate out the adverse health risks specific to each occupation from the general health consequences of lifestyles associated with those occupations (Leete and Fox, 1977). The identity of a man's occupation with his lifestyle is therefore taken for granted, but the parallel identity for a woman's occupation is less likely to be assumed.

Research on women's and children's health has generally assumed that the occupation of the head of household (usually defined as the husband) influences the health status and health behaviour of all family members. For example, analyses of infant mortality by social class in the UK are based on the occupation of the father (MacFarlane and Mugford, 1984); a practice which is becoming increasingly problematic as the proportion of illegitimate births increases in many European countries. At issue is whether the family is the appropriate unit of analysis for studies of life chances and, if so, whether the family's class should be measured by the occupational class of the head of household.

The definition of social class used in the *Inequalities in Health* report (DHSS, 1980, p.13) is based on Townsend (1979) who argues that 'social classes may be said to be segments of the population showing broadly similar types and levels of resources, with broadly similar styles of living' (p. 370). Goldthorpe (1983; 1984) argues that, despite the increased labour force participation of women, a woman's attachment to the labour market is weak and conditioned by her husband's class, and that wives are dependent on their husbands for the determination of their life chances. Thus, inequalities in married women's health would be expected to reflect their husband's rather than their own occupations.

Opposition to this 'conventional' view has been vociferous particularly from feminists (Stanworth, 1984) and in Equal Opportunities Commission publications (Nissel, 1980; Hunt, 1980). The evidence cited includes the fact that nearly 60 per cent of married women are in paid work (Beacham, 1984), that women's employment and incomes are crucial to the family budget and influence the family's lifestyle, and that it is no longer socially or politically acceptable for women to be considered an appendage of men, with their class position derived from their husbands (Arber, Dale and Gilbert, 1986).

An individualistic approach is advocated which classifies a woman on the basis of her own current or last occupation. However, the option of measuring class based on the woman's last job is often not available because this information may not be collected for women without paid employment, for example at death registration and in the UK census. Even where details of last occupation are available, as in the GHS, there is frequently no indication of the length of time since the job was held, or whether the last job was full-time or part-time. A previous full-time job may be a better indicator of a woman's current class than a part-time one. Similarly, a job held prior to the birth of a woman's first child may be a better indicator of class position than one taken on after a woman has children. In summary, an individualistic approach assumes that last occupation is as good an indicator of class position for women not in employment as for men not currently employed, even though some women may not have worked for many years.

The distinction between an individualistic approach and a household-based approach is clarified by Hart (1983; 1986) who contrasts an individualistic (or distributional) model of class with a structural model. Hart characterises Stern (1983a, 1983b) and others, who emphasise social mobility as a major mechanism for health selection, as conceptualising class primarily as a sorting mechanism producing a series of strata as part of a ranked hierarchy. She contrasts this with a structural model of class which emphasises the unequal distribution of control over resources and power, which shapes and creates the social distribution of health. In the latter model life chances are influenced primarily by the social and economic circumstances of the household. These structural inequalities influence the likelihood and consequences of unemployment, and the likelihood of other social stressors which have health consequences. Thus, in a structural model, the primary measure of class must be a household-based measure. If a household-based measure is accepted, the issue becomes one of determining the most appropriate household-based measure of social class.

Marsh (1986) reminds us that there is no single best way to define class; the most appropriate measure depends on the theoretical purposes of the research. Therefore, whether women should be analysed in terms of their own occupation or in terms of the class of the family depends on the topic under study. Although the appropriate unit of analysis is primarily a theoretical question, one task of the researcher is to answer the empirical question 'which measures is the best discriminator in terms of distinguishing the healthy from the unhealthy?'. It is surprising that so little empirical research on women's health has contrasted the alternatives of an individualistic model of class which classifies women by their own occupation, and a structural model in which women are categorised by a household-level characteristic, such as their husband's occupation.

This chapter considers whether life chances in the form of health are primarily determined by the actions and experiences of the individual woman in the labour market, or are to a greater extent influenced by the social and material circumstances of the family. Research on differentials in mortality and morbidity for women will be reviewed, before analysing class differences in women's morbidity using data from the General Household Survey.

Occupational class and women's mortality and morbidity

Analyses of class inequalities in mortality among women have assumed that women's mortality is primarily influenced by the lifestyle of the family, measured by the husband's occupational class. The class gradient in mortality for men is slightly steeper than for married women classified by their husband's occupational class (DHSS, 1980; OPCS, 1978). Single women are classified by their own occupation in the *Decennial Supplement*. The gradient is slightly less for single women than for men and there is a somewhat different pattern – for example, single women in class I have an above-average mortality (McDowall, 1983). However, Koskinnen (1985, p. 4) suggests that mortality data for single women is less reliable because many have no occupation recorded at census.

There has been recent interest in an individualistic approach – analysing women's mortality using their own occupation (Roman, Beral and Inskip, 1985; OPCS, 1985; Moser and Goldblatt, 1985). McDowall (1983) argues that it is problematic to use the *Decennial Supplement* for this purpose, because although 49 per cent of women aged 15–64 had their occupation recorded in the 1971 Census, only 20 per cent could be so classified from death registrations between 1970 and 1972. He states 'This discrepancy makes mortality rates by occupation [for women] meaningless, using the *Decennial Supplement* method, and it is likely to be biased between occupations' (McDowall, 1983, p. 25). However, Roman, Beral and Inskip (1985) analysed women's mortality for 1970–72 using this method.

The *OPCS Longitudinal Study* (Moser and Goldblatt, 1985) provides a partial solution to the lack of information collected at death registration about women's previous occupation. The 1971 Census collected information on main employment last week or on the most recent job, if retired or out of work. Housewives who did not have a job last week were not asked about their most recent job. In the *Longitudinal Study*, 62 per cent of women aged 15–59 were assigned a class at census based on their own occupation. Moser and Goldblatt (1985) analysed the mortality of these women between 1971 and 1981 and found a much weaker mortality gradient for women than for men, but a clear difference between women in non-manual and manual occupations. Unlike for men, there was no gradient *within* either non-manual or manual classes. Indeed, they report 'the main anomaly is the low relative mortality of women in Social Class V (SMR of 86) in 1971' (p. 24). (The SMR for all women in employment in 1971 and aged 15–59 at death was 81 for deaths 1971–75 and 87 for deaths 1976–81.) Moser and Goldblatt do not analyse class differences in women's mortality by marital status or by whether the woman is working full-time or part-time.

There is very little other work on mortality differences based on women's own occupation. Lynge, Anderson and Horte (Chapter 8), in a comparison of women's occupational mortality within Scandinavian countries (Norway, Sweden, Finland and Denmark) using census-based linkage, found smaller differentials between occupational groups for women than for men. Women teachers in each country exhibited considerably lower mortality than three other occupations – administrative and clerical work, textile work and restaurant work. However, these smaller differentials for women are complex to interpret because they refer to all women in employment, irrespective of family status and hours of work. The latter factors influence the nature of women's labour force participation and therefore the likely extent and pattern of health inequalities.

Valkonen (1983) using census-linked mortality data from Finland uses an alternative way of classifying women into social classes. Women are classified by their own occupation if in paid employment at the time of the census, but by their husband's occupation if they are economically dependent. However, there is gender-bias in the treatment of those without paid employment, since men are always classified by their most recent occupation. Using this 'employment-based' approach class differences in mortality are greater for men than for women. This method of analysis combines an individualistic approach for employed women and a household approach for housewives. It is therefore impossible to assess the relative effects of the difference in mode of classification for economically active and inactive women on the extent of inequalities revealed.

In the UK, research on class differences in morbidity among women has been based primarily on the 'conventional' approach; for example, the General Household Survey classifies women with husbands by their husband's occupation and all other women by their own current or last occupation. This 'conventional' approach reveals comparable, or slightly smaller, health differentials for women than for men. It has the advantage of classifying *all* women, unlike most studies of mortality which only analyse women in certain marital statuses or only analyse employed women, but has the disadvantage of combining two gender-differentiated class structures into one. Married women, irrespective of their own employment status or occupational level, are classed by their husband's occupation. This has implications because men's occupations are differently distributed from women's occupations (Hakim, 1979).

There have been few studies of women's health based on their own occupation, partly because any meaningful analysis must disentangle the effects of marital status and employment status (Arber, Gilbert and Dale 1985). These problems do not arise in research on the health of young adults. Power, Fogelman and Fox (Chapter 16) considered a range of health measures and found that the gradient for women's own class is as strong or slightly stronger than for men at age 23. For both young men and young women, their own class at age 23 was somewhat more closely associated with their health status than their class of origin.

Data and methods

The General Household Survey (GHS) is based on an annual nationally representative sample of about 12,000 private households (OPCS, 1984). GHS data for 1981 and 1982 have been combined to provide a larger sample for analysis and therefore more reliable estimates of the differentials in ill-health among the non-institutionalised British population. The response rate was 84 per cent in 1981 and 1982. The analysis considers the age-range 20–59: about 28,000 men and women.

The measure of occupational class used in the GHS is based on 19 socio-economic groups (OPCS, 1984). In the GHS Annual Reports these are usually collapsed into six socio-economic groups (SEGs), which for men's occupations are broadly similar to the Registrar General's (RG) social classes (CSO, 1975). However, there are considerable differences betwen the RG's classes and collapsed SEG for women's occupations. For example, lower professionals, such as nurses, teachers and social workers, are classified in RG's class II (managers, employers and technical) but in the GHS *Annual Reports* are placed in collapsed SEG 3 (intermediate and junior non-manual). Thus, two-thirds of men in RG's Social Class II are also coded in SEG 2, but this is the case for under a third of women. Although collapsed SEG and the RG's classes tend to be used interchangeably there are a number of differences with regard to the classification of women, particularly women working part-time in manual and personal service occupations (Arber, Dale and Gilbert, 1986).

To simplify the present analysis we have used collapsed SEG as in the published GHS reports, but have divided SEG 3 (intermediate and

junior non-manual) into SEG 3a (containing socio-economic group 5.1
– mainly lower professionals) and SEG 3b (containing socio-economic
groups 5.2 and 6 – supervisory non-manual, clerical and secretarial).
We shall show later that lower professional women in SEG 3a report
considerably better health than women in SEG 2 and SEG 3b, a
difference which is hidden in both the GHS collapsed socio-economic
groups and in RG social class.

The GHS data on self-reported illness are based on individuals'
perceptions of their ill-health as well as their willingness and ability to
report it to interviewers (Blaxter, Chapter 10). There is no research
evidence of variations between social groups in their willingness to
report ill-health. The paper uses 'limiting long-standing illness' (LLI)
as a measure of health status. The respondent is asked 'have you any
long-standing illness, disability or infirmity', and if so, whether it
'limits your activities in any way' (OPCS, 1984). This measure of
limiting long-standing illness is identified by Blaxter (Chapter 10) as a
measure of functional health status.

This conventional method of comparing inequalities in mortality is
to use Standardised Mortality Ratios, which enable comparisons after
taking into account differences in the age structure of each occupation
or class. It is surprising that researchers who have analysed morbidity
using GHS data have not standardised for differences in the age
structure of occupational groups. The *Inequalities in Health* report
relied heavily on the GHS for documenting class differences in
morbidity but simply presented figures from published GHS reports
broken down into very broad age categories: under 16, 16–44, 45–64
and 65 and over (DHSS, 1980). This chapter uses the indirect method
of standardisation to calculate 'standardised limiting long-standing
illness' (SLLI) ratios using 10-year-age groups: 20–29, 30–39, 40–49
and 50–59.

Occupational class and women's health

The linear gradient between ill-health and occupational class is well
established (DHSS, 1980; Hart, 1985b; 1986), and is clearly evident
in the 1981–82 GHS data. Table 12.1 (a) shows that under 10 per cent
of men in higher professional occupations (SEG 1) report a limiting
long-standing illness compared with 24 per cent of unskilled men
(SEG 6). Health differentials for women are comparable with those for
men, using the 'conventional' approach, which classifies married
women by their husband's occupation and all other women by their
own current (or last) occupation, Table 12.1 (b). This approach has
the disadvantage of combining two distinct occupational structures.
Men's occupations are differently distributed from women's with a
much higher proportion of men in professional and managerial

Table 12.1   *Percentage with limiting long-standing illness by socio-economic group and sex (ages 20–59)*

	Socio-economic group							
	Non-manual				Manual			All
	1	2	3a	3b	4	5	6	
(a) Men – own	9.7%	11.7%	10.9%	13.3%	15.6%	18.5%	23.6%	14.9%
class	(753)	(2208)	(996)	(1364)	(5665)	(2231)	(537)	(13754)
(b) Women –	10.0%	13.7%	12.3%	14.8%	16.0%	19.8%	22.8%	15.8%
conventional	(650)	(2187)	(1202)	(2233)	(4755)	(2465)	(552)	(14044)
class+								
(c) Women –	6.6%	14.5%	11.4%	13.7%	17.3%	18.7%	20.2%	15.7%
own class	(106)	(691)	(1705)	(5498)	(1147)	(3756)	(1194)	(14097)

Socio-economic group

1 Higher professional
2 Employers and managers
3a Lower professional
3b Supervisory and junior non-manual

4 Skilled manual and own account
5 Semi-skilled manual and personal service
6 Unskilled manual

+ Women with husbands are classified by their husband's occupation, women of other marital statuses are attributed to their own (current or last) occupational class.

Source: *General Household Survey*, 1981–82

occupations (SEG 1 and 2) and skilled manual occupations (SEG 4), whereas women are concentrated in routine non-manual jobs (SEG 3), personal service and semi-skilled work (SEG 5), and working part-time in unskilled cleaning work (SEG 6). The 'conventional' approach thus combines two gender-differentiated occupational structures.

An individualistic approach which classifies women by their current (or last) occupation yields only a slightly weaker class gradient than the 'conventional' approach, Table 12.1 (c). The proportion of women reporting a limiting long-standing illness increases from 7 per cent of the small number of women working in the higher professions to 20 per cent of women in unskilled jobs. Women in lower professional occupations (SEG 3a) report somewhat less limiting long-standing illness, 11.4 per cent, than women who are managers or employers (SEG 2), 14.5 per cent.

Because health status deteriorates with age, and members of some occupational classes are, on average, older than others, it is necessary to standardise for differences between the age structure of classes to obtain precise comparisons of class inequalities in ill-health. Table 12.2 shows limiting long-standing illness expressed as standardised (SLLI) ratios and the data are presented graphically in Figure 12.1. The SLLI ratios for men vary from 66 for higher professional, (SEG

Table 12.2   *Standardised limiting long-standing illness ratios by socio-economic group and sex (a) men – own occupation, (b) women – conventional SEG, i.e. husband's occupation if married, (c) women – own occupation, (d) women – own occupation if in employment, if not conventional SEG*

| | Socio-economic group | | | | | | | |
| | Non-manual | | | | Manual | | | All |
	1	2	3a	3b	4	5	6	
(a) *Men*								
– own occupation	66	73	78	97	105	124	155	100
(b) *Women*								
– conventional								
SEG+	63	82	84	104	101	121	127	100
(c) *Women*								
– own occupation	52*	102	77	91	107	117	113	100
(current or last)								
(d) *Women*								
– own occupation	74	92	78	85	128	112	106	100
If in employment++								

Socio-economic group

1 Higher professional
2 Employers and managers
3a Lower professional
3b Supervisory and junior non-manual

4 Skilled manual and own account
5 Semi-skilled manual and personal service
6 Unskilled manual

* Expected frequency < 10

+ Women with husbands are classified by their husband's occupation, women of other marital statuses are attributed to their own (current or last) occupational class.

++ Married women in employment are classified by their own occupation, otherwise by their husband's occupation. Women of other marital statuses are attributed their own occupational class.

Source: *General Household Survey*, 1981–82

1) to 155 for unskilled men (SEG 6), (Table 12.2 (a)). Thus, higher professional men are 34 per cent less likely and unskilled men are 55 per cent more likely to have a limiting long-standing illness than the average for all men. Using the 'conventional' approach the gradient is similar for women to that for men, except that the health of women classified as unskilled (SEG 6) is not as poor (127) as for men (155) (Table 12.2 (b)). The gradient is not perfectly linear, women in the lower professional class (SEG 3a) have an SLLI ratio of 83, whereas women in the routine non-manual group (SEG 3b) have an above average SLLI ratio of 104, which is slightly higher than for women in the skilled manual class, 101 (SEG 4).

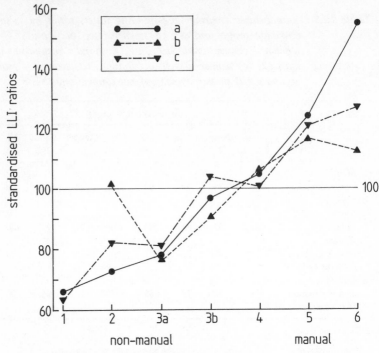

Figure 12.1   Standardised limiting long-standing illness ratios by socio-economic group (SEG) and sex (a) men (b) women – own SEG (c) women – husband's SEG if married.

An individualistic approach which classifies women according to their present or most recent occupation produces a class gradient which is weaker than the 'conventional' approach and in which two classes deviate somewhat from the linear pattern (see Table 12.2 (c) and Figure 12.1). Limiting long-standing illness is slightly lower among women in unskilled occupations, (113 for SEG 6), compared with women classified as semi-skilled, (117 for SEG 5), and women who are managers or employers (SEG 2) report a considerably higher level of long-term illness, 102, than any other non-manual group. The apparently better health of women working in unskilled occupations compared with those in semi-skilled occupations was also observed in relation to mortality in the *Longitudinal Study* (Moser and Goldblatt, 1985).

An 'employment-based' approach uses the woman's occupation if she is in employment, but the husband's for women who are economically dependent (Valkonen, 1983). This approach combines information about women's and men's occupations, but only uses the

Table 12.3   *Standardised Mortality Ratios by social class using Decennial Supplement method, Great Britain, 1979–80, 1982–83 (All men/all women = 100)*

	Social class						
	I	II	IIIN	IIIM	IV	V	All
Men aged 20–64	66	76	94	106	116	165	100
Women+ aged 20–59	69	78	87	100	110	134	100

* These data are subject to serious bias and do not represent usable estimates of mortality by social class. The table is included only to illustrate the discussion of the validity of the social class data in this report.

+ Married women classified by husband's social class.

Source: OPCS (1986) *Occupational Mortality*, Series DS, no. 6, Table 4.8.

latter for women out of the labour force. Women out of the labour force have been shown to report poorer health; over 50 per cent more housewives than employed women report a limiting long-standing illness (Arber, 1987). Because few women but a high proportion of men work in skilled manual occupations (SEG 4) the 'employment' approach reveals a high level of chronic illness for women classified in the skilled manual class, who are mainly housewives, (an SLLI ratio of 128, see Table 12.2 (d)). This is an artefact of the method of classification which only uses men's occupations for women out of the labour force – many of whom have been selected out because of ill-health. The corollary is that classes which contain a high proportion of women's occupations compared to men's show relatively better health. This is part of the reason for the somewhat better health of women classified as unskilled (SEG 6) using the 'employment' approach. This method of classifying women by class will not be discussed further because of the problem of interpreting class differentials where there is confounding of employment status with the use of men's or women's occupations.

Class differences in chronic illness measured using standardised ratios in the 1981–82 GHS (Table 12.2a and b) are remarkably similar to the Standardised Mortality Ratios for both men and women reported in the *Decennial Supplement on Occupational Mortality* for 1979–83 (OPCS, 1986). The relevant table is reproduced as Table 12.3. The authors of the *Decennial Supplement* are at great pains to point out that 'SMRs on class are subject to considerable bias' (p. 42). The major bias is said to be the 'numerator/denominator bias' in which some men are assigned to a different class at census and at death registration. This is said to occur particularly for men in Social Class

V (unskilled). Because of these biases, the *Decennial Supplement* concludes that the social class SMRs are unreliable and discounts the apparently widening class differential shown in 1979–83 compared to 1970–72.

General Household Survey data do not suffer from any biases based on 'numerator/denominator' inconsistencies, because the data about ill-health and about social class are obtained at the same time from the same individual. Therefore, the class gradient for age-standardised limiting long-standing illness which is found in the GHS cannot be dismissed as a methodological artefact. The remarkable similarity of this class gradient in the GHS and the mortality gradient in the *Decennial Supplement* suggests that the class data in the latter should not be treated with the scepticism accorded by the authors of that report.

The association of marital status and employment status with class differences in women's health

Women who lack employment, whether they are unemployed or housewives, report more long-standing illness than the employed (Arber, 1987). In addition, married women report better health than the single or previously married.

The 'conventional' approach combines different information about groups of women depending on their marital status. Married women report considerably better health (SLLI ratio 93) compared with single women and previously married women (SLLI ratios of 118 and 141 respectively). Table 12.4 and Figure 12.2 disaggregate the relationship between class and health for women according to marital status. The strongest gradient is found for single women, from a SLLI ratio of 62 for higher professional women (SEG 1) to 155 for skilled manual (SEG 4) and unskilled women (SEG 6). There is a clear non-manual/manual health divide; single women working in non-manual occupations report as good, or better, health than married women working in non-manual occupations, but single women in manual jobs report considerably poorer health than married women in manual jobs. This difference partly reflects health selection operating in both the employment and the marriage market. Single women in non-manual jobs are more likely to have made a conscious choice to remain single 'career' women, whereas single women in manual jobs may have been less likely to marry because of poor health. Also, they are likely to suffer from the adverse health consequences of manual work. Married women in manual jobs report only slightly worse health than their non-manual counterparts. This is partly because of the occupational downgrading of married women in the labour market, particularly women in part-time jobs (Martin and Roberts, 1984). Previously

Table 12.4   Standardised limiting long-standing illness ratios by socio-economic group by marital status and sex (ages 20–59)

	Socio-economic group							
		Non-manual				Manual		All
	1	2	3a	3b	4	5	6	
Women								
Married								
– Husbands SEG	65	81	83	86	98	109	107	93
– Own SEG	56*	92	75	84	91	108	102	92
Single:								
– Own SEG	62*	95+	78	79	155+	136	155*	118
No Longer								
Married:								
– Own SEG	–	114+	100	126	190	156	156	141
Men								
Married:	69	72	75	93	108	113	157	98
Single:	52+	70	79	102	85	146	145	103
No longer								
Married:	44*	102+	61*	131*	111	172	173+	122

Socio-economic group

1 Higher professional
2 Employers and managers
3a Lower professional
3b Supervisory and junior non-manual

4 Skilled manual and own account
5 Semi-skilled manual and personal service
6 Unskilled manual

* Expected frequency < 10
+ Expected frequency < 20

Source: *General Household Survey*, 1981–82

married women working in manual occupations also report very poor health.

Thus, single and previously married women in manual jobs report very poor health, and in the 'conventional' approach are combined with married women classified by their husband's occupation. The latter are healthier overall and those in manual classes do not report such poor health – indeed married women in skilled manual occupations (SEG 4) have below-average long-standing illness (SLLI ratio of 91 for their own class and 98 for husband's class). Comparing Table 12.2 (b) and Table 12.4, we can see that the strength of the class gradient based on the 'conventional' approach is largely because of the poor health of single and previously married women in manual occupations, since the gradient for married women classified by their husband's occupation is much weaker.

Among women working in non-manual occupations, irrespective of

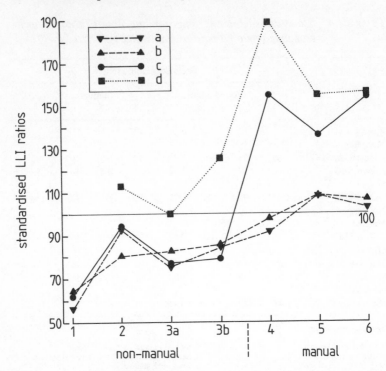

Figure 12.2   Standardised limiting long-standing illness ratios for women by socio-economic group (SEG) (a) married – own SEG (b) married – husbands SEG (c) single – own SEG (d) no longer married – own SEG.

marital status, women in SEG 2 (managers and employers) report poorer health than other non-manual women. This is not the case for women married to men in SEG 2 (classified by their husband's occupation). The consistency of the pattern suggests that the meaning of some occupational classes, such as managerial occupations (SEG 2) differs for men and for women. For women SEG 2 either results in, or selects people with, poorer health, but for men this is not the case. An alternative explanation might be that the composition of men's and women's occupations classified in SEG 2 differs causing this different pattern. Whatever the explanation, the key point to note is that the same occupational class for men and for women may have different meanings and thus is associated with health in a different way.

The class gradient is strong for men irrespective of marital status, although the gradient is not linear for single and previously married men (see Table 12.4 and Figure 12.3). The health of unmarried men

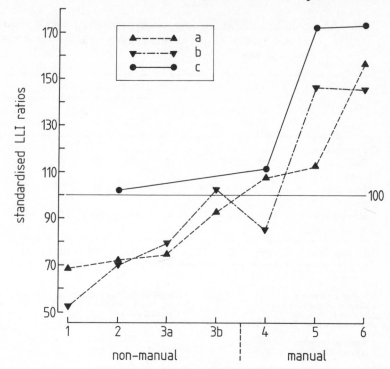

Figure 12.3   Standardised limiting long-standing illness ratios for men by socio-economic group and marital status (a) married men (b) single men (c) no longer married men

in both semi-skilled and unskilled occupations (SEG 5 and 6) is equally poor; among the semi-skilled and unskilled, the SLLI for single men is 145–6 and for previously married men is 172–3.

For married women, the class gradient is nearly as strong using the 'individualistic' approach as by using the 'conventional' approach which classifies women by their husband's occupation. The interpretation of the class gradient using the woman's own (current or last) occupation is clarified by disaggregating the gradient into its component parts. Table 12.5 and Figure 12.4 show the way in which class inequalities in health, using women's own occupation, are the aggregate of inequalities by class for married women working full-time, part-time and women not in employment, classified by their last occupation. The class gradient for married women in employment is very small and is not linear. The least long-standing illness is reported by married women working in routine non-manual jobs (SEG 3b) for women working full-time and part-time (SLLI ratio 65), and the most

Table 12.5   Standardised limiting long-standing illness ratios for married women by own socio-economic group by employment status ages (20–59)

	Socio-economic group							
	Non-manual					Manual		All
	1	2	3a	3b	4	5	6	
Own occupation								
– Full-time: current	79*	93	71	65	74	87	81+	75
– Part-time: current	–	40+	65	65	86	75	78	70
– Housewives: last occupation	109*	129+	78	104	104	130	139	114
All – own SEG	56*	92	75	84	91	108	102	92

Socio-economic group

1 Higher professional
2 Employers and managers
3a Lower professional
3b Supervisory and junior non-manual

4 Skilled manual and own account
5 Semi-skilled manual and personal service
6 Unskilled manual

* Expected frequency < 10
+ Expected frequency < 20

Source: *General Household Survey*, 1981–82

long-standing illness is reported by women working full-time in SEG 2 (SLLI ratio 93) and women working part-time in skilled manual occupations (SLLI ratio of 86, SEG 4). A full explanation of these patterns is beyond the scope of this study. Married women who work are more likely to take jobs which do not reflect their abilities, skills and lifestyle, and this is particularly the case for women working part-time in semi-skilled and unskilled jobs (SEGs 5 and 6). Martin and Roberts (1984) show that, for the majority of women, the overriding factor influencing labour force participation is the woman's primary responsibility for her family. Thus, jobs are taken because they can be accommodated within childcare arrangements or school hours, and are convenient to home. Since a high proportion of women, particularly those with children, 'underachieve' in terms of occupational attainment, class based upon own occupation is less likely to reflect a woman's educational level and health status than is the case for a man.

The health of housewives classified by their most recent occupation shows a somewhat clearer gradient than for employed married women classified by their current occupation. Housewives all report more long-standing illness than the national average, except those who last

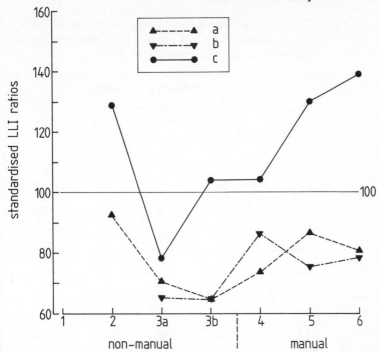

Figure 12.4   Standardised limiting long-standing illness ratios for married women by employment status and own socio-economic group (a) full-time (b) part-time (c) housewives – last job

worked in a semi-professional job (SEG 3a have an SLLI ratio of 78). Married women who last worked in an unskilled job have an SLLI ratio of 139. The class gradient may reflect poorer health resulting from working in certain occupations – e.g. SEG 5, 6, and 2 – or may be because married women with poor health are less likely to return to work after a period of childrearing, or are more likely to leave work because of health factors. Thus, the healthy worker effect is particularly likely to operate for married women.

Ill-health and the class of husbands and wives

Traditionally class differences in women's health have been analysed by their husband's occupational class, but more recently an individualistic approach has been advocated. We have shown that, for married women, a slightly stronger class gradient is found using the conventional rather than an individualistic approach. It is also important to consider whether the occupations of both spouses are associated with the health of each partner. The level of limiting long-standing illness

*Table 12.6   Standardised limiting long-standing illness ratios by own
socio-economic group and spouse's socio-economic group by
sex (married men and women ages 20–59)*

		Husband's socio-economic group			
		Higher 1,2,3a	Middle 3b,4	Lower 5,6	All
Men Wife's SEG					
	Higher 1,2,3a	74	65	90	72
	Middle 3b,4	85	100	114	104
	Lower 5,6	110+	115	124	120
All		80	90	113	97
Women Wife's SEG					
	Higher 1,2,3a	76	80	145+	80
	Middle 3b,4	74	91	95	85
	Lower 5,6	94	105	113	106
	All	78	95	109	92

+ Expected frequency less than 20

Source: *General Household Survey*, 1981–2

of married men and women will be examined using a cross-classification of husband's and wife's occupational class (see Table 12.6).
Occupational class has been grouped into three categories – 'higher'
which corresponds to SEG 1, 2 and 3a, 'middle' which corresponds to
SEG 3b and 4, and 'lower' which corresponds to the semi-skilled and
unskilled, SEG 5 and 6. Occupational class is based on last occupation
for those not currently in paid employment. The marginals on Table
12.6 show that *both* the husband's and wife's occupational class are
associated with the health of each spouse. The gradients for standardised LLI ratios are approximately the same, but somewhat higher
gradients are found for the association of the wife's occupational class
with her husband's health. Men married to women in a 'higher' class
have an SLLI ratio of 72 compared to 120 for men married to women

in a 'lower' class. The influence of a woman's occupational class on her husband's health is consistent for men in each occupational class. In each occupational class, men married to women in a 'low' class have an SLLI ratio at least 40 per cent higher than men married to women in a 'high' class. For women the differentials are not so pronounced, but it is clear that the occupational class of both spouses influence women's health.

Britten and Heath (1983) suggest the use of 'composite' measures of class which incorporate information about the husband's and wife's occupation. However, despite the clear pattern of association shown in Table 12.6, it is unlikely that composite measures will be used in analysing inequalities in health for a number of reasons. The analysis of health inequalities using a cross-classification of husband's and wife's occupation could not be done with the full six classes traditionally used in analyses of class inequalities, because there would be only a small number of cases in some cells. Also, the approach may be appropriate for the traditional family of a married couple, with or without dependent children, but is not relevant for other family forms, such as single-parent or single-person households.

An alternative approach, which retains the advantage of a household-based measure and is available for all women, but which takes cognisance of the fact that over half married women are in employment, is to use an approach which characterises the household by the occupation of the spouse who is economically dominant (Erickson, 1984; Goldthorpe and Payne, 1986). Where both husband and wife are in employment the household is classified by the partner with the higher occupational class, on the assumption that the market situation and life chances of the family are more dependent on the work position of the partner with the higher occupational class. It is therefore irrelevant which partner has the dominant position. Where only one partner is in employment the occupation of that partner is used to classify the household. The approach is therefore not gender-biased because, where the husband is unemployed and the wife is working, her occupation will be used to classify the household, unlike in the 'conventional' approach. The 'dominance' approach will produce somewhat different class distributions to the 'conventional' approach, but they are unlikely to be radically different, because of the lower occupational attainment of women which to a considerable extent reflects the sexual division of labour in which married women are defined as having primary responsibility for the family with paid employment being a secondary role (Martin and Roberts, 1984).

Very similar class gradients are found for married couples using the 'dominance' approach to those found using 'conventional' class measures (see Table 12.7). For married women using 'dominance' the

Table 12.7   *Standardised limiting long-standing illness ratios by socio-economic group for married men and women (a) own socio-economic group, (b) socio-economic group of the occupationally dominant spouse★, (c) husband's socio-economic group (for women) (ages 20–59).*

| | Socio-economic group | | | | | | | |
| | Non-manual | | | | Manual | | | All |
	1	2	3a	3b	4	5	6	
Married men								
(a) Own SEG	69	72	75	93	108	113	157	98
(b) Dominance★ (SEG of dominant spouse)	68	72	82	103	107	129	154	98
Married women								
(a) Own SEG	56+	92	75	84	91	108	102	92
(b) Dominance★ (SEG of dominant spouse)	65	82	79	81	107	111	110	92
(c) Husband's SEG	65	81	83	86	98	109	107	93

Socio-economic group

1 Higher professional
2 Employers and managers
3a Lower professional
3b Supervisory and junior non-manual

4 Skilled manual and own account
5 Semi-skilled manual and personal service
6 Unskilled manual

★ Dominance – if only one spouse is employed – SEG of that spouse;
     – if both or neither are employed – SEG of occupationally higher spouse

★ Expected frequency < 10

Source: *General Household Survey*, 1981–82

range of SLLI ratios is from 65 for SEG 1 to 110 for SEG 6, and using the 'conventional' approach of classifying married women by their husband's occupation is from 65 for SEG 1 to 107 for SEG 6 (see Table 12.7). The level of inequalities among manual classes is somewhat greater using 'dominance' than using either the conventional or individualistic approach. This suggests that, where women are currently working in an occupational class which is higher than that of their manual husband, the health of these women is better than for comparable women who are not in employment or who work in a lower occupational class. Women married to semi-skilled and unskilled men have somewhat better health if they themselves are working in a higher occupational class.

The advantages of the 'dominance' approach include the following: it is applicable to all households irrespective of the number or composition of household members; it is relatively easy to calculate; and it allows the continued use of the full range of occupational classes. We have shown that the 'dominance' approach reveals a slightly stronger class gradient than the conventional approach for married women. The 'dominance' approach should be considered for use in analysing women's health, as it is a household-based measure which unlike the conventional approach, is not gender-biased.

Inequalities in health among women using other socio-economic indicators

The complications of measuring class within an occupation-based framework may lead to a consideration of other individual-based measures, such as education; and household-based measures, such as housing tenure and car ownership, which are easier to collect and are applicable to all households irrespective of their size, characteristics or composition.

Educational attainment is particularly useful for comparing the extent and pattern of inequalities among men and women (Valkonen, Chapter 7), because it is equally applicable for both men and women, and is unchanging over the lifespan, unlike occupational class. Valkonen argues that educational attainment, based on number of years of education, is more useful in international comparisons than occupation-based classifications which are difficult to compare because of differences in the occupational structure. However, educational attainment has proved to be of less use in the UK primarily because educational qualifications and age left full-time education have a very skewed distribution with the bulk of the population having no qualifications, or leaving at the minimum school-leaving age. In addition, comparison between age cohorts is complicated by changes in the educational system, the growth in higher education, and the raising of the minimum school-leaving age. Also, it is retrospective information and may not be accurately recalled. Fox and Goldblatt (1982), using the *Longitudinal Study*, found a clear inverse gradient between level of educational qualifications and mortality rates for men, but found no gradient for women. Women with degrees and 'A' levels had the same mortality rates as women with no qualifications. However, the *Longitudinal Study* analyses are restricted to those with 'A' levels or above, which in the 1971 Census was less than 20 per cent of the population.

Using the 1981–82 General Household Survey, highest educational qualifications show a clear linear gradient for both men and women, with the least limiting long-standing illness among those with degrees,

*Table 12.8   Standardised limiting long-standing illness ratios by highest
educational qualifications and sex (ages 20–59)*

	SLLI Ratios		% Distribution	
	Men	Women	Men	Women
Degree or teaching qualification	66	74	9.9	6.5
A levels, HNC/HND, nursing qualification	85	82	18.0	9.1
O levels	83	87	13.7	17.3
CSE, apprenticeship, clerical qualifications+	96	97	15.7	14.9
No qualifications	119	110	42.6	52.2
All	101	101	100%	100%
N			(13113)	(14214)

+ Includes foreign and other qualifications

Source: *General Household Survey*, 1981–82.

SLLI ratios of 66 for men and 74 for women (see Table 12.8). Despite the increase in educational qualifications over recent years, in 1981–82 in the UK, about half of men and women aged 20–59 had no qualifications. Those with no qualifications, especially men, report poorer health (SLLI ratio for men of 119 and for women 110). Since most research on inequalities in health is concerned with understanding the factors associated with adverse health, educational qualifications as an indicator is insufficient for this purpose, because such a large proportion of the population have no qualifications or leave school at the minimum age.

Housing tenure is a household-based measure which reflects the lifestyle of the family. It has the advantages of being available for all members of the population and is equally applicable, with the same meaning, for men and women. Other advantages over occupational class are that it is easier to collect, and divides the population into larger groups than is the case for occupational class measures which concentrate on the health differentials between two relatively small categories, Classes I and V. Fox and Goldblatt (1982) found high mortality for both men and women in local authority accommodation and the lowest mortality for owner-occupiers. Moser and Goldblatt (1985) show that tenure provides more discriminatory power for women's mortality than social class based on the woman's own occupation. There is little research on morbidity and housing tenure – indeed, Blaxter (Chapter 10) notes that the GHS has not used tenure

Table 12.9 Percentage reporting limiting, long-standing illness by housing tenure, age and sex

	Owner-occupiers	Privately rented	Local authority	Ratio Local authority/ owner-occupiers
Men				
20–29	7.6%	8.4%	10.3%	1.36
30–39	10.1%	10.9%	16.3%	1.61
40–49	13.7%	18.5%	24.4%	1.78
50–59	21.1%	22.8%	31.3%	1.48
All	12.2%	12.7%	18.2%	1.49
N	(9193)	(1645)	(4715)	
Women				
20–29	7.0%	7.6%	10.9%	1.56
30–39	10.1%	14.7%	18.4%	1.82
40–49	14.8%	21.7%	26.0%	1.76
50–59	21.3%	27.5%	32.2%	1.51
All	12.3%	14.1%	20.4%	1.66
N	(9400)	(1608)	(5034)	

Source: *General Household Survey*, 1981–82.

as a variable in health analyses since the early 1970s, and at that time reported higher chronic illness among those in privately rented than local authority rented accommodation. The housing market has changed markedly in the UK since the early 1970s with a growth in owner-occupation at the expense of both the privately rented and the local authority sectors. The privately rented sector is increasingly becoming an intermediary sector, occupied at transitional life-cycle stages (Jones, 1986), and the council sector is increasingly becoming a residual sector for those whose structural circumstances make it impossible for them to be owner-occupiers (Byrne *et al.*, 1986a). Thus, we would expect local authority tenants to have poorer health, and that the tenure-health differential will continue to widen in the foreseeable future.

Men and women in local authority accommodation report more limiting long-standing illness than owner-occupiers, with local authority tenants aged 30–49 reporting nearly 80 per cent more long-standing illness than owner-occupiers (see Table 12.9). In each age group, those in privately rented accommodation occupy an intermediate position, but for younger adults their health status is similar to owner-occupiers. The tenure differential for men and women is roughly the same, although women in council housing appear to be

Table 12.10   Standardised limiting long-standing illness ratios by housing tenure, car ownership and sex (ages 20–59)

	Owner occupiers	Privately rented	Local authority	All
Men				
One or more cars	81	80	114	88
No car in household	125	124	158	146
All	86	95	134	100
Women				
One or more cars	80	86	125	90
No car in household	97	146	145	131
All	83	109	135	100
% Distribution	59.5%	10.4%	30.1%	100%
N men and women				(28370)

Source: *General Household Survey*, 1981—82.

slightly more disadvantaged than men. This differential is clear from the standardised LLI ratios, which vary from 83 for women owner-occupiers to 135 for women council tenants (Table 12.10). The equivalent ratios for men are 86 for owner-occupiers and 134 for those living in council housing. Thus, housing tenure reveals slightly *larger* inequalities in health for women than for men, unlike occupational class where there are greater class differentials for men than women using existing class scales.

Data from the OPCS *Longitudinal Study* also demonstrate the strength of association between car-ownership and mortality, and how mortality varies with the cross-classification of tenure and car-ownership. Moser and Goldblatt (1985) emphasise the size of the differential between the two 'extreme' groups – owner-occupiers with a car and local authority tenants without a car. For women aged 15–59 the SMR was 77 and 136 for these two groups respectively. The 1981–82 GHS data for standardised limiting long-standing illness show remarkably similar but slightly larger differentials, perhaps reflecting the residualising of council housing since 1971. Table 12.10 shows that, for men, the differential between these two 'extreme' groups is from an SLLI ratio of 81 for owner-occupiers with cars to 158 for local authority tenants without cars. For women the differential is slightly smaller, from an SLLI ratio of 80 to 145 respectively. The pattern of ill-health in Table 12.10 shows that men in privately rented accommodation have equivalent levels of LLI to owner-occupiers among both car owners and non-owners. However, the pattern differs for women; women in privately rented accommodation without cars report as poor health as those in council housing without cars. Thus, there may be gender differences in the use and meaning of the privately rented sector.

The GHS data on morbidity differentials therefore support the findings of Fox and Goldblatt (1982) that housing tenure and car-ownership are strongly associated with health inequalities in mortality for both men and women. However, the explanations for these associations have not been fully explored. Housing tenure is a key aspect of the structural definition of social class, since it measures control over resources and wealth (Byrne *et al.*, 1986a). Car-owner-ship is both a measure of assets but is also partially dependent on health status; those in poorer health are less likely to be able to drive and therefore to own a car. The health selection effects associated with car-ownership are more probable for men than for women, since car-driving and car-ownership is differentiated by gender (Dale, 1986). The GHS data gives partial confirmation of this since the health differential with car ownership is greater for men than for women: for men the SLLI ratio is 88 for car owners compared to 146 where there is no car in the household, the comparable SLLI ratios are 90 and 131 for women. Byrne *et al.*, (1986b) suggest that it is necessary to distinguish those in local authority housing into the 'central' working class and the 'residual' working class. This distinction is based on the form and degree of dependence of households on state benefits. Their analysis, of a very small and unrepresentative sample, shows that state benefit-dependent households report poorer health than those living in council accommodation who are not dependent on state benefits.

It is important to assess the extent to which council accommodation and lack of car-ownership provide good indicators of the disadvan-taged structural position of some groups in society, which is reflected in the poor health status of these groups. One factor which may partially explain these findings is that a higher proportion of local authority tenants are out of employment, either as unemployed, long-term sick, or retired, and that these groups have poor health. Men and women in council accommodation report worse health irrespective of their employment status (see Table 12.11). However, the unemployed and housewives in local authority housing appear to be particularly disadvantaged. Unemployed men who are owner-occupiers have an SLLI ratio of 114 compared with a ratio of 162 for local authority tenants. The differentials are even greater for women who are housewives, with an SLLI rate of 96 for owner-occupiers compared to 164 for council house tenants. Thus, although housing tenure is associated with employment status, this cannot explain the poorer

*Table 12.11   Standardised limiting long-standing illness ratios by housing
tenure, employment status and sex (ages 20–59)*

	Owner-occupiers	Privately rented	Local authority	All	N
Men					
– employed	77	78	95	82	(11983)
– unemployed	114	113	162	142	(1332)
Women					
– employed:					
– full-time	71	92	100	81	(4831)
– part-time	65	76	96	76	(3885)
– unemployed	104	86+	132	115	(705)
– housewives	96	126	164	122	(4618)

+ Expected number < 20

Source: *General Household Survey*, 1981–82

health overall of local authority tenants. It might be that unemployment has a lesser impact for owner-occupiers who have more alternative resources and bases of self-esteem than local authority tenants.

Conclusion

The analysis of class inequalities in health among women has provided insights into the reasons for, and pattern of, health inequalities for both women and men. The traditional way of characterising the class of the household by the occupation of the head of household, usually defined as the husband, may no longer be appropriate in the late 1980s. However, class differentials in women's health using the 'conventional' approach were found to be greater than using an individualistic approach based on the woman's own (current or last) occupation.

It is suggested that the appropriate unit of analysis for studying health inequalities is the household rather than the individual – therefore household-based measures should be used.

An alternative occupation-based measure which can be used to study inequalities in health is the class of the occupationally 'dominant' member of the household. Using the 'dominance' approach produces similar class gradients in ill-health to the conventional approach for both married women and men, but is applicable to all households and is not gender-biased. In addition, the wife's occupational class was shown to have a clear impact on the husband's health, irrespective of his class. Findings from the 'dominance' approach, and from an analysis of health based on the cross-classification of husband's and wife's class, lend support to structural–materialist explanations of health. Health status is influenced by the class position of the household which is the result of the combination of the roles of both spouses in the labour market.

Alternative household-based measures of class were examined. Asset-based measures, such as housing tenure and car-ownership, were confirmed as strongly associated with the health of both men and women. Health differentials for women are as large as for men using these measures, unlike for occupational class. For all analyses of class inequalities, whether using occupation-based measures or asset-based measures, it is important to be aware of how these variables are associated with employment status. The unemployed and housewives have poorer health. They are also more likely not to be married, to be in a lower occupational class, to live in council housing and not have a car. Therefore, when assessing class inequalities it is important to separate out the effects of employment status and marital status from class. These associations suggest that adverse health is concentrated among those whose material circumstances and employment position are least good.

Acknowledgements

I would like to thank the Office of Population Censuses and Surveys (OPCS) for permission to use the General Household Survey, and the ESRC Data Archive for their role in supplying the data. The ESRC provided support for the preparation of the 1981 and 1982 GHS into SPSS and SIR files (Grant no. H0023050), prepared by P Truscott, N Gilbert, A Dale and S Arber. My colleagues Angela Dale and Nigel Gilbert were co-researchers on some of the work on which this paper is based; their help has been invaluable.

References

Arber, S., Gilbert, G.N. and Dale, A. (1985), 'Paid employment and women's health: a benefit or a source of role strain?', *Sociology of Health and Illness*, **7**, (3), pp. 375–400.

Arber, S., Dale, A. and Gilbert, G.N. (1986), 'The limitations of existing social class classifications for women' in A. Jacoby (ed.), *The Measurement of Social Class*, Social Research Association.

Arber, S. (1987), 'Social class, non-employment and chronic illness: continuing the inequalities in health debate', *British Medical Journal* **294**, (i), pp. 1069–73.

Beacham, R. (1984), 'Economic activity: Britain's workforce 1971–1981', *Population Trends*, **37**, pp. 6–13.

Britten, N. and Heath, A. (1983), 'Women, Men and Social Class' in E. Garmarnikov *et al.* (eds), *Gender, Class and Work*, London: Heinemann.

Brown, G. and Harris, T. (1978), *Social Origins of Depression*, London: Tavistock.

Byrne, D. *et al.* (1986a), *Housing and Health*, Aldershot: Gower.

Byrne, D., McCarthy, P., Keithley, J. and Harrison, S. (1986b), 'Housing, class and health: an example of an attempt at doing socialist research', *Critical Social Policy*, **13**, pp. 49–72.

Central Statistical Office (1975), 'Social commentary: social class, *Social Trends*, no. 6, London: HMSO.

Dale, A. (1986), 'A note on differences in car usage for married men and married women: A further response to Taylor-Gooby', *Sociology*, **20**, (1), pp. 91–2.

Department of Health and Social Security (1980), *Inequalities in Health*, London: DHSS.

Erickson, R. (1984), 'Social class of men, women and families', *Sociology*, **18**, (4), pp. 500–14.

Fox, A.J., and Goldblatt P.O. (1982), *Socio-demographic mortality differentials from the OPCS Longitudinal Study 1971–75* (series LS no. 1), London: HMSO.

Fox, A.J., Goldblatt P.O., and Jones D.R. (1985), 'Social class mortality differentials: artefact, selection or life circumstances?, *Journal of Epidemiology and Community Health*, **39**, (1), pp. 1–18.

Goldthorpe, J.H., (1983), 'Women and class analysis: In defence of the conventional view', *Sociology*, **17**, (4), pp. 465–88.

Goldthorpe, J.H., (1984), 'Women and class analysis: A reply to the replies', *Sociology*, **18**, (4), pp. 491–9.

Goldthorpe, J.H. and Payne, C. (1986), 'On the class mobility of women; Results from different approaches to the analysis of recent British data', *Sociology*, **20**, (4), pp. 531–55.

Gove, W.R. (1978), 'Sex differences in mental illness among adult men and women: An evaluation of four questions regarding the evidence of the higher rates of women', *Social Science and Medicine*, **12B**, pp. 187–98.

Gove, W.R. and Hughes, M. (1979), 'Possible causes of the apparent sex differences in physical health: an empirical investigation', *American Sociological Review*, **44**, pp. 126–46.

Gove, R. and Tudor, F. (1973), 'Adult sex roles and mental illness', *American Journal of Sociology*, **78**, pp. 812–35.

Hakim, C. (1979), *Occupational Segregation*, Department of Employment Research Paper, no. 9, London: Department of Employment.

Hart, N. (1983), 'Understanding debates about health inequality', Paper presented to the Joint Meeting of Health Economists and Medical Sociologists, University of York, July.

Hart, N. (1985), *The Sociology of Health and Medicine*, Causeway Press.

Hart, N. (1986) 'Inequalities in health: the individual versus the environment, *Journal of the Royal Statistical Society*, **149**, (3), pp. 228–48.

Hunt, A. (1980), 'Some Gaps and Problems arising from Government Statistics on Women at Work', *Equal Opportunities Commission Research Bulletin*, no. 4, pp. 29–42.

Jones, G. (1986), *Youth in the Social Structure: Transitions to Adulthood and their Stratification by Class and Gender*, unpublished PhD thesis, University of Surrey.

Koskinnen, S. (1985), 'Time trends in cause-specific mortality by occupational class in England and Wales', Paper presented to the IUSSP XX General Conference, Florence, Italy, June.

Leete, R. and Fox, A.J. (1977), 'Registrar General's social classes: origins and uses', *Population Trends*, no. 8, pp. 1–7.

McDowall, M. (1983), 'Measuring women's occupational mortality', *Population Trends*, **34**, pp. 25–9.

MacFarlane, A. and Mugford, M. (1984), *Birth Counts: Statistics of Pregnancy and Childbirth*, London: HMSO.

Marsh, C. (1986), 'Social class and occupation' in R.G. Burgess (ed.), *Key Variables in Social Investigation*, London: Routledge and Kegan Paul.

Martin, J. and Roberts, C. (1984), *Women and Employment: A Lifetime Perspective*, Department of Employment/OPCS, London: HMSO.

Mechanic, D. (1978), 'Sex, illness behaviour, and the use of health services', *Social Science and Medicine*, **12B**, pp. 207–14.

Moser, K.A., Fox, A.J. Jones, D.R. (1984), 'Unemployment and mortality in the OPCS *Longitudinal Study*', *Lancet*, 8 December, pp. 1324–9.

Moser, K.A., Goldblatt, P.O. (1985), 'Mortality of women in the OPCS *Longitudinal Study*: Differentials by own occupation and household and housing characteristics', Social Statistics Research Unit Working Paper no. 26, London: City University.

Nathanson, C. (1975), 'Illness and the feminine role: a theoretical review', *Social Science and Medicine*, **9**, pp. 57–62.

Nathanson, C. (1977) 'Sex, illness and medical care: a review of data, theory and method', *Social Science and Medicine*, **11**, pp. 13–25.

Nathanson, C. (1980), 'Social roles and health status among women: the significance of employment', *Social Science and Medicine*, **14A**, pp. 463–71.

Nissel, M. (1980), 'Women in government statistics: basic concepts and assumptions', *Equal Opportunities Commission Research Bulletin*, no. 4, pp. 5–28.

Office of Population Censuses and Surveys (1978), *Occupational Mortality 1970–72*, London: HMSO.

Office of Population Censuses and Surveys (1984), *General Household Survey 1982*, London: HMSO.

Office of Population Censuses and Surveys (1985), 'Women's occupational mortality, 1970–72', *OPCS Monitor*, DH1 85/1. Written by E. Roman, H Inskip, V Beral.

Office of Population Censuses and Surveys, (1986), *Occupational Mortality: The Registrar General's Decennial Supplement for Great Britain, 1979–80, 1982–83*, London: HMSO.

Roman, E., Beral, V., Inskip, H. (1985), 'Occupational mortality of women in England and Wales', *British Medical Journal*, **291**, pp. 194–6.

Stanworth, M. (1984), 'Women and class analysis: a reply to John Goldthorpe', *Sociology*, **18**, (2), pp. 59–70.

Stern, J. (1983a), 'The relationship between unemployment and morbidity and mortality in Britain', *Population Studies*, **37**, pp. 61–74.

Stern, J. (1983b), 'Social mobility and the interpretation of social class mortality differentials', *Journal of Social Policy*, **12**, (1), pp. 27–49.

Townsend, P. (1979), *Poverty in the United Kingdom*, Harmondsworth: Penguin.

Valkonen, T. (1983), 'Socio-economic mortality differentials in Finland' in M Lagergren (ed.), *Halsa for alla i Norden ar 2000*, Nordic School of Public Health, Rapport NHW 1983: 1.

Verbrugge, L.M. (1979), 'Females and illness: recent trends in sex differences in the United States', *Journal of Health and Social Behaviour*, **17**, pp. 387–403.

Waldron, E. (1976), 'Why do women live longer than men?', *Journal of Human Stress*, **2**, pp. 2–13.

Waldron, E. (1980), 'Employment and women's health: an analysis of causal relationships', *International Journal of Health Services*, **10**, pp. 435–54.

Waldron, E. (1983), 'Sex differences in illness incidence prognosis and mortality: issues and evidence', *Social Science and Medicine*, **17**, pp. 1107–23.

Warr, P., Parry, G. (1982), 'Paid employment and women's psychological wellbeing', *Psychological Bulletin*, **91**, pp. 498–516.

13 Inequalities in prognosis: socio-economic differences in cancer and heart disease survival
David Leon and Richard G. Wilkinson

Introduction
Although the existence of wide social class differences in death rates is well known, very little is known of the relative contributions of disparities in the incidence and survival of the major causes of death. In Britain, the *Black Report* on inequalities in health appears to have overlooked the possibility that socio-economic differentials in mortality may not arise simply from differentials in exposure to the risk factors associated with the incidence of disease. This chapter examines the evidence of social class differences in survival and looks in particular at cancer and heart disease which together account for approximately half of all deaths.

New evidence of class differences in the survival of cancers in England and Wales is presented from the OPCS Longitudinal Study (*LS*). Following this the chapter goes on to review published evidence on socio-economic differences in cancer and heart disease survival more generally.

Data and methods
The OPCS Longitudinal Study
The OPCS Longitudinal Study population examined here is a 1 per cent sample of people enumerated at the 1971 Census of England and Wales. Entry into the study sample was determined according to date of birth stated on the census schedule; all those whose birth dates fell on one of four sample days spread evenly throughout the year were selected into the sample. This resulted in a study population which comprises 250,588 males and 262,484 females.

Cancer registrations
In the period from census day to the end of 1975 a total of 8,195 study members were notified as having been registered with cancer. Their cancer registrations were derived from the National Cancer Registration Scheme (NCRS) which covers the whole population of England and Wales. During the period 1971–75, data collected by the NCRS is known to have been incomplete; case ascertainment during this time

Table 13.1 *Deaths from all causes in 1971–76 among LS members registered with cancer in 1971–75*

	Males	Females	Total
Malignant neoplasms registered 1971–75	4,190	4,005	8,195
Deaths amongst cases 1971–76	3,047	2,367	5,414

is thought to have been somewhere between 70 per cent and 90 per cent. As a consequence, not all members of the OPCS Longitudinal Study (*LS*) diagnosed with cancer were subsequently registered as such. However, the mechanism for identifying LS members amongst those cases that were registered at the NCRS was highly efficient, achieving a linkage rate of over 98 per cent. Cancer registration data in the LS is therefore representative of the data collected by the NCRS, although it does not include every cancer diagnosed in an LS member.

Survival/fatality

In addition to the routine notification of cancer registrations, the deaths occurring to members of the LS population are notified to the study. As well as permitting direct analyses of mortality, this allows the survival of LS members registered with cancer to be investigated.

By the end of 1976 a total of 5,414 fatalities had occurred amongst the 8,195 LS members registered with cancer in the period 1971–75, as shown in Table 13.1. Males had accrued a survival rate of 27 per cent and females a rate of 41 per cent.

Socio-economic characteristics

Using characteristics recorded at the 1971 Census, members of the LS population may be classified using a number of different measures of socio-economic position. In these analyses, two of the measures are employed – namely social class (based on own occupation) and housing tenure. Social class was derived using the Registrar General's schema, shown below:

Social Classes	Residual Groups
I Professional etc. occupations	Armed forces
II Intermediate occupations	Inadequately described occupations
IIIN Skilled occupations (non-manual)	Unoccupied
IIIM Skilled occupations (manual)	
IV Partly skilled occupations	
V Unskilled occupations	

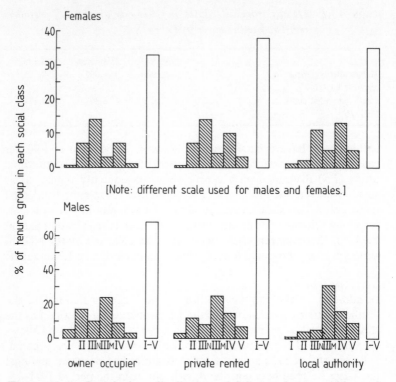

Figure 13.1　Social class distribution of LS population within each housing tenure group (males and females, own social class at census)

Housing tenure is a household characteristic that may be applied to individual household members. It is determined according to the ownership of the household residence in which each individual was enumerated. It has three main categories and one residual group, comprising those enumerated in hospitals and other forms of non-private household. These four categories are as follows:

- Owner occupation
- Private rented
- Local authority
- Non-private households

Although they are used separately in the present analyses, it should be noted that social class and housing tenure are interrelated measures. This is shown in Figure 13.1, where the social class distribution of males and females in each of the three main private tenure categories is presented. In both sexes, although more pronounced in the case of males, the distributions by class varies between tenure categories. The population of local authority tenants is heavily weighted towards those in the manual 'classes compared to those enumerated in owner-occupied housing, who are weighted more towards Social Classes I and II. Although not shown, the distribution of people within social classes by tenure shows similar features; i.e. the non-manual classes (I–IIIN) are weighted towards owner occupiers, while the manual classes (IIIM–V) are weighted towards local authority tenants.

One final point should be made. The proportion of women who were able to be classified to a social class on the basis of their own occupation is relatively small. Whereas 90 per cent of all males aged 15 or over at census were assigned to a social class, the equivalent figure for females was only 45 per cent.

Measuring differentials in fatality

Socio-economic differentials in survival from cancer have been measured by comparing the fatality rates of registered cancer cases in different social classes and housing tenure categories as classified at the 1971 Census.

Comparisons of fatality have been made by calculating an indirectly standardised rate ratio – the standardised fatality ratio (SFR). This is calculated in a similar fashion to the more familiar SMR, although in addition to standardising for age, the SFR also takes into account variation of fatality rates with length of follow-up from time of registration.

In formal terms, the expected number of deaths from all causes has been calculated by applying age, sex and survival period specific fatality rates for *all* LS members registered with the cancer being considered, to the person-days-at risk in each social class or housing tenure category. The SFR therefore expresses the fatality of a particular population sub-group compared to the fatality of all LS members of the same sex registered with the same single or aggregate group of cancers. An SFR of greater than 100 indicates higher fatality than the average – and hence poorer survival – while an SFR of below 100 indicates the opposite, i.e., lower than average fatality and better than average survival.

Confidence intervals

Confidence intervals for the fatality rate ratios have been calculated using the method described by Vandenbrouke (1982). These intervals should be interpreted with caution: as the random variation associated with the estimate of the standard rates is not taken into account in their calculation, they tend to be too narrow.

Table 13.2 'All cause' fatalities, 1971–76, amongst LS members registered with a malignant neoplasm, by own social class at census, sex and period (in days) since registration: Standardised Fatality Ratios* and approximate 95 per cent confidence intervals

Own social class at 1971 Census	Males Period (in days) since registration 1–183	184+	Total (all periods)	Females Period (in days) since registration 1–183	184+	Total (all periods)
Non-manual (I-IIIN)	87 (475) 80–96	83 (270) 74–94	86 (745) 80–92	93 (160) 79–108	87 (145) 73–103	90 (305) 80–101
Manual (IIIM-V)	103 (1107) 97–109	108 (616) 100–117	105 (1723) 110–110	97 (190) 84–112	113 (188) 97–130	104 (378) 94–115
Indequately described Unoccupied Armed forces	119 (235) 104–135	107 (108) 87–128	115 (343) 103–128	102 (860) 95–109	100 (604) 92–108	101 (1464) 96–107

Notes:
Figures in brackets are observed numbers of fatalities.

*Expected fatalities calculated using age, sex and survival period-specific fatality rates for all LS members registered with a malignant neoplasm.

Results
All malignant neoplasms
In Table 13.2, standardised fatality ratios for the aggregate of all malignant neoplasms are presented by sex according to own social class and the period (in days) since cancer registration.

For both sexes the SFRs in the manual category are consistently higher than those in the non-manual category, regardless of time since registration. However, the non-manual/manual differentials are most pronounced for males. The other notable feature of the data for males is the high ratio for the residual groups in the early follow-up period (SFR = 119).

Table 13.3 presents similar data by housing tenure. For males the SFRs show a negative gradient in both follow-up periods, from a low amongst those enumerated in owner-occupied property to a high for those in local authority housing; the private rented occupying an intermediate position.

A similar pattern is seen amongst females in the early follow-up period. However, in the later period (184+ days), the private rented do not occupy an intermediate position, although the local authority SFR is still greater than that for owner-occupiers.

Table 13.3 *'All cause' fatalities, 1971–76, amongst LS members registered with a malignant neoplasm 1971–75, by housing tenure at census, sex and period (in days) since registration: Standardised Fatality Ratios* and approximate 96 per cent confidence intervals*

Housing tenure at 1971 Census	Males			Females		
	Period (in days) since registration		Total (all periods)	Period (in days) since registration		Total (all periods)
	1–183	184+		1–183	184+	
Owner occupation	93 (813) 87–100	92 (461) 83–101	93 (1274) 87–98	91 (564) 83–98	93 (468) 84–101	91 (1032) 86–97
Private rented	104 (371) 94–115	103 (196) 89–118	104 (567) 95–113	101 (232) 88–115	111 (185) 95–128	105 (417) 95–116
Local authority	106 (580) 98–116	114 (323) 101–127	109 (903) 102–116	117 (373) 105–129	104 (255) 91–117	111 (628) 102–120
Non-private households	112 (59) 85–144	106 (29) 70–149	110 (88) 88–135	105 (46) 76–138	137 (37) 95–185	117 (83) 93–144

Notes:
Figures in brackets are observed numbers of fatalities.

*Expected fatalities calculated using age, sex and survival period-specific fatality rates for all LS members registered with a malignant neoplasm.

It should be noted that the fatality ratios shown in Tables 13.2 and 13.3 do not take into account socio-economic differences in the site composition of the aggregate of all malignant neoplasms. Despite this, they can be interpreted as expressing the relative burden of cancer-related fatality, part of which may be attributed to differences between socio-economic categories in the composition of the total incidence by site. Ratios standardised for site of registration are presented in a later section.

Site-specific ratios

Turning to site-specific data, Figures 13.2 to 13.5 represent the SFRs for a variety of sites of registration, for males and females separately according to social class and housing tenure. For both socio-economic measures, ratios are presented for two categories only, designated as 'high' and 'low'. In the case of social class, the 'high' category are those in the non-manual classes, while the 'low' are those in the manual classes. For housing tenure, owner occupation is considered to be the 'high' category and local authority to be the 'low'.

Of the sixteen site-specific comparisons of SFRs made for males (Figures 13.2 and 13.3), in only two instances are the SFRs for the

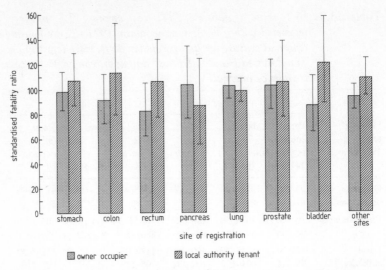

Figure 13.2   '*All causes' fatalities 1971–76, amongst males registered
            with a malignant neoplasm, 1971–75, by site of registration
            and housing tenure at census (Standardised Fatality
            Ratios* and approximate 95 per cent confidence intervals)*

*Expected fatalities calculated using age and survival period specific fatality rates for LS males
registered with the neoplasm concerned.

'high' category greater than the SFRs for the 'low' category. The
situation for females (Figures 13.4 and 13.5), is only slightly more
heterogeneous with four out of the eighteen comparisons showing the
'high' SFR to be greater than the SFR for the 'low'.

For the majority of comparisons, the confidence intervals for the
SFRs are extremely wide, reflecting the relatively small numbers of
fatalities upon which the ratios are based. As a consequence, it is
difficult to draw any reliable conclusions concerning the variation in
the magnitude of the differentials from site to site.

Amongst females, colon and breast cancer both have SFRs that are
greatest in the 'low' categories of social class and housing tenure. For
these two sites, the ratio of the cumulative observed and expected
fatalities are presented in Figures 13.6 and 13.7 by tenure category
according to period since registration. For both sites the differentials
between the owner-occupiers and local authority tenants are established within the first eighteen months of follow-up and thereafter
remain almost constant. In the case of breast cancer the tenure
differentials are established particularly rapidly. However, it should
be noted that due to the termination of follow-up at the end of 1976,
the ratios for successive years of follow-up are based on progressively

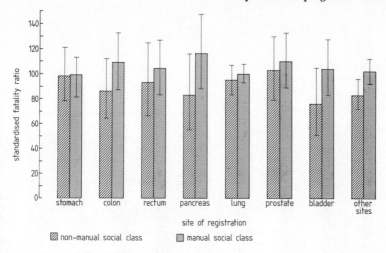

Figure 13.3 'All causes' fatalities 1971–76, amongst males registered
with a malignant neoplasm, 1971–75, by site of registration
and own social class at census (Standardised Fatality
Ratios* and approximate 95 per cent confidence intervals)

*Expected fatalities calculated using age and survival period specific fatality rates for LS members
registered with the neoplasm concerned.

smaller numbers of registrations and subsequent fatalities. For
instance, while ratios for periods under one year are based on the
experience of cancer cases registered in all five years (1971–75), the
ratios for the later period of four years and more are based only on
registrations for 1971.

All malignant neoplasms (site-standardised)

As discussed above, the all malignant neoplasm fatality ratios shown
in Tables 13.2 and 13.3 take no account of socio-economic differences
in the site composition of this aggregate category. This presents a
problem. The incidence of many different cancers is related to socio-
economic position. For instance, owner-occupiers have lower rates of
stomach and lung cancer than those in local authority housing.
Similarly, these two sites have incidence rates that are lower in the
non-manual than the manual social classes. Furthermore, of the major
malignancies, lung and stomach cancer both have particularly poor
survival. Thus crude comparisons of fatality rates for all malignant
neoplasms may provide a misleading estimate of socio-economic
differences in survival/fatality.

To overcome this difficulty, fatality ratios, standardised for site of
registration, have been produced for all malignant neoplasms com-

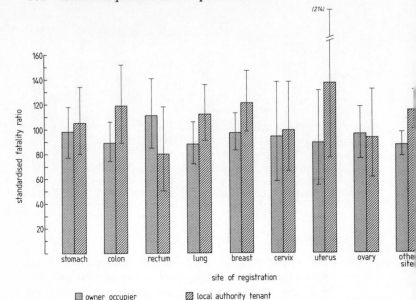

Figure 13.4   'All causes' fatalities 1971–76, amongst females registered
with a malignant neoplasm, 1971–75, by site of registration
and housing tenure at census (Standardised Fatality Ratios*
and approximate 95 per cent confidence intervals).

*Expected fatalities calculated using age and survival period specific fatality rates for LS females
registered with the neoplasm concerned.

bined (Tables 13.4 and 13.5). These standardised ratios have been
calculated in a similar fashion to the crude fatality ratios, as described
in the Data and Methods section, with the difference that the expected
registrations are derived by applying age, sex, survival period *and* site
of registration-specific fatality rates for all LS members to the
corresponding person-days at risk.

As may be seen from Tables 13.4 and 13.5, standardisation by site
of registration produces a narrowing of differentials between the
'high' and 'low' socio-economic categories, this effect being most
pronounced for males. However, in both sexes, fatality ratios for the
'low' (manual, local authority) socio-economic categories continue to
be consistently greater than those in the 'high' categories (non-
manual, owner-occupied).

Discussion

The data from the OPCS Longitudinal Study are consistent with the
results of studies in other countries showing that people registered

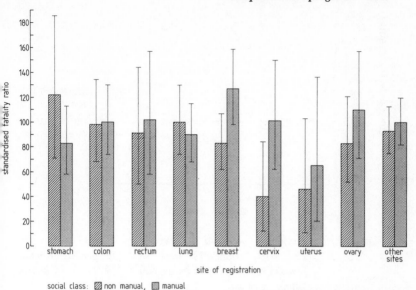

Figure 13.5 '*All causes' fatalities 1971–76, amongst females registered with a malignant neoplasm, 1971–75, by site of registration and own social class at census (Standardised Fatality Ratios* and approximate 95 per cent confidence intervals)*

*Expected fatalities calculated using age and survival period specific rates for LS females registered with the neoplasm concerned.

with cancer fared worse if they were from lower rather than higher socio-economic categories. In the USA Lipworth *et al.*, (1970) showed that people from poorer neighbourhoods had lower 3-year survival rates for 11 of the 15 sex- and site-specific cancers which he looked at. Using the Massachusetts and Connecticut State Cancer Registries, he reported that, among patients attending non-private hospitals, people from poorer neighbourhoods had a combined 'all sites' 3-year survival rate of 41 per cent compared to 46 per cent for people from better-off neighbourhoods (after adjusting for differences in the proportion of cancers at different sites in each class). In a subsequent study of all cancer patients treated in Boston hospitals, Lipworth compared survival rates for private and non-private patients (Lipworth and Bennett, 1972). Two months after diagnosis 13 of the 15 sex- and site-specific survival rates were higher among the private patients. Within each treatment group, survival rates were about twice as high for private as for non-private patients.

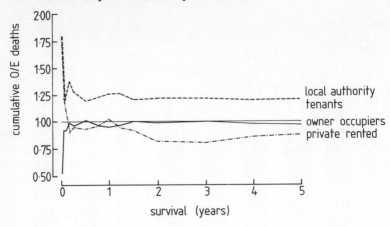

Figure 13.6   Ratio of observed to expected deaths (all causes,
1971–76), cumulated over survival period, amongst
females registered with breast cancer (1971–75) by housing
tenure at census*

*Expected deaths based on age and survival period specific mortality of all LS females registered
with breast cancer.

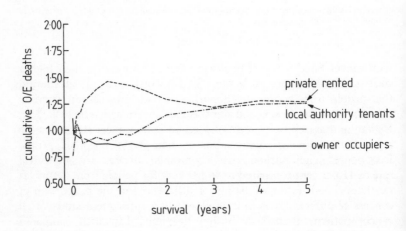

Figure 13.7   Ratio of observed to expected deaths (all causes,
1971–76), cumulated over survival period, amongst
females registered with cancer of the colon (1971–75) by
housing tenure at census*

*Expected deaths based on age and survival specific mortality of all LS females registered with
cancer of the colon.

Table 13.4 'All causes' fatalities, 1971–76, amongst LS members registered with a malignant neoplasm 1971–75, by own social class at census and sex: fatality ratios (and approximate 95 per cent confidence intervals) with and without standardisation for site of registration

	Males		Females	
	Non-manual	Manual	Non-manual	Manual
Without site	86	105	90	104
standardisation	80–92	100–110	80–101	94–115
With site	90	102	90	101
standardisation*	84–97	98–107	80–101	94–116

*Standardised using sex- age- and period-specific fatality rates for sites/site aggregates specified in Figures 13.2 to 13.5.

Table 13.5 'All causes' fatalities, 1971–76, amongst LS members registered with a malignant neoplasm 1971–75, by housing tenure at census and sex: fatality ratios (and approximate 95 per cent confidence intervals) with and without standardisation for site of registration

	Males		Females	
	Owner-Occupied	Local Authority	Owner-Occupied	Local Authority
Without site	93	109	91	111
standardisation	87–98	102–116	86–97	102–120
With site	96	103	92	111
standardisation*	91–102	97–110	86–98	103–120

*Standardised using sex- age- and period-specific fatality rates for sites/site aggregates specified in Figures 13.2 to 13.5.

Socio-economic differences in cancer survival rates such as these may arise from four sources:

1. differences in delay prior to treatment;
2. differences in the efficacy of treatment;
3. differences in histological type of tumour; and
4. socio-economic influences on host resistance.

While the LS data presented here lack the information needed to sort out the relative importance of these four factors, they do have the advantage of employing direct measures of individuals' socio-economic position. Similar direct measures are not usually available in those data sets which include information on delays in seeking treatment, on the stage of development which cancers have reached at diagnosis and on the type of treatment used. Instead proxy measures of socio-economic position, such as race, patients' health insurance status, or area of residence were used in most of the studies we cite. Even so, the survival findings are sufficiently similar to allow us to draw a few tentative conclusions.

Staging

Stage differences were the preferred explanation for the large differences in skin cancer survival rates between white- and blue-collar workers found in a Swedish study (Vagero Persson, 1984); but, in the absence of staging data, the hypothesis could not be tested. However Hackett *et al*. (1973) have shown that there is a significant tendency for cancer patients from lower social classes to delay seeking treatment for longer after first noticing symptoms than upper class patients. It has also been demonstrated, at least for breast cancer, that early detection (in this case resulting from breast self-examination) improves survival (Foster and Costanza, 1984).

Class differences in delay and the degree to which survival chances improve with early treatment differ from one cancer site to another. In the two Lipworth studies mentioned above, the survival differences given are adjusted for stage. In general, differences in stage made only minor contributions to class differences in survival. Another large American study by Berg *et al*. (1977) comes to similar conclusions: 21 of 22 cancer sites showed only very minor staging contributions to socio-economic differences in survival. Only for cervical cancer was stage an important factor. Among studies of cancer at single sites, Dayal and Chui (1982) found that, after controlling for stage, the black prostatic cancer survival rate was 41 per cent compared to the white rate of 51 per cent. Differences in survival of gastro-intestinal cancers between Israelis born in Europe and those born elsewhere (which were thought to be at least partly socio-economic in origin) remained after allowing for differences in staging (Modan and Kallnes, 1971). However, as one might expect, survival differences were concentrated among those diagnosed at the earlier, treatable stages, rather than among those whose illness was already in the terminal stages. Since comparisons of breast cancer survival might be thought to be particularly vulnerable to staging differences, it is therefore of interest that Young *et al*. (1984) found breast cancer survival to be lower for black than white American women at every stage of the disease.

Thus the impression is that, while variations in the stage cancers have reached at first diagnosis do make a small contribution to socio-economic differences in survival, another explanation has to be found for most of the disadvantages suffered by lower-class patients.

Treatment

The role of differences in treatment is particularly difficult to assess. A study of US Veterans Administration cancer patients which, unlike other studies, found no significant racial differences in cancer survival (with the single exception of bladder cancer), concluded that this was because all patients received the same standard of treatment at Veterans Administration hospitals (Page and Kuntz, 1980). The authors did however recognise that this sub-group of the Veterans Administration population was relatively poor and may not have spanned a sufficiently wide socio-economic range to demonstrate the differences reported in other studies. This point was taken up by Dayal as a possible explanation of why his findings on prostatic cancer differed from those of the Veterans Administration Study (Dayal and Chui, 1982).

While the problem of socio-economic or racial differences in treatment is probably larger in the United States than in some other countries, in a study of cancer patients attending a single hospital (University of Iowa Hospital) Berg *et al.*, (1977) claim to have established that socio-economic differences are not primarily due to variations in treatment. Berg examined survival rates in three different patient categories: 'private', 'clinic-pay' and 'indigent'. The findings of the study hang on the authors' assertion that while the three groups were socio-economically distinct, the 'clinic-pay' and 'indigent' patients received the same treatment from the same clinical teams. For all but one of 22 cancer sites – for which private patients had at least a 40 per cent survival rate – the indigent survival rates were at least 10 per cent below the 'clinic-pay' rates. After adjusting for stage, the indigent group did substantially worse in the first five years in every cancer group which had a reasonable expectation of cure. The average of the 39 sex- and site-specific 5-year survival rates was 51 per cent for the private patients, 45 per cent for the 'clinic-pay' and 35 per cent for the indigents. The authors conclude that because the larger difference between the indigent and 'clinic-pay' survival rates cannot be ascribed to treatment, it must reflect socio-economic factors which then also become the most likely explanation for the smaller difference between the private and 'clinic-pay' patients. Confidence that the survival differences were not in fact due to treatment is strengthened by the fact that the survival differences were as large in the 1940s, when treatment was less effective, as they were in the 1960s.

At least four studies control in different ways for fairly crude differences in treatment by comparing survival rates for people treated by surgery, chemotherapy, radiation or some combination of these (Modan and Kallner, 1971; McWhirter *et al.*; 1983; Lipworth *et al.*, 1970; Lipworth and Bennett, 1972). Socio-economic differences in survival appeared within almost all treatment groups. Interestingly, Lipworth found that, in 9 of his 14 sex- and site-specific cancers, it was the patients from the poorer neighbourhoods who were most likely to be treated with surgery or radiotherapy.

While the balance of the evidence suggests that socio-economic differences in survival rates are not due to major differences in treatment, none of the studies exclude the possibility that there were influential minor differences in treatment within the broad therapeutic categories defined.

Tumour type and grade

Histological differences in the type of tumour found at each site can have important implications for survival. There is, however, very little evidence of socio-economic variations in the type of tumour which patients are likely to develop. Among the few studies with data on tumour type, Modan (1971) concluded that the survival advantage of European-born Israelis was primarily due to the type of gastric tumour they developed. On the other hand, Dayal and Chui (1982) found that although the histological grade of the tumour was highly prognostic, it did not account for the black/white differences in prostatic cancer survival. Despite the scarcity of evidence, we can take some comfort from the fact that, where differences in tumour grade are highly prognostic, they are also likely to be highly correlated with stage at diagnosis – as indeed they were in the Dayal study. This means that those studies which control for stage will simultaneously be controlling for some of the effect of differences in tumour grade. While there is potentially a problem of tumour type at all sites, at some of the most common cancer sites the predominance of one histological type means that the problem may be of little practical importance.

Host resistance

One of the most important clues as to what lies behind the socio-economic differences in case fatality rates is the fact that the lower-class disadvantage is so general across cancers at different sites. In the OPCS Longitudinal Study data classified by housing tenure, the lower socio-economic groups suffered a survival disadvantage in 13 of the 17 sex- and site-specific comparisons. Using the manual/non-manual classification, 15 of the 17 comparisons show worse survival in the lower-class group. The study by Berg *et al.* (1977) and the two by

Lipworth, give much the same picture. Even for cancers such as breast cancer, where incidence is higher in higher classes, the lower classes still have the lowest survival rates.

Such a general phenomenon suggests the influence of one overriding factor rather than the coincidence of a number of separate ones. This consideration alone weighs against a primary explanation in terms of differences in treatment, staging, or tumour type, none of which would be expected to influence more than a few sites. After recognising that these factors are likely to make only minor contributions, we necessarily fall back for the rest of the explanation on the unsatisfactory notion of unknown environmental influences on people's ability to survive cancers.

The most plausible mechanism through which such an influence could make itself felt is a reduced immune-response leading to a more rapid tumour spread and growth. The main merit of such an explanation is that it would appear to operate at the right level of generality. The main candidates for the cause of such differences are nutrition and psychosocial factors. Both Lipworth and Berg mentioned reduced host resistance as the most likely explanation of the survival differences and suggested the possibility of a nutritional origin. So far, however, this hypothesis has not been investigated. In contrast the influence of psychosocial factors in prognosis have been investigated and the results are very mixed. Results from the OPCS Longitudinal Study suggest that the death of a spouse makes at most only a small difference to cancer survival rates (Jones *et al.*, 1984). Prospective studies of individual psychological attributes and cancer survival have produced conflicting results (Cassileth *et al.*, 1985; Derogatis *et al.*, 1979).

Differentials in ischaemic heart disease survival

Most of the studies of socio-economic differences in heart disease survival are studies of survival after myocardial infarction. As with the cancer studies, there are rather few of them and several use race as a proxy for socio-economic position. There is however a good deal of consistency in the results which show survival differences very much like the ones seen for cancer. A few examples will give an idea of the scale of survival differences which have been found.

Shapiro *et al.* (1970) reported that, in New York, the mortality of blue-collar workers was 1.6 times that of white-collar workers over a three-and-a-half year period following a myocardial infarction. Of US Veterans Administration patients who survived the first six months after hospital admission with a diagnosis of coronary heart disease, white men in professional occupations had a crude 18-year survival rate of 50 per cent compared with only 34 per cent for those in nonprofessional occupations (Hrubec and Zukel, 1971). Mortality between six months and five years was 8 per cent for the professionals and 15 per cent for others. A Finnish study found a one-year survival rate of 67 per cent for the 'higher professional classes' compared to 57 per cent for unskilled workers (Koskenvuo *et al.*, 1981). At a one-year follow-up of myocardial infarction patients discharged from a North Carolina hospital, it was found that while there had been no deaths or reinfarctions among people in Social Classes I and II, some 26 per cent of Social Class V had died or had a reinfarction (Kottke *et al.*, 1980). Lastly, male survivors of myocardial infarction in the Health Insurance Plan of New York with less than nine years of education had a 3-year mortality rate of 20 per cent compared to 15 per cent for those with nine or more years' education. There seems to be no published studies suggesting that lower socio-economic groups do not suffer a survival disadvantage.

The factors which might influence survival – and so socio-economic differences in survival – after an acute event such as myocardial infarction are rather different from those which influence cancer survival. While differences in aspects of hospital treatment such as defibrillation may influence short-term survival in the period immediately after a heart attack, there is no equivalent to the intensive long-term hospital treatment which cancer patients undergo. Differences in initial hospital treatment are unlikely to have an impact on the longer-term survival differences with which most studies are concerned. Although the causes of the reported survival differences are largely unknown, the risk differential can sometimes be narrowed down to a well defined sub-group of the population. Shapiro *et al.* (1972) found that the poorer survival of the blue-collar workers was confined to those with hypertension at first myocardial infarction. This group were less likely to be taking antihypertensive drugs and had a reinfarction rate 2.5 times as high as white-collar hypertensives. Kottke (1980) showed that much of the survival differential among North Carolina hospital patients could be explained in terms of the differing incidence of diabetes and hypertension but, like Shapiro, he also found that reinfarction rates among hypertensive patients remained significantly higher in the lower- than in the upper-class patients. He concluded that the poorer prognosis in lower classes is due primarily to what he called 'comorbidity' in the form of diabetes and hypertension and said that hypertension is more likely to remain uncontrolled in the lower classes. Among factors which do not seem to affect prognosis – at least after the first six months – Shapiro lists age, prior physical activity, cigarette smoking and cholesterol levels.

It is hard to judge the importance of Weinblatt's (1978) findings (using Health Insurance Plan of NY data) that a higher risk of sudden death after myocardial infarction was concentrated exclusively among those who were both poorly educated and found to have a particular ventricular arrythmia during initial monitoring. Though the risk of sudden death was over three times as high for this group, its effect on longer-term survival was largely offset by later deaths among the better educated. The authors' clinically oriented conclusion was that low education was probably a marker for circumstances which caused a chronic stable arrythmia to change to a lethal ventricular fibrillation. However, commenting on Weinblatt's finding Jenkins (1978) suggested that part of the explanation might be that an inadequate education not only makes it more likely that people will have to cope with more stressful life events, but that they will be less well equipped to deal with them.

Several researchers have suggested various social factors which might contribute to survival differences. Kottke thought that financial barriers to medical care were likely to have been part of the reason why hypertension was less well controlled among lower social classes. He and Shapiro pointed out that fewer lower-class patients return to work after infarction and suggest that this may be because of the greater metabolic demands of manual work. In general, heart disease caused the greatest lifestyle changes in the social groups least likely to have the necessary resources to cushion them.

The demonstration that coronary risk factors are responsive to relaxation therapy (Patel *et al.*, 1985) suggests that there may be a psychosocial contribution to the survival differences between classes.

It is worth noting that a class gradient in ischaemic heart disease survival does not necessarily imply that treatment is of less benefit to people in lower classes. What evidence there is suggests that treatment improves survival rates by the same amount in all classes. Assessing the results of coronary artery bypass grafting at the Walter Reed Army Medical Centre, Sterling (1984) found no difference in the immediate operative mortality for blacks and whites but said that long-term prognosis might be slightly better for blacks. Similarly, among patients recruited into a double-blind control trial of long-term use of beta blockers after myocardial infarction, the proportional reduction in mortality of the treatment compared to placebo groups was at least as great for blacks and whites (Haywood, 1984). This was so despite the fact that the usual black/white survival differences were present in both groups. Lastly, on the preventive side, the Multiple Risk Factor Intervention Trial counselled a selected high-risk population on behavioural factors related to coronary heart disease and anti-hypertensive drug use. Apparently unaffected by the major differences in education and income, the 7-year follow-up showed that '. . . the effects of intervention in reducing risk factors were almost identical in black and white participants'.

Incidence, survival and mortality

Survival from cancer and heart disease appears to be consistently better amongst those at the upper end of the socio-economic scale. Among cancers, the lower-class survival disadvantage may be more consistent than the incidence disadvantage. The incidence of cancers of the breast, ovary and testis is greater in the 'high' compared to the 'low' socio-economic categories, while for cancers of the lung, stomach and cervix the reverse is true. The incidence of cancer at other sites, such as the rectum and pancreas seem to show no consistent relationship to socio-economic factors.

Turning to mortality, socio-economic differences in death rates reflect the combined influence of socio-economic differences in incidence and fatality rates. From a public health perspective there arises the question of the relative contribution of these two components to differences in mortality. Providing a precise answer to this question is beyond the scope of this chapter. To do so would require a knowledge of the life expectancy of survivors at the end of follow-up. As the follow-up time is short, many apparent survivors will go on to die of their cancers in the immediate post-follow-up period, while others will make a full recovery. We do not know whether the class differences in case fatality rates represent merely a slower rate of progress of the disease process, ending with similar proportions failing to recover, or whether they represent differences in the proportions who recover and go on to enjoy some years of normal life. For this reason it is impossible to say what contribution the observed class differences in case fatality rates make to class differences in mortality.

Conclusion

While the evidence reviewed here is suggestive rather than conclusive, it does reveal some of the difficulties in understanding the determinants of class differences in mortality. Risk factors for contracting a disease may be different from risk factors for dying of it, while the two together determine the overall rate of death from the disease. However, although amongst the sick those in the lower socio-economic categories generally tend to fare the worst, the shortness of the follow-up period over which case fatality rates are measured means that these data cannot be used to estimate the contribution of case fatality differences to mortality differentials.

Note

David Leon was supported in the Social Statistics Research Unit at City University by the Cancer Research Campaign to analyse cancer incidence and survival using the Office of Population Censuses and Surveys' *Longitudinal Study*. Data were provided by the Office of Population Censuses and Surveys. The views expressed here are those of the authors. Crown copyright is reserved.

References

Berg, J.W., Ross, R. and Latourette, H.B. (1977), 'Economic status and survival of cancer patients', *Cancer*, **39**, pp. 467–77.

Cassileth, B.R., Lusk, J., Miller, D.S. *et al.* (1985), 'Psychological correlates of survival in advanced malignant disease?', *New England Journal of Medicine*, **312** (24), pp. 1551–5.

Connett, J.E. and Stamler, J. (1984), 'Responses of black and white males to special intervention program of multiple risk factor intervention trial', *American Heart Journal*, **108**, pp. 839–48.

Dayal, H.H. and Chui, C. (1982), 'Factors associated with racial differences in survival for prostatic carcinoma', *Journal of Chronic Diseases*, **35**, pp. 553–60.

Derogatis, L.R., Abeloff, M.D. and Melisaratos, N. (1979), 'Psychological coping mechanisms and survival time in metastatic breast cancer', *Journal of the American Association*, **242** (14), pp. 1504–8.

Foster, R.S. and Costanza, M.C. (1984), 'Breast self examination practices and breast cancer survival', *Cancer*, **53**, pp. 999–1005.

Gillum, R.F. and Grant, C.T. (1982), 'CHD in black populations I & II: risk factors', *American Heart Journal*, **104**, pp. 839–52.

Hackett, T.P., Cassem, N.H. and Raker, J.W. (1973), 'Patient delay in cancer', *New England Journal of Medicine*, **289**, pp. 14–20.

Haywood, L.J. (1984), 'CHD mortality/morbidity and risk in blacks', *American Heart Journal*, **108**, pp. 787–96.

Hrubec, Z. and Zukel, W.J. (1971), 'Socio-economic differentials in prognosis following episodes of CHD', *Journal of Chronic Diseases*, **23** (12) pp. 881–9.

Jenkins, C.D. (1978), 'Low education: a risk factor for death, (editorial), *New England Journal of Medicine*, **299**, pp. 95–7.

Jones, D.R., Goldblatt, P.O. and Leon, D.A. (1984), 'Bereavement and cancer: some data on deaths of spouses from the Longitudinal study of OPCS', *British Medical Journal*, **289**, pp. 461–4.

Keller, A.Z. (1969), 'Survivorship with mouth and pharynx cancers and their association with cirrhosis of the liver, marital status and residence', *American Journal of Public Health*, **59** (7), pp. 1139–53.

Koskenvuo, M., Kaprio, J., Romo, M. and Langinvanio, H. (1981), 'Incidence and prognosis of IHD with respect to marital status and social class', *Journal of Epidemiology and Community Health*, **35**, pp. 192–6.

Kottke, T.E., Young, D.T. and McCall, M.M. (1980), 'Effect of social class on recovery from myocardial infarction', *Minnesota Medicine*, **63** (8), pp. 590–7.

Langford, H.G., Oberman, A. *et al.*, (1984), 'Black–White comparisons of indices of CHD and myocardial infarction in the stepped-care cohort of the hypertension detection and follow-up program', *American Heart Journal*, **108**, pp. 797–801.

Linden G, (1969), 'The influence of social class in the survival of cancer patients', *American Journal of Public Health*, **59**, pp. 267–74.

Lipworth, L., Abelin, T. and Connelly, R.R. (1970), 'Socio-economic factors in the prognosis of cancer patients, *Journal of Chronic Diseases*, **23**, pp. 105–16.

Lipworth, L. and Bennett, B. (1972), 'Prognosis of non-private patients', *Journal National Cancer Institute*, **48**, pp. 11–16.

McWhirter, W.R., Smith, H. and McWhirter, K.M. (1983), 'Social class as a prognostic variable in acute lymphoblastic leukaemia', *Medical Journal of Australia*, **2** (7), pp. 318–21.

Modan, B. and Kallner, H. (1971), 'Gastrointestinal cancer in Israel', *Israeli Journal of Medical Science*, **7** (12), pp. 1475–8.

Morrison, A.S. (1978), 'Sequential pathogenic components of rates', *American Journal of Epidemiology*, **109**, pp. 709–18.

Oberman, A. and Cutter, G. (1984), 'Issues in the natural history and treatment of CHD in black populations: surgical treatment', *American Heart Journal*, 108, pp. 688–94.

Page, W.F. and Kuntz, A.J. (1980), 'Racial and socio-economic factors in cancer survival', *Cancer*, 45 (5), pp. 1029–40.

Patel, C., Marmot, M.G., Terry, D.J. *et al*. (1985), 'Trial of relaxation in reducing coronary risk – 4 year follow up', *British Medical Journal*, 290, pp. 1103–6.

Shapiro, S., Weinblatt, E., Frank, C.W. and Sager, R.V. (1970), 'Social factors in the prognosis of men following first myocardial infarction', *Milbank Memorial Fund Quarterly*, 48, pp. 37–50.

Shapiro, S., Weinblatt, E. and Frank, E.W. (1972), 'Return to work after first myocardial infarction', *Archives of Environmental Health*, 24, pp. 17–26.

Shaw, H.M., McGovern, V.J. and Farago, G.A. (1981), 'Cutaneous malignant melanoma: occupation and prognosis', *Medical Journal of Australia*, I, (1), pp. 37–8.

Smith, J.W. (1980), 'Mortality after recovery from myocardial infarction', *Journal of Chronic Diseases*, 33, pp. 1–4.

Sterling, R.P., Graeber, G.M. *et al*. (1984), 'Results of myocardial revascularization in black males', *American Heart Journal*, 108, pp. 695–9.

Vagero, D. and Persson, G. (1984), 'Risks, survival and trends of malignant melanoma among white and blue collar workers in Sweden', *Social Science and Medicine*, 19 (4), pp. 475–8.

Vandenbrouke, J.P. (1982), 'A shortcut method for calculating the 95% confidence interval of the SMR', *American Journal of Epidemiology*, 115, pp. 303–4.

Watkins, L., Gardner, K., Gott, V. and Gardner, T.J. (1983), 'CHD and bypass surgery in urban blacks', *Journal of the National Medical Association*, 75, pp. 381–3.

Weinblatt, E., Ruberman, W., Goldberg, J.D. *et al*. (1978), 'Relation of education to sudden death after myocardial infarction', *New England Journal of Medicine*, 299, pp. 60–5.

Young, J.L., Ries, L.G. and Pollack, E.S. (1984), 'Cancer patient survival among ethnic groups in the USA', *Journal of the National Cancer Institute*, 763 (2), pp. 341–52.

14 Social health inequalities in South European countries: is it a different problem?
Oriol Ramis-Juan and Katerina Sokou

Introduction
Accepted assumptions on the relationship between social distribution of wealth and health

Most of the existing empirical research on social inequalities looks at the distribution of wealth, especially income, within socieities. The implicit assumption is that income is the main determinant of, or at least is closely correlated to, the rest of the components of wealth and desirable goods. Some countries show a wider wealth distribution than others where it tends to concentrate in smaller proportions of the population. Policies designed to reduce inequality in wealth distribution have existed in Europe particularly since the onset of the welfare state. The impact of such policies is still a matter for discussion (Le Grand, 1982; Atkinson, 1979).

Although the association between poverty and poor health is obvious, occurring through mechanisms such as poorer nutrition, a worse environment and less ability to cope with this environment (Antonovsky, Chapter 19 in this volume), there is no clear model to relate distribution of wealth and distribution of health. Moreover, the available methodologies and empirical evidence, however convincing they might be, are far from clearly established (Scrivens and Holland, 1983; Le Grand, Chapter 4 in this volume).

The early theorists of the welfare state implicitly assumed that wealth inequalities did not automatically determine health inequalities. They believed direct intervention in the health sector could reduce health inequalities without changing the distribution of wealth. Some maternal and child health care policies were probably successful in reducing a proportion of inequalities. However, researchers from different persuasions deny the possibility of eradicating health inequalities without simultaneously tackling wealth distribution. Some of these claim that priority has to be given to wealth redistribution: equity in other desirable goods such as health would logically follow (for example, Gough, 1979). Others say that economic development and general enrichment of a society is a prerequisite for an equitable distribution of health and still others stand for a more careful design of social policies with attainable objectives (DHSS, 1980; Le Grand, 1982).

Accepted assumptions about the position of Southern Europe inside the developed world

The geographic delimitation of Southern Europe* is unclear. The UN Report on *Level and Trends of Mortality* (UN, 1982) listed Spain, Portugal, Italy, Yugoslavia, Greece, Albania, Cyprus and Israel; the WHO Regional Office for Europe added Turkey and Morocco and excluded Israel (WHO, 1985). Since 1986 Israel has been included and Morocco has been excluded; the European Community is obviously talking only about its country members, namely, Italy, Greece, Spain and Portugal. Although some of the points discussed here may apply to other countries, this chapter will focus on the Southern EEC countries. Most of the present discussions on social policy in international forums assume that Southern Europe is poorer, its wealth distribution more inegalitarian and its health indicators worse than in Northern Europe. These assumptions are usually based on the consideration of a few crude global indicators, especially GNP per capita and crude or age-specific mortality rates. The belief that wealth distribution is less egalitarian is probably based on the known underdevelopment of redistribution and welfare policies in these countries. It is then concluded that inequalities in the distribution of health between different income or wealth strata are also greater than in the western and northern countries. As the relationships between social distribution of wealth and health are far from well understood there is neither a clear deductive model to allow for such a conclusion nor are data and methods available to test it empirically.

This chapter aims to discuss some of these assumptions, which are summarised in the following questions:

1. Are Southern European countries still poorer than northern and western countries?
2. Is Southern Europe still unhealthier compared with the rest of Europe?
3. Is the wealth of Southern European countries more inequitably distributed than in northern and western countries?
4. Are the existing social inequalities more associated with an unequal distribution of health indicators than they are in the rest of Europe?
5. What rational forecast can be made for the next years and what can be done?

* Very small countries or territories such as Andorra, Gibraltar, Monaco, San Marino, Vatican City and Malta are not considered.

Table 14.1 GNP per capita in US $ in selected European countries

	1978	1981	1983	1983*
Greece	3450	5750	3505	5512
Spain	3960	6876	4136	6976
Italy	4600	8534	6208	8711
UK	5720	7944	8068	9861
France	8880	11408	9539	11269
Netherlands	9200	8931	9203	10246
Belgium	9700	10239	8126	10689
Germany	10300	9924	10646	11455
Sweden	10540	15743	11024	13508

Notes:
(*) Those estimations based in purchasing power parity of the US $. The rest based on exchange rates.

Sources: 1978 *World Tables*, Baltimore: World Bank, 1983
1981, 1983, (*) OECD, op. cit.

The wealth of Southern Europe

The definition of a country's wealth can not be discussed here. There are both conceptual and measurement problems in the use of the Gross National Product (GNP) per capita, the indicator most often used. Although comparisons inside the EEC show less differences than when these countries are compared with the Third World or Eastern countries, they still need to be considered. Development, as measured by increases in GNP per capita, is usually associated with factors which are likely to improve health and welfare such as a good food supply or correct environmental hygiene. However, evidence exists to show that rapid growth of GNP per capita in some countries is not correlated with those factors and indeed is at times inversely correlated. Countries with lower GNP per capita are more likely to under-report economic activities such as own-consumption agriculture or non-accountable economy. This will tend to exaggerate the gap between countries. However, GNP per capita is probably the only available existing summary figure for making cross-national comparison and there is still a clear GNP per capita gradient between Northern and Southern Europe (see Table 14.1). These differences hold even when measured in purchasing power units to avoid erratic currency exchange rates. (OECD, 1985).

The health of Southern Europe

Definition, measurement, and comparison of health presents even more problems than those encountered when studying wealth. Mortality levels are usually used for international comparisons as they are often the only available, comparable indicator. Other health measurements, related or not to social development, may show better indicators in the Southern countries because of different exposure to risk factors through different cultural habits, natural environment and genetic capacities. Unfortunately those indicators are not available or standardised for international comparisons (Blaxter, Chapter 10 in this volume). However, some conclusions can be drawn from mortality data alone. Reductions in overall mortality and infant mortality rates in Southern Europe in the last 30 years have been far more impressive than those in the North and the West. The present differences in overall mortality and infant mortality between Northern/Western and Southern/Eastern countries are only a small part of what they were in 1950 (see Table 14.2). Greece, Spain and Italy, but not Portugal, are relatively well-placed in the world ranking of life expectancy at birth for males, following countries such as Sweden or Norway, and before Germany FR and Scotland (see Table 14.3). Female life expectancy at birth has also improved more in Southern Europe than in the North and the West but the advantage over the male mortality decline was smaller than the values described in the North (see Table 14.4). Rapid changes, such as incorporation of women into the workforce and disruption of family networks may have played a role in the difference.

Comparisons of cause-specific mortality rates must be studied with caution as low rates in the 1950s and 1960s may have been caused by relevant proportions of undefined causes in those years. However, Southern European countries have always been characterised by their low rate of male cardiovascular mortality. Unlike Northern and Western Europe, where the general trend was a deterioration in the 1960s followed by a slight improvement in the 1970s, cardiovascular mortality rates among male populations have increased in most of the Southern European countries (see Table 14.5).

Increase in tobacco consumption in the Southern European countries could explain the deterioration of lung cancer mortality rates among young (25–44) males and females. Southern Europe still has lower rates of cancer and cardiovascular diseases, the most important causes of mortality in the developed world (see Tables 14.5 and 14.6). This advantage is likely to be lost if the increasing prevalence of well known risk factors is not kept under control (Domenech and Gispert, 1984; Balaguer-Vintro and Sans, 1985; Symposium, 1984).

Although the well known correlation between GNP per capita and infant mortality rates is still found in Europe, since Albania and Turkey still show low GNP per capita and high infant mortality rates, all the remaining countries are now on the right side of the curve where the correlation diminishes and other factors must be taken into

Table 14.2 *Expectation of life at birth around 1950 and in the 1970s in selected European and developed countries and regions**

Region and Country	Around 1950 Period	Around 1950 Males	Around 1950 Females	1970s Period	1970s Males	1970s Females
Northern America		65.9	71.6		69.0	76.7
Regional increase in % 1970s/1950s:					+4.7	+7.1
Canada	1950–2	66.3	70.8	1970–2	69.3	76.4
US	1950–4	65.9	71.7	1976	69.0	76.7
Japan	1949–50	56.2	59.6	1977	72.7	78.0
Increase in % 1970s/1950s					+29.4	30.9
Europe						
Eastern:		59.6	64.4		67.4	73.6
Regional increase in % 1970s/1950s					+13.1	14.3
Bulgaria	1946–47	53.3	56.4	1969–71	68.6	73.9
Hungary	1948–49	58.3	63.2	1974	66.5	72.4
Romania	1956	61.5	65.0	1974–76	67.4	72.0
Northern:		66.7	71.4		69.7	75.9
Regional increase in % 1970s/1950s:					+4.5	9.6
Denmark	1946–50	67.8	70.1	1975–76	71.1	76.8
Finland	1946–50	58.6	65.9	1975	67.4	75.9
Norway	1946–50	69.3	72.7	1975–76	71.9	78.1
Sweden	1946–50	69.0	71.6	1976	72.1	77.9
England+Wales	1950–54	67.1	72.3	1974–76	69.6	75.8
Northern Ire.	1950–52	65.5	68.8	1973–75	67.2	73.6
Scotland	1950–54	65.0	69.5	1973–75	67.4	73.9
Southern[1]:		61.4	65.4		69.0	74.6
Regional increase in % 1970s/1950s					+12.4	14.1
Greece	1950	63.4	66.7	1970	70.1	73.6
Italy	1950–53	63.8	67.3	1970–72	69.0	74.9
Portugal	1949–52	55.5	60.5	1974	65.3	72.0
Spain	1950	58.8	63.5	1970	69.7	75.0
Southern:		60.5	63.6		68.4	73.9
Regional increase in % 1970s/1950s:					+13.1	16.2
Western:		64.4	68.9		68.8	75.8
Regional increase in % 1970s/1950s:					+6.8	10.0
Austria	1949–51	61.9	67.0	1976	68.1	75.1
Belgium	1946–49	62.0	67.3	1968–72	67.8	74.2
France	1950–51	63.6	69.3	1968–72	69.0	76.9
Germany F.R.	1949–51	64.6	68.5	1974–76	68.3	74.8
Netherlands	1947–49	69.4	71.5	1971–75	71.2	77.2
USSR	1954–55	61	67	1971–72	64	74
					+4.9	10.4

Notes
* The regional averages include Czechoslovakia, The German DR, and Poland (Eastern region), Iceland and Ireland (Northern region), Albania, Malta and Yugoslavia (Southern region), Luxembourg and Switzerland (Western region), in addition to the countries shown in the table.
[1] Southern EEC countries only.

Source: Compiled from United Nations, *Level and Trends of Mortality since 1950 . . .*, 1982, p. 9.

account to explain discrepancies. Even if diverse *ad hoc* comparative

Table 14.3   Ranking of more developed countries according to expectation of life at birth for males 1950s–70s

	1950s			1970s		Average annual increase (years)
1.	Iceland	69.4	1.	Japan	72.7	.60
2.	Netherlands	69.4	2.	Sweden	72.1	.11
3.	Norway	69.3	3.	Norway	71.9	.09
4.	Sweden	69.0	4.	Iceland	71.6	.09
6.	Israel	67.2	6.	Denmark	71.1	.12
7.	New Zealand	67.2	7.	Israel	70.3	.13
8.	England+Wales	67.1	8.	Switzerland	70.3	.20
9.	Switzerland	66.4	9.	GREECE	70.1	.34
10.	Canada	66.3	10.	Cyprus	70.0	.27
11.	Australia	66.1	11.	SPAIN	69.7	.55
12.	USA	65.9	12.	England+Wales	69.6	.11
13.	N. Ireland	65.5	13.	Canada	69.3	.15
14.	GDR	65.1	14.	USA	69.0	.16
15.	Scotland	65.0	15.	ITALY	69.0	.27
16.	German FR	64.6	16.	France	69.0	.23
17.	Ireland	64.5	17.	Australia	68.9	.10
18.	ITALY	63.8	18.	German DR	68.8	.16
19.	Cyprus	63.6	19.	Bulgaria	68.6	.65
20.	France	63.6	20.	Ireland	68.6	.27
21.	GREECE	63.4	21.	New Zealand	68.6	.07
22.	Belgium	62.0	22.	Malta	68.4	.46
23.	Austria	61.9	23.	German FR	68.3	.15
24.	Luxembourg	61.7	24.	Austria	68.1	.24
25.	Romania	61.7	25.	Belgium	67.8	.26
26.	USSR	61	26.	Scotland	67.4	.11
27.	Czechoslovakia	60.9	27.	Finland	67.4	.33
28.	SPAIN	58.8	28.	Romania	67.4	.31
29.	Finland	58.6	29.	N. Ireland	67.2	.07
30.	Hungary	58.3	30.	Luxembourg	67.0	.22
31.	Yugoslavia	56.9	31.	Poland	67.0	.42
32.	Japan	56.2	32.	Czechoslovakia	66.9	.24
33.	Malta	55.7	33.	Albania	66.5	.73
34.	Poland	55.5	34.	Hungary	66.5	.31
35.	PORTUGAL	55.5	35.	Yugoslavia	65.6	.47
36.	Bulgaria	53.3	36.	PORTUGAL	65.3	.42
37.	Albania	52.6	37.	USSR	64	.18

Source: UN, op. cit., 1982.

studies show no differences in low birthweight proportions between Northern and Southern samples, differences still exist in neonatal mortality rates between them (Table 14.7).

Inequity and distribution of wealth in Southern Europe
While income is a potential spending-power measure, the pattern of expenditure, and therefore its effect on health, is determined by those

Table 14.4   *Ranking of more developed countries according to expectation of life at birth for females 1950s–70s*

	1950s			1970s		Average annual increase (years)
1.	Iceland	73.5	1.	Norway	78.1	.20
2.	Norway	72.7	2.	Japan	78.0	.67
3.	England+Wales	72.3	3.	Sweden	77.9	.23
4.	USA	71.7	4.	Iceland	77.5	.16
5.	Sweden	71.6	5.	Netherlands	77.2	.23
6.	Netherlands	71.5	6.	France	76.9	.32
7.	New Zealand	71.3	7.	Denmark	76.8	.24
8.	Switzerland	70.9	8.	USA	76.7	.25
9.	Canada	70.8	9.	Canada	76.4	.28
10.	Australia	70.6	10.	Switzerland	76.2	.27
11.	Israel	70.1	11.	Finland	75.9	.37
12.	Denmark	70.1	12.	Australia	75.9	.19
13.	Scotland	69.5	13.	England+Wales	75.8	.15
14.	France	69.3	14.	Austria	75.1	.31
15.	German DR	69.1	15.	SPAIN	75.0	.58
16.	Cyprus	68.8	16.	ITALY	74.9	.39
17.	N. Ireland	68.8	17.	Germany FR	74.8	.25
18.	Germany FR	68.5	18.	New Zealand	74.6	.17
19.	ITALY	67.3	19.	German DR	74.4	.23
20.	Belgium	67.3	20.	Poland	74.3	.44
21.	Ireland	67.1	21.	Belgium	74.2	.31
22.	Austria	67.0	22.	USSR	74.0	.41
23.	USSR	67.0	23.	Luxembourg	73.9	.34
24.	GREECE	66.7	24.	Israel	73.9	.17
25.	Finland	65.9	25.	Scotland	73.9	.20
26.	Luxembourg	65.8	26.	Czechoslovakia	73.9	.34
27.	Czechoslovakia	65.5	27.	Bulgaria	73.9	.74
28.	Romania	65.0	28.	GREECE	73.6	.35
29.	SPAIN	63.5	29.	N. Ireland	73.6	.21
30.	Hungary	63.2	30.	Cyprus	72.9	.17
31.	Poland	62.5	31.	Ireland	72.9	.39
32.	PORTUGAL	60.5	32.	Malta	72.9	.55
33.	Japan	59.6	33.	Hungary	72.4	.36
34.	Yugoslavia	59.3	34.	PORTUGAL	72.0	.49
35.	Malta	57.7	35.	Romania	72.0	.37
36.	Bulgaria	56.4	36.	Yugoslavia	70.4	.60
37.	Albania	54.4	37.	Albania	70.4	.84

Source: UN, op. cit., 1982.

factors usually associated with wealth and social class (for example, education, cultural habits, and the rest). However, income is still the most available measure and its unequal distribution has been mea-

Table 14.5   Trends in death rates from cardiovascular diseases in middle-aged males in selected developed countries

Rates per 100,000 population
45–64 years, males

	1960	1970	1976	decline 1960–76
Northern America:				
Canada	762	684	635	16.7
USA	909	839	712	21.7
Japan:	582	455	334	42.6
Europe:				
Eastern:	465	562	598	+28.6
Bulgaria	351	436	521	+48.4
Hungary	512	632	665	+29.9
Romania	–	509	525	
Northern:	629	676	671	+6.7
Denmark	498	506	548	+10.0
Finland	840	1001	962	+14.5
Norway	455	553	515	+13.2
Sweden	465	448	479	+3.0
England+Wales	665	696	678	+2.0
Scotland	851	853	844	0.8
Southern:	411	443	450	+9.5
Greece	252	298	327	+29.8
Italy	482	446	442	8.3
Portugal	440	485	511	+16.1
Spain	363	394	404	+11.3
Yugoslavia	370	428	488	+31.9
Western:	482	502	473	1.8
Austria	556	585	532	4.3
Belgium	576	590	532	7.6
France	403	367	366	9.2
Germany FR	515	542	523	+1.6
Netherlands	387	534	491	+26.9

Source: UN, op. cit., 1982.

sured using different methods and indicators (Sen, 1973; Sawyer, 1976; Atkinson, 1979). No single indicator can claim to be the best summary of income inequality as each one tends to stress particular aspects of inequality (Le Grand, Chapter 4 in this volume). However, comparisons of the proportion of the national income owned by each population decile, ranked according to its wealth, gives a reasonable description. The World Bank uses the percentage of income received by the poorest 20 per cent of households and the percentage of income received by the richest 5 per cent to compare internal wealth

Table 14.6   Trends in death rates from neoplasms in middle-aged males in selected developed countries

Rates per 100,000 population
45–64 years, males

	1960	1970	1976	decline 1960–76
Northern America:				
Canada	281	320	325	+15.7
USA	326	360	359	+10.1
Japan:	346	327	314	9.3
Europe:				
Eastern:	352	354	376	+6.0
Bulgaria	337	294	295	12.5
Hungary	340	356	398	+17.1
Romania	–	311	331	
Northern:	353	350	346	+2.0
Denmark	310	328	335	+8.1
Finland	452	418	393	13.1
Norway	247	258	268	+8.5
Sweden	241	239	252	+4.6
England+Wales	417	407	392	6.0
Scotland	456	453	436	4.4
Southern:	275	292	303	+10.0
Greece	277	282	298	+7.6
Italy	349	382	397	+13.8
Portugal	246	272	273	+11.0
Spain	270	286	298	+10.4
Yugoslavia	250	272	298	+19.2
Western:	374	383	390	4.0
Austria	422	380	365	13.5
Belgium	389	414	413	+6.2
France	387	405	447	+15.5
Germany FR	370	357	364	1.6
Netherlands	345	395	384	+11.3

Source: UN, op. cit., 1982.

distribution between countries (see Table 14.8). More complete but older figures were published by Sawyer (1976) and Atkinson (1979). Even if some Northern countries tend to be more egalitarian in income distribution than Southern countries using those indicators, the general assumption that poorer Southern countries have a clearly less egalitarian wealth distribution than other developed countries can hardly be supported with the available data. Given its unreliability it would be very dangerous to draw any definite conclusion about the relationship between the distribution of earnings and the level of

Table 14.7   Neonatal mortality rates and percentage of low birthweight babies in Northern and Southern European countries

	*Percentage of babies weighting 2500 grms or less at birth	Neonatal mortality rate ** (per 1000 livebirths)
Sweden	4.1	3.7
Finland	4.7	4.2
Norway	4.9	3.8
Netherlands	5.5	4.2
Denmark	5.6	3.6
France	5.6	4.2
Great Britain	6.5	5.0
Belgium	n/a	6.9
German FR	n/a	4.8
Italy	5.1	10.3
Spain	5.4	8.0+
Greece	5.8	8.3

Sources: *Data from Boldman and Reed, see Reed and Stanley, *The Epidemiology of Prematurity*, 1977, except for Spain and Greece see Ramis-Juan (own data) and T. Bakoula: personal communication). For other countries, sources see Boldman and Reed's appendix.
**World Health Statistics*, WHO, Geneva, 1984.

Table 14.8   Percentage of income received by the poorest 20 per cent and the richest 10 per cent of households

	Lowest 20%	Highest 10%
Greece	5.7	n/a
Spain	6.0	18.5
Italy	6.2	n/a
France	5.3	n/a
Germany FR	6.9	18.2
Sweden	7.2	16.8
UK	7.4	13.7
Denmark	7.4	n/a
Netherlands	8.1	22.0
Belgium	n/a	n/a

Source: *World Tables*, Baltimore: World Bank, 1983.

development (Atkinson, 1979). Moreover, even if this indicator (i.e. the proportion of the national income belonging to the bottom 20 per cent of households) is considered, rich countries such as the USA or France show a less egalitarian distribution than most of the Southern European countries (Sawyer, 1976). However, the lowest deciles in the poorest countries may get less resources even if their relative share of the national income is the same as in richer countries. The incidence of poverty, in whatever way is defined, may be higher and its effects on health inequalities greater.

Social health inequalities in Southern Europe

If it is difficult to show that Southern Europe is less egalitarian than the North it is even more difficult to show whether health is more evenly distributed across income groups or not. In the Southern European countries, where there is no tradition of routine health registers using socio-economic groups, only *ad hoc* surveys or individual-based inequality measures can be used to assess the extent of health inequalities. Use of individual-based inequality measures (for example, Gini Coefficient, Atkinson Index or other summary measures) (Le Grand, Chapter 4) will probably be a step forward in Southern countries as they allow for a relatively sophisticated inequality measure using very crude data. However, the methodology must be properly validated before it can be used and *ad hoc* surveys will still be needed. Some of the available epidemiological and sociological studies report differences across social classes, occupational groups or educational groups in those countries (Ramis-Juan, 1982; Sokou, 1985). As socio-stratification classifications derived from occupation or education have seldom gone through a validation process, non-differential misclassification can be expected (Rothman, 1985). These errors can only be assumed to underestimate the observed differences, which are similar to those seen in countries where classifications have been properly validated (for example Tables 14.9 and 14.10).

Rational forecasts on health inequity in Southern Europe

These provisional and scarce findings suggest that differences in some aspects of health, usually mortality, between social classes may be similar in the South to the North in spite of both a poorer national income in terms of GNP per capita and slightly worse national mortality rates. It would be interesting to see if the overall relative advantages in the Southern countries in indicators such as cardiovascular and cancer mortality is associated with less social differences in those causes of death. While a more extensive and vigorous consideration of these findings should be tackled in the near future, an interesting set of plausible forecasts can be formulated.

Table 14.9   Perinatal mortality rates by occupational groups

England and Wales (1983)*			Spain (1979)	
Social Class	I	3.8	Professionals	6.3
	II	4.6	Managers	6.3
	IIINM	5.2	White Collar	7.9
	IIIM	5.5	Blue Collar	8.2
	IV	6.9	Rural Workers	12.6
	V	7.0	Spain	8.5
Armed Forces Students Retired Unclassif.	}	7.6		
Illegitimate		7.4		
England and Wales		5.7		

Note:
* English data are presented according to the Registrar General Classification of Social Classes ranging from I (e.g. professionals) to V (e.g. labourers).

Source: Spain: *Movimiento Natural de la Poblacion 1979*, INE, Madrid 1981.
England and Wales: OPCS *Monitor*, London, 1985.

Table 14.10   Neonatal mortality rates by occupational class

Barcelona, Spain (1984)	Occupational Class Mother Rate (C.I.–95%)	Occupational Class Father Rate (C.I.–95%)
Low (5–6)	10.0 (16.4–6.1)	8.0 (14.0–4.6)
Mid (4–3)	5.7 (8.2–4.0)	5.4 (7.5–5.0)
High (2–1)	5.3 (9.2–3.1)	6.8 (9.5–4.9)
Unclassified (9)	9.8 (11.5–8.4)	29.5 (42.3–20.6)
Total	8.0	8.0

Source: Ramis-Juan O., *Neonatal Mortality in Barcelona* (forthcoming).

First, it could be suggested that extensive social and family support still exists in all social groups in these countries, compensating for a scarcer availability of health and welfare services and the adverse effects of low national income. Should this hypothesis be correct, a deterioration of health differentials can be expected in those countries as extended social networks disappear, even in rural areas, through rapid geographical mobility, the relatively fast incorporation of women into the workforce and the decline of extended families.

Logically, these changes must adversely affect the health of the low-income groups to a greater extent.

A second hypothesis could be based on the *Black Report's* preliminary hypothesis on the evolution of health inequalities between social classes (DHSS, 1980). Without providing convincing empirical evidence, the Report suggested that, although general health standards have improved nationwide in England and Wales in the last 40 years, the health of the richest population groups improved more than that of the poorest classes and therefore social differences increased.

Further evidence is provided by research on health promotion as overall reduction in risk factors, such as tobacco consumption, has been associated with increased social inequality in smoking habits: the affluent groups tend to adhere to healthier lifestyles, which both improve overall rates and increase the gradient between social classes (Scrivens and Holland, 1983; DHSS, 1980). If these hypotheses were also true for Southern countries, increasing differences between income groups could also be predicted for the near future.

Thirdly, increasing unemployment among the young has very little welfare policy coverage and is likely to put large sectors of young adults into the lower-income groups for a long time.

Finally, the *Black Report* explanation relied very heavily on defects of welfare measures. A careful study of the impact of social and health policy measures on health inequalities between the different income groups in the Northern countries, where data are available, will help to define new policies in the South and to avoid the errors made in the implementation of policies in the North. Equity is currently an implicit objective of the current policy developments in Southern Europe, especially NHS reforms in Spain, Greece and Italy, and also in the new developments in social services and education. To operationalise equity as an objective, effort should be made to scrutinise planned reforms and to assess their impact on equity, especially because, unlike Northern Europe, those reforms are tackled in a time of a cold economic climate.

References

Atkinson, (1979), *The Economics of Inequality*, Oxford University Press.

Balaguer-Vintro, I. and Sans, S. (1985), 'Coronary heart disease mortality trends and related factors in Spain' in *Cardiology*, 72, pp. 97–104.

DHSS (1980), *Inequalities in Health* (The *Black Report*), London,

Domenech, J. and Gispert, R. (1984), 'Mortality Trends in Catalonia 1975–79' (Tendencias de Mortalidad en Catalunya 1975–1979), paper presented to the Ier Congreso Nacional de Salud Publica, Barcelona, mimeo.

Gough, I. (1979), *The Political Economy of the Welfare State*, London: Macmillan Press.

Le Grand, J. (1982), *The Strategy of Equality*, London: George Allen and Unwin.

OECD (1985), *Health Care Expenditure*, Paris: OECD.

Ramis-Juan, O. (1982), 'Poverty 1982: unemployment and health: the case of Spain', unpublished paper presented to the WHO Consultation Meeting on Poverty,

Inequality and Health, Aberdeen.

Reed, D. and Stanley, F. (1977), *The Epidemiology of Prematurity*, Baltimore and Munich: Urban and Schwarzenberg.

Rothman, K. (1985), *Modern Epidemiology*, Chestnut Hill: New England Epidemiology Institute.

Sawyer, A. (1976), 'Income Distribution in OECD Countries' in *OECD, Overlook*.

Scrivens, E. and Holland, W. (1983), 'Inequalities in Health in Britain: A Critique of the Report of a Research Working Group', in *Effective Health Care* 1 (2), pp. 97–107.

Sen, A. (1973), *On Economic Inequality*, Oxford: Clarendon Press.

Sokou, K. (1985), Report in WHO Office for Europe: 'The Burden of Health Inequalities', Copenhagen, mimeo.

Symposium on Smoking and Health in the South European Countries (1985), Generalitat of Cataluna Publishers, Barcelona.

United Nations (1982), *Level and Trends of Mortality Since 1950: A Joint Survey by the United Nations and the World Health Organisation*, New York: United Nations.

WHO Seminar on Health Promotion in the Southern European Countries, Barcelona, 1985.

World Tables (1983), Baltimore, London: The World Bank.

PART IV
EXPLANATIONS

15 The role of health services in relation to inequalities in health in Europe
Sally Macintyre

Introduction

In discussions of inequalities in health it is very common for health care to be equated with health. Aiach and Carr-Hill (Chapter 2 in this volume) noted, for example, that when they circulated a questionnaire on debates about inequalities in *health* many of their respondents replied only in terms of inequalities in *health care*, or health care *resources*. Similarly, reviews of particular patterns of ill-health often start by arguing that their causes lie outside the health care sector, but then proceed, in the policy section, to recommend changes in health care provision without explaining why this should be an appropriate type of remedy (Black, 1980; Short, 1980; NBHW, 1985.)

The linking of health care with health is frequently implicit rather than explicit. Many authors who appear to treat them as automatically equated would doubtless agree, if challenged, that the two are not necessarily the same. It is therefore curious how consistent and universal is the apparent assumption that patterns of health care and patterns of health are the same thing. The pervasiveness of this assumption means that examination of the actual or possible links between health care and health tends to be neglected, with potentially serious consequences for debates about medical and social policy.

In this chapter I review arguments about, firstly, the relationship between health services and health in general, and, secondly, the relationship between health services and inequalities in health. I then review material on inequalities both in health care and in health in Europe, and extract some common themes. I conclude by arguing that we need to make clearer distinctions than we currently do about the different functions the health services might have in relation to inequalities in health in Europe.

Health services and aggregate morbidity and mortality

As is well known, McKeown (1965; 1976) has argued that the decline in mortality that occurred in Western Europe from the early nineteenth century was due to a rising standard of living, the control of the physical environment, and favourable trends in the relationship between infectious agent and human host. This thesis has frequently been extended by others to suggest that health services have little influence on aggregate levels of morbidity or mortality.[1] This is actually a major extension to McKeown's thesis, his point being that specific therapies were not important in reducing aggregate mortality until the beginning of the twentieth century, not that they are never important (1965; 1976). He is, however, almost universally cited as the authority for the view that health services are relatively unimportant in determining the health and life expectancy of a population.

There is, however, as little evidence for this extension-to-McKeown argument as there is for the contrary, and probably more prevalent, view that the provision and use of health services are automatically effective and beneficial. It is this latter view which appears to be manifest in the way consumption of health services is equated with health, or the equalisation of health service use is seen as a remedy for inequalities in health.

The two views – that health services have little impact on a population's health, or that health services are the major contributor to a population's health – are differentially fashionable among different professional and scholarly groups, among different political parties, and at different times. Both positions are characterised by a lack of clear empirical evidence and repeated appeals to the same small number of authorities or examples, such as McKeown (1965; 1976) and Cochrane (1972) to support the former position, and French, Swedish or Finnish antenatal care to support the latter.

The problem with both assumptions tends to be in their rather blanket approach, that is, their tendency to generalise from one or two examples to the whole of health care or to all types of health. However, it is logically (and empirically) possible for some components of health care to do good for some conditions or for some people; others to do harm for some conditions or some people; and others to have no effects, or a mixture of harm and good. Just because survival after heart attack may be as good with care at home as with care in an intensive care unit (Mather *et al.*, 1971), it does not mean that most of us would choose to be without polio vaccine, antibiotics, and hip joint replacements. Furthermore, the same component of health care may be effective at some levels but harmful at others. For example, while there is currently concern about the rising rate of caesarian sections in many developed countries, few people would argue that *no* caesarian sections should ever be performed.

Just as arguments about nature versus nurture, or selection versus social causation, are most unproductive when carried on at a global level, arguments about whether health services matter may be particularly useless when conducted at too generalised a level. It is also probably true that the global question 'do health services matter for aggregate health or life expectancy?' is in any case not a popular one to address. Whatever health care's demonstrable effect, or lack of it, on aggregate outcome measures, there is clearly a demand for health care from individuals, professionals, and communities which it would be impolitic for governments, and unprofitable for private medicine, to deny. Since health services of some kind or another are not likely to wither away, scrutiny of how they can do most good is more productive than worrying about whether they do any good at all. For these reasons we should be looking to research which examines the effectiveness of specific interventions or forms of care – whether at the primary, secondary or tertiary levels of disease prevention – in relation to specified types of morbidity or mortality.

Another argument for narrowing down research concerns the inferential problems involved in much of the data typically available; for example, either cross-sectional correlational data (that is, percentage GNP spent on health care in different countries related to outcomes such as infant mortality rates) or time series data (for example, changes in intervention rates over time related to changes in some outcome measures). There are so many confounding variables that it is difficult to reach valid conclusions from such data. Most of the strategies for overcoming such problems seem to involve focusing on very specific health service inputs and equally specific 'outputs'.[2]

For example, Beaglehole (1986) has studied in detail the contribution of specific interventions (resuscitation before admission to hospital, coronary care units, treatment with beta blockers, coronary artery bypass surgery and the treatment of hypertension) to the decline in mortality from coronary heart disease in Auckland between 1974 and 1981, and was able to conclude that these interventions accounted for 40 per cent of the lowered mortality. Similarly detailed scrutiny of individual deaths has of course been carried out in maternal or perinatal mortality surveys (DHSS, 1979; McIlwaine *et al.*, 1979). Another strategy is to exploit naturally occurring quasi-experimental situations. Goldthorp and Richman (1974) looked at domiciliary confinements that occurred because of a strike of hospital workers. Hemminki (1983) showed that, in Finland as a whole, increasing rates of high technology interventions in labour and delivery were accompanied by decreasing rates of perinatal mortality. However, examination of hospitals or counties with differing obstetric policies and practices revealed that perinatal mortality decreased at roughly the same rate in all of them, suggesting that the high technology interventions could not explain the lowered mortality rates.

Another strategy was that used by Hall *et al.* (1980; 1985) in assessing the effectiveness of antenatal care. Rather than using gross outcomes (such as perinatal mortality rates) and gross inputs (such as number of antenatal visits), she undertook a detailed examination: 'of the rate at which asymptomatic problems are diagnosed, missed and overdiagnosed in an antenatal clinic, and the extent to which problems occur despite routine antenatal care' (Hall *et al.*, 1980 p. 78). A final strategy worth mentioning is that of examining what Rutstein *et al.* (1976) have called 'unnecessary untimely mortality', that is, deaths from conditions from which death is thought to be avoidable by health care interventions. In a recent paper it was claimed that mortality from such 'avoidable' causes had declined faster, in six industrialised countries in which health service expenditure had increased over the period, than had mortality from other causes (Charlton and Velez, 1986).[3]

Thus, rather than trying to address the global question 'do health services matter?', I suggest that we should be investigating the circumstances in which particular components of health care can do harm or good to specific conditions or social groups.

Health services and inequalities in health

The role of health services in relation to inequalities in health is a separate, though related, issue to that of their role in relationship to aggregate morbidity or mortality. A reduction in aggregate mortality in a country could mask a widening of mortality differentials between groups. Conversely, reducing inequalities between groups may have little impact on aggregate mortality (and may therefore be of little interest to some clinicians or planners).

As Mooney (1983) has pointed out, the concept of equity in health care is complex. He suggested seven possible definitions of equity in an attempt to clarify various senses of the concept: equality of expenditure per capita; equality of input for equal need; equality of (opportunity of) access for equal need; equality of utilisation for equal need; equality of marginal met need; and equality of health. Mooney examines the issues surrounding these definitions and points out that the seventh definition, that of equality of health, requires much greater positive discrimination in health care provision than any of the input-orientated definitions, and would involve an extremely unequal distribution of health care resources. He also stresses the need to distinguish between supply factors (which influence equality of access) and demand or need factors (which influence utilisation rates).

Another type of distinction is posed by Blaxter (1983; 1985), who suggests that, on the one hand, we may be interested in some overall continuum (for example, of social class or income), or, on the other hand, in particularly disadvantaged sub-groups of the population (such as the long term unemployed, the unskilled, members of large or one-parent families, the elderly, etc.). Both our measurement and conceptualisation of inequalities in health, and our concerns with the role of health services in relation to these inequalities, may depend on which of these we are interested in.

Health services could influence the distribution of disease or death across social groups at each of the three levels of prevention – primary, secondary and tertiary. Preventive procedures, such as immunisation, could influence the incidence of disease among different social groups if differentially available or used; screening and treatment procedures could influence cure or survival rates among different social groups if differentially available, used, or effective; and rehabilitative and after-care services could influence the consequences of disease among different social groups, again if differentially available, used, and effective. Unfortunately the distinction between these three levels is frequently not made. There is a particularly common tendency to confuse the possible role of health services in generating health inequalities in the first place with their role in ameliorating the consequences of health inequalities once generated from other sources. Discussions of use of primary health care are often muddled in this regard, it being unclear whether, for example, under-use of primary health care is seen as the *cause* of high rates of disease, or simply as unfair given *existing* high rates of disease among those under-using the services.

The question 'what effect do health services have on inequalities in health?' presents similar difficulties to the question 'do health services matter at an aggregate level?'. The first problem is that the data that would be required to answer it are unavailable or non-comparable, and the second is the difficulty of inferring cause and effect from such data as do exist.

In order to address this question in the European context it would be necessary to have comparable data from European countries both about the distribution of health services (primary, secondary and tertiary) by various social groups (men/women, social classes, regions, etc.), and about the distribution of various indices of health by these same social groups. However, not only is there little such comparable data across countries, but in many countries no data is available at all on these *distributional* aspects of health or health care. A common theme running through the papers presented on 15 European countries at the WHO meeting on the Health Burden of Social Inequities, (Copenhagen, December 1984) was that little systematic national data were available on these distributional aspects, and that the authors had to rely on small scale, or *ad hoc*, studies (Illsley and Svensson, 1986).

Even if comparable data were available and showed that, for example, countries with more equal distributions of health care had more equal distributions of health, it would be difficult to conclude from these data alone that the two were causally connected (in either direction). Equalities (or inequalities) in health and in health care could both be the outcome of other factors such as the wealth or stage of socio-economic development of the countries in question. One of the problems with much existing work on distributional aspects of health care provision or use is that no clear link with outcome is suggested or demonstrated.[4] In the UK, for example, there is a lot of interesting work on social class variations in access to, use of, and quality of health care which, though excellent in itself, fails to address the question of whether any of these variations matter for health, as opposed to general principles of fairness (Macintyre, 1986).

Some solutions to these problems of inference may be found in the sorts of approaches outlined in the previous section. The contribution made by specific interventions to aggregate coronary heart disease mortality (Beaglehole, 1986) could be extended to look at differential mortality. This would allow one to explore the relative contribution to the differentials of, on the one hand, treatment or other health care factors and, on the other hand, factors such as delay in seeking treatment, differences in incidence, differences in host resistance, etc, (Leon and Wilkinson, Chapter 13 in this volume). Similarly, studies of the diagnosis, missing or overdiagnosis of asymptomatic pregnancy complications at antenatal clinics – and of the consequences of these diagnoses – could be extended to examine the comparative reliability and validity of diagnosis across social groups (Hall *et al.* 1980; 1985).

Charlton *et al.* (1983) extended the use of the concept of 'unnecessary untimely mortality' to examine, within England and Wales, regional variations in mortality from conditions amenable to medical intervention. Socio-economic factors are associated with the incidence of, and case fatality from, these conditions, so the authors examined the extent to which variation in mortality was associated with crude socio-economic indicators (car-ownership, housing tenure, proportion of unskilled workers) and then treated the considerable remaining variation between areas as being due to health service factors.

In general there seems to be a need for much more of this type of work, looking at the distribution of specific types of medical intervention or health care provision in relation to specified outcomes. Detailed studies should be conducted of primary, secondary and tertiary prevention. A broader picture of the role of health services in relation to inequalities in health in Europe can then be built up from these individual pieces of evidence. In addition, there is a need for national data to be routinely collected on the distribution of health care resources and of various health outcomes. Thus I suggest that, instead of asking the global question, 'Do health services matter for inequalities in health?', we should be asking, 'under what circumstances do which specific components of health care (whether at the primary, secondary or tertiary level of prevention) increase or decrease inequalities in which conditions between which social groups?'.

Inequalities in health care and in health in Europe

The remainder of this paper reviews some common themes emerging from papers presented to the 1984 WHO Meeting on the Health Burden of Social Inequities. Papers were prepared on 15 European countries.[5] Each author was asked to present material on: characteristics of the country and its health services; social inequalities in various measures of death, ill-health or self-reported health; and the availability and use of health services. They therefore appeared to comprise a reasonably comprehensive and up-to-date comparative source of data about inequalities in health care and health in Europe.

I started by attempting a systematic comparison between the data contained in each paper, but found this extremely difficult even for summary statistics for each country, and virtually impossible for any statistics about the distribution of care. The only datum available for nearly all the countries was the proportion of the population covered by compulsory health insurance or a state medical care system. Since for all the countries (except Ireland), well over 90 per cent of the total population is covered either by an insurance or state system,[6] this comparison was not particularly illuminating. I tried listing five summary statistics for all the countries; the percentage of GNP spent on health services, the number of physicians per 100,000 population, the number of hospital beds per 100,000 population, and life expectancy for males and females at birth. The problem with these comparisons for the purposes of this chapter is threefold: the absence of data from some countries; the non-comparability of some of the data (variations in how 'physician' or 'hospital bed' is defined, for example); and the fact that none of the material refers to the distribution of these variables across different social groups in the population. Thus, even if the missing data were found and the existing data made comparable, they would still not shed light on the question of inequalities in health or in health care. I therefore abandoned the attempt to compare figures across the countries, and instead I have picked out four themes that seemed to recur in several of the papers.

Regional variations in health care

Several papers mention regional disparities in the provision of care and either state or imply that these might generate or exacerbate regional variations in morbidity or mortality.

In the Federal Republic of Germany, hospital and physician services are distributed unequally between urban and rural localities. The sick funds provide more medical services per capita in urban areas than in rural areas, and the city districts of urban areas have a higher density of medical services than their rural outskirts (Gerhardt and Kirchgassler, 1986).

The urban–rural disparity is extremely marked in Greece. Seventy-two per cent of all specialists work in Athens or Thessalonika. There are 457.6 physicians per 100,000 population in Athens, and 436.3 in Thessalonika, compared with 125.8 in the rest of Greece; in Athens there are 9.5 hospital beds per 100 inhabitants compared to a range from 2.6 to 7.6 in the counties (Sokou, 1986). Ireland and Poland show a similar centralisation of physician services. In Ireland 49 per cent of all consultants (accredited specialists) practise in the Eastern Health Board Area, which includes Dublin. The ratio of paediatricians to the child population was 1: 15,300 in the Eastern Health Board District and 1:58,000 in the South East while nationally the ratio was 1:21,900 (O'Hare, 1986). While Poland has a relatively good overall number of physicians (18.8 per 10,000 population in 1983), there are widespread problems of maldistribution and shortage of physicians. There are reported to be 43.8 doctors per 10,000 population in Warsaw and 32.0 in Krakov, compared with 9.1 in Zamosc voivodship and 9.0 in Siedlice township (Sokolowska and Duch, 1986). Similarly, in Switzerland there are significant rural–urban differences in health care resources. While only 43.3 per cent of the population are urban residents, 68.4 per cent of all physicians and 82.3 per cent of specialists practise in urban areas (Haour-Knipe, 1986).

Other health care facilities are also distributed or used differentially between urban and rural areas. In Ireland only nine family planning clinics are licensed to provide information and advice on all methods of family planning, and only one of these is in a rural area, thus effectively confining access to family planning services to city dwellers (O'Hare, 1986). In Portugal more diagnostic tests (X-rays, ECGs, blood tests, etc.) are performed per capita on urban than rural residents: in 1981 the national average was 2.2 per person, while for Lisbon residents it was 4.0 and for the inhabitants of Braganca, 0.5. In 1979 10 per cent of deliveries in Portugal occurred without professional assistance. In Lisbon the percentage was 1.5 while in Villa Real, a rural Northern District, 43.6 per cent of deliveries were unassisted (Santos Lucas, 1984).

Such figures illustrate obvious regional disparities in the availability or use of certain types of health care, particularly between rural and urban areas. However, it is not clear what the implications are for regional variations in health. In the Federal Republic of Germany and in Greece, early mortality rates are higher in urban than in rural areas: between 1970 and 1980 neonatal mortality rates in Greece were 20.30/1,000 in urban areas, 13.06/1,000 in semi-urban areas and 12.06/1,000 in rural areas (Sokou, 1986). Is this because health services are concentrated in the cities, in spite of health services being concentrated in the cities, or quite unconnected? The issue becomes even more problematic when we learn that in Greece, at least, adult mortality has the opposite rural–urban gradient: in 1981 the mortality per 1,000 population was 7.57 in urban areas, 8.52 in semi-urban areas, and 11.32 in rural areas (Sokou, 1986).

Special groups

Most of the papers mention sub-groups of their national populations which are regarded as being especially vulnerable, either because of their lack of access to health care or because of their poor health.

In Belgium three sub-groups are singled out for special attention. The sub-proletariat have higher morbidity risks but have a lower consumption of medical care than the rest of the population, this underconsumption being attributed to ignorance, feelings of inferiority and financial barriers. Foreign workers have heightened risks of TB, VD, occupational diseases and work-related accidents, and it is suggested that they and the elderly (the third group mentioned), may have less access to health care (Van Wanseele, 1986).

In Greece there are 'hard-to-reach' populations within urban centres, composed of migrant workers, recent rural-to-urban migrants and ethnic minorities. 'These populations often live under disadvantaged conditions in polluted areas, often without adequate sanitation facilities, lacking knowledge about existing services and information about their health rights. As a consequence, they may receive even less adequate care than their rural counterparts' (Sokou, 1986).

In Ireland the young unemployed (31 per cent of those aged 15–24 were unemployed in February 1985), the elderly living alone, travellers,[7] single mothers, and the single homeless are singled out as groups at risk of particular health problems and for whom traditional medical approaches may not be appropriate (O'Hare, 1986).

Foreign workers, ethnic minorities and gypsies are mentioned in relation to several countries. In the Federal Republic of Germany women of non-German nationality, especially Turkish women, show poor utilisation of health services as well as higher perinatal mortality (Gerhardt and Kirchgassler, 1986). In Switzerland 14.2 per cent of the total population is foreign, comprising a mixture of refugees, seasonal migrant workers, longer-term migrant workers and upper-level management in international organisations. There are a number of problems relating to health and to health care among each of these groups (Haour-Knipe, 1986). In Israel, while only 2 per cent of the Jewish population is not covered by health insurance, 26 per cent of the non-Jewish population is not insured; there are higher rates of adult and infant mortality among the non-Jewish population than among the Jewish population (Shuval, 1986). In Hungary the difference between the Hungarian and the gypsy population in average duration of life is about 20 years for both sexes, to the gypsies' disadvantage (Csaszi, 1986).[8]

Similar groups are thus pinpointed in many countries as being problematic, either because their access to health care is legally, culturally or financially restricted, because they under-use available health care, or because they have particular health risks. It is not always clear, however, whether the focus is on inequalities in use of health care as an inequity which should *per se* be remedied, or whether the inequalities in health care are assumed to explain the observed health disadvantages of these groups.

Use of health services – secondary or tertiary services

Several countries report that people from lower social classes visit doctors more frequently than people in higher social classes, but that when morbidity is kept constant their consultation rates are relatively less than their higher-class counterparts. This is reported from Finland (Lahelma, 1986), Ireland (O'Hare, 1986), Portugal (Santos Lucas, 1984) and Sweden (Vagero, 1986).[9] In Portugal it is reported that working-class people are 2.3 times more frequently out of work, have a 2.1 times higher probability of being confined to bed because of illness, and more often have days of restricted activity, than people in the service class. Nevertheless the use of physician services by the Lisbon adult working-class population only exceeds that of the service class by 0.2 (Santos Lucas, 1984).

From the Federal Republic of Germany it is reported that persons whose income is less than 60 per cent of the national average visit physicians less frequently than those with higher incomes. On average their length of stay in hospital is longer, but they receive less specialised medical services (Gerhardt and Kirchgassler, 1986). In a 1976 survey in Finland special analyses were made of groups thought to be vulnerable because they used health services less than other segments of the population. These were the 8 per cent of the population living in remote rural areas, the 13 per cent active in agriculture and forestry, and the 20 per cent earning low incomes (there is substantial overlap between these). Respondents were asked about barriers to consultations with GPs; 45 per cent mentioned poor availability of GP services and 21 per cent mentioned financial barriers. A higher level of health care utilisation is reported in urban communities and in South Finland, as compared with rural areas and North Finland, and the authors comment that this does not correspond to the observed variations in morbidity or mortality, the highest death rates being found in the East, North, and in less developed areas (Lahelma, 1986).

In Israel, long-term care for the chronic sick is not covered by general health insurance. The elderly are in greatest need of long-term care or nursing facilities, which are only partially provided by public bodies; 24 per cent of such care is paid for directly by the elderly and their families. There are more doctor visits per capita among Jews than among non-Jews. In 1981, for males, the figures for visits per annum to general or family practitioners, internists or paediatricians were 6.0 for Jews and 1.8 for non-Jews. Thirty per cent of family expenditure on health in Israel goes to private practice. More affluent and Israeli-born families are more likely to use private health services (Shuval, 1986). In Poland too, the higher the educational level the more frequent is the use of private or cooperative forms of medical care as distinct from the state system (Sokolowaska and Duch, 1986).

Thus it is commonly reported from these European countries that lower social class people, or those with low incomes or little education, use physician services less than their higher-class counterparts, either absolutely or relative to some concept of need. Rural dwellers and ethnic minorities are, similarly, commonly reported to 'under-use' physician services. Unfortunately it is often not clear whether the relative under-use of physician services on the part of some group is being attributed to 'supply' factors, or to 'demand' factors, or to some combination of the two.[10]

Use of health services – *primary prevention*
Use of preventive health care (such as dental care, pre- or postnatal care and immunisation) is consistently reported to be associated with social class, income, and education.

In Belgium, for example, consumption of dental care is reported to be highly income-elastic (Van Wanseele, 1986). In Denmark the lower-income groups and lower social classes have the lowest dental care utilisation rates; 40 per cent of farmers and unskilled workers, 25 per cent of skilled workers and 12 per cent of lower white collar workers never go to the dentist (Holstein, 1984). In Greece significantly more dental health services are used by higher socio-economic strata; higher socio-economic groups use dental care primarily for preventive purposes, while lower socio-economic groups use them on an emergency basis (Sokou, 1986). In Israel dental care is hardly covered by health insurance and 92 per cent of the population are estimated to obtain dental care through private practitioners. Use of dental care is reported to be highly income-dependent (Shuval, 1986). Similarly, in Norway, dental care is provided on a fee-for-service basis and it is reported that 44 per cent of the lowest income group have their own teeth compared with 86 per cent of the highest income group (Maseide, 1986).

In Germany the Bremen/Lower Saxony Perinatal Mortality Study found significant differences between lower-class and middle- or upper-class women in physician contact during pregnancy (Gerhardt and Kirchgassler, 1986). Similarly, in Greece, social class is reported to be related to the use of prenatal health care (Sokou, 1986). In Israel prenatal and postnatal maternal and child care services are used almost universally, but use of other preventive or screening services shows a gradient by education, socio-economic status and ethnic origin (Shuval, 1986). Although only briefly mentioned in this collection of papers, it is worth noting here that health education campaigns and the provision of preventive services tend to be successful first among the more educated and advantaged groups of the population (Blaxter, 1983).

Use of preventive services rather than general medical care often forms a more obvious link between lower consumption and higher rates of morbidity or mortality, usually because both the preventive measures and the health outcomes are specified more closely (for example, the relationship between polio vaccine and incidence of polio, or between use of dental services and edentulousness). It also seems easier to determine the relative importance of supply and demand factors than it is for general medical care, since in many countries the supply of preventive services (for example, availability and cost of immunisations) is easier to measure.

Summary and conclusions

The question 'do inequalities in health care influence inequalities in health?', is an extremely difficult one to answer because of lack of comparable and relevant data and the existence of so many other factors that might be related to the distribution of health care or of health. Nevertheless, inequalities in health care and inequalities in health are often equated with each other in a rather uncritical fashion. From a practical point of view, it seems important to decide whether we are mainly interested in inequalities in health care *per se*, regarding these as wrong or inequitable on principle, or mainly interested in them as they might contribute to inequalities in health. If we are interested in the latter it is also important to distinguish between inequalities in health care that might generate inequalities in health in the first place (primary prevention), those that might influence cure or survival rates (secondary prevention), and those relating to rehabilitation or nursing care (tertiary prevention).

If we are mainly interested in some concept of justice involving equality of opportunity for health care then we may be content with one of the first four of Mooney's definitions of equity: equality of expenditure per capita, equality of inputs per capita, equality of input for equal need or equality of (opportunity of) access for equal need (1983). But if we are mainly concerned with producing equalities in health, or at least reducing inequalities in health, we have to recognise, from the experience of welfare states, that equalising access to care need not equalise either use of care or health. Indeed, those already healthy or wealthy may gain most from equally accessible health or welfare services (Le Grand, 1982). We would then need to adopt one of the last three of Mooney's definitions of equality; equality of utilisation for equal need, equality of marginal met need, or equality of health (1983). If we adopted any of these, we would be faced with three problems: firstly that we do not know how to reach these goals; secondly that they would involve very unequal distribution of resources; and thirdly that some of the causes of social differentiation in health are not only not caused by health service factors but also may not be remedied by them.

Certain common concerns emerge from a review of the European literature. In most countries there are disparities in the availability or use of all or some aspects of health care between urban and rural areas and between different social classes or socio-economic strata. In most cases, these disparities follow the 'inverse care law' (Tudor Hart, 1971) that is, those with higher morbidity or mortality rates have less care. The same is true of certain sub-groups of the population who are at high risk of ill-health and who have little contact with official health services – the sub-proletariat, ethnic minorities, migrant workers, gypsies, etc. Rarely, however, is the magnitude of the disparities in health care sufficient to explain the disparities in health or death rates. For other reasons, too, it is difficult to conclude that disparities in health care are a, or the, cause of the disparities in health,[11] not least because both use of health services and health may separately be related to third factors such as income, employment, or social integration, either at an individual or an aggregate level. There is a need for better national statistics on the distribution of health care and of various health 'outputs', and for further study of the circumstances in which health care could remedy inequalities in health.

Notes

1. It has further been extended by others to argue that health services can have an adverse effect on aggregate morbidity and mortality (Illich, 1976).
2. In theory, the ideal way of examining the effect of health services would be to

conduct randomised controlled trials. Given that people believe that health services do good and that individuals have a right of access to them, it is difficult to envisage consent being granted for such RCTs. I therefore do not discuss them further.

3. Unfortunately we are not told what happened to mortality from these 'avoidable' causes in countries in which health services expenditure had not increased over the period.

4. Apparently declining inequalities in health in some Scandinavian countries during the last 20 years have been attributed both to features of the health care system and to features of the socio-economic–political system (Blaxter, 1983). It is perfectly possible for shallow gradients in health, high health service coverage, and a certain socio-economic–political system to be related to each other and all be 'caused' by high per capita wealth.

5. Austria, Belgium, Denmark, Finland, France, Federal Republic of Germany, Greece, Hungary, Ireland, Israel, Norway, Poland, Portugal, Sweden and Switzerland.

6. Proportion of the population stated to be covered by health insurance or a national health service: Austria 99.5 per cent; Belgium 'virtually the entire population'; Denmark 95 per cent chose free medical care paid by health insurance'; F.R.G. 99.7 per cent; Finland 100 per cent; France 99.2 per cent (1982); Greece 95 per cent; Hungary 100 per cent; Ireland 38 per cent completely, 47 per cent mostly, 15 per cent partially covered; Israel 94.5 per cent (1984); Norway 100 per cent; Poland 100 per cent; Portugal not stated; Sweden 100 per cent; Switzerland 97.4 per cent (1982); UK 100 per cent.

7. Also known as tinkers or gypsies.

8. I am unclear from the paper whether the gypsy population has different entitlement or access to care compared with the rest of the population.

9. This is also true of the UK. Blaxter (1983) quotes a ratio of specialist consultation/perceived chronic illness (derived from the *General Household Survey*, 1976) of 1.56 in Social Class I compared with 0.49 in Social Class V. The British *Morbidity Statistics from General Practice 1970–71* shows, for all adults and all causes of death taken together, a much steeper social class gradient in Standardised Mortality Ratios than for Standardised Patient Consulting Ratios (RCGP, 1982). Blaxter (1984) offers a detailed analysis of these consultation data by social class, sex, and different conditions. She also provides a succinct review of the British debates on equity and consultation rates in general practice.

10. To a sociologist the concept of 'supply' and 'demand' sometimes appear artificially distinct when applied to health care, but I believe that Mooney (1983) is correct in emphasising the distinction as a means of clarifying what we mean by 'equity' in health care.

11. Readers will note that, although I have referred in general to 'health' throughout, nearly all the empirical examples have been of 'death' of some kind or another. This is awkward since, as Kohn and White point out, 'It is a moot point whether mortality is to be considered as an outcome of, or an input measure into, a health service system' (1976, 1979). However, if there is a paucity of comparable data on the distribution of mortality, there is an even greater dearth of comparable data on the distribution of health (Blaxter, 1985).

References

Aiach, P. (1986), 'France' in Illsley, R. and Svensson, P.G. *The Health Burden of Social Inequities*, Copenhagen: WHO.

Beaglehole, R. (1986), 'Medical management and the decline in mortality from coronary heart disease', *British Medical Journal*, **292**, pp. 33–5.

Black, Sir D. (1980), *Working Party on Inequalities in Health*, DHSS, London: HMSO.

Blaxter, M. (1983), 'Health services as a defence against the consequences of poverty in industrialised societies', *Social Science and Medicine*, 17 (16) pp. 1139–48.

Blaxter, M. (1984), 'Equity and consultation rates in general practice', *British Medical Journal*, 288, pp. 1963–67.

Charlton, J., Hartley, R., Silver, R. and Holland, W. (1983), 'Geographical variation in mortality from conditions amenable to medical intervention in England and Wales', *Lancet*, 26 March, pp. 691–996.

Charlton, J. and Velez, R. (1986), 'Some international comparisons of mortality amenable to medical interventions', *British Medical Journal*, 292, pp. 295–301.

Cochrane, A.L. (1972), *Effectiveness and Efficiency: Random Reflections on the NHS*, London: National Provincial Hospitals Trust.

Csaszi, L. (1986), 'Hungary' in Illsley, R. and Svensson, P.G. (eds), *The Health Burden of Social Inequities*, Copenhagen: WHO.

DHSS (1979), *Report on Confidential Enquiries into Maternal Deaths in England and Wales 1973–5*: London: HMSO.

Gerhardt, U. and Kirchgassler, K. (1986), 'Federal Republic of Germany' in Illsley, R. and Svensson, P.G. op. cit.

Goldthorpe, W.O. and Richman, J. (1974), 'Maternal attitudes to unintended home confinements', *Practitioner*, 212, p. 845.

Hall, M., Chng, P. and Macgillivray, I. (1980), 'Is routine antenatal care worthwhile?', *Lancet*, 12 July pp. 78–80.

Hall, M., Macintyre, S. and Porter, M. (1985), *Antenatal Care Assessed*, Aberdeen: Aberdeen University Press.

Haour-Knipe, M. (1986), 'Switzerland' in Illsley, R. and Svensson, P.G. op. cit.

Hemminki, E. (1983), 'Obstetric practice in Finland 1950–1980: changes in technology and its relation to health', *Medical Care*, 21, (12), pp. 1131–43.

Holstein, B.E. (1984), 'Denmark' in Illsley, R. and Svensson, P.G. op. cit.

Illich, I. (1976), *Medical Nemesis: The Expropriation of Health*, New York: Random House.

Illsley, R. and Svensson, P.G. (eds) (1986), *The Health Burden of Social Inequities*, Copenhagen: WHO.

Kohn, R. and White, K.L. (1976), *Health Care: An International Study Report of the WHO/International Collaborative Study of Medical Care Utilization*, London: Oxford University Press.

Lahelma, E. (1986), 'Finland' in Illsley, R. and Svensson, P.G. op. cit.

Le Grand, J. (1982), *The Strategy of Equality: Redistribution and the Social Services*, London: Allen & Unwin.

McIlwaine, G., Howat, R., Dunn, F. and Macnaughton, M. (1979), 'The Scottish Perinatal Mortality Survey', *British Medical Journal* 2 p. 1103.

Macintyre, S. (1986), 'The patterning of health by social position in contemporary Britain: directions for sociological research', *Social Science and Medicine*, 23 (4), pp. 393–415.

Mckeown, T. (1965), *Medicine in Modern Society*, London: Allen & Unwin.

Mckeown, T. (1976), *The Role of Medicine: Dream, Mirage or Nemesis*, London: Nuffield Provincial Hospitals Trust.

Maseide, P.C. (1986), 'Norway' in Illsley, R. and Svensson, P.G. op. cit.

Mather, H., Pearson, W.G., Read, K., Shaw D., Steed, G., Thorne M., Jones, S., Guerrier, C., Eraut, C., McHugh, P., Chowdhury, N., Jafary, M. and Wallace, T. (1971), 'Acute myocardial infarction: home and hospital treatment, *British Medical Journal*, 3, p. 334.

Mooney, G. (1983), 'Equity in health care: confronting the confusion', *Effective Health Care* 1 (4), pp. 179–84.

National Board of Health and Welfare, Sweden (1985), HS90: *The Swedish Health Services in the 1990s*, Stockholm: Liber Tryck.

O'Hare, A. (1986), 'Ireland' in Illsley, R. and Svensson, P.G. op.cit.

Pelikan, J.M. (1986), 'Austria' in Illsley, R. and Svensson, P.G. op. cit.

Royal College of General Practitioners, Office of Population Censuses and Surveys and

Department of Health and Social Security (1982), *Morbidity Statistics from General Practice 1970–71: Socio-Economic Analysis*, Studies on Medical and Population Subjects, **46**, HMSO.

Rutstein, D., Berenberg, W., Chalmers, T., Child, C., Fishman, A. and Perrin, E. (1976), 'Measuring the quality of medical care: a clinical method', *New England Journal of Medicine*, **294**, pp. 582–8.

Santos Lucas, J. (1984), 'Portugal', Paper prepared for the WHO Meeting on the Health Burden of Social Inequities, Copenhagen, 5–7 December.

Short, R. (1980), *Second Report from the Select Committee on the Social Services: Perinatal and Neonatal Mortality*, London: HMSO.

Shuval, J.T. (1986), 'Israel' in Illsley, R. and Svensson, P.G. op. cit.

Sokolowaska, M. and Duch, D. (1986), 'Poland' in Illsley, R. and Svensson, P.G. op. cit.

Sokou, K. (1986), 'Greece', Paper prepared for the WHO Meeting on the Health Burden of Social Inequities, Copenhagen: 5–7 December.

Tudor Hart, J. (1971), 'The Inverse Care Law', *Lancet* 1, p. 405.

Vagero, D. (1986), 'Sweden' in Illsley, R. and Svensson, P.G. op. cit.

Van Wanseele, C. (1986), 'Belgium' in Illsley, R. and Svensson, P.G. op. cit.

16 Class and tenure mobility: do they explain social inequalities in health among young adults in Britain?
K. Fogelman, A. J. Fox and C. Power

Abstract
We have used housing tenure as an index of socio-economic status in extending our previous analyses of the relationships between socio-economic differences in health at age 23 and socio-economic circumstances earlier in life. By focusing separately on subjects whose circumstances remained stable, we have investigated whether health-related social mobility occurs, its magnitude and its importance to net differences observed at age 23. These analyses support hypotheses that subjects who have been upwardly mobile between ages 16 and 23, in terms of social class or housing tenure, are on the whole healthier than those subjects who had been downwardly mobile. This was most marked for emotional health ('malaise') and self-rated health. Weaker evidence is found supporting hypotheses that young adults whose parents were upwardly mobile before the subject was 16 were healthier than those whose parents were not. These findings do not, however, explain the socio-economic differences observed at age 23. Indeed, the health of subjects whose circumstances were stable were found to differ between socio-economic groups as much as, if not more than, that of those who were mobile.

Introduction
The debate about mechanisms underlying social inequalities in health has gathered momentum since the publication of the *Black Report* (DHSS, 1980) and a new decennial supplement on occupational mortality (OPCS, 1986). Both reports contain evidence which suggests that differences in mortality between social classes are as wide, if not wider, now than at any time this century. The *Black Report* indicated that health differences between social classes are usually attributed to a combination of artefact, social selection, material circumstances and health behaviour. These groupings have been elaborated upon by a number of authors (for example, Carr-Hill, 1985; Illsley, 1986; Wilkinson, 1986). The debate is principally concerned with which explanation is the most important and what are the policy implications for those wishing to reduce these differences.

In an earlier paper, we suggested a model of influences upon an individual's health which incorporates a wide range of circumstances and experiences (Power *et al.*, 1986). These influences are grouped under the headings of 'inheritance' at birth, socio-economic circumstances, education and training, and health behaviour. A complex network of interactions is envisaged with causal paths operating within and between influences in both directions, not only between each set of factors, but also between each of them and the individual's health status. We also suggested that the relative weighting of each set of explanations should be expected to vary with the individual's age.

We have explored this model using data from the National Child Development Study (NCDS), a longitudinal study of a cohort of young adults born in one week in March 1958. This source allows us to look at relationships during childhood and early adulthood using a variety of different indicators of both socio-economic circumstances and health. Our previous paper investigated the contribution of selective social mobility to the development of inequalities in health in early adulthood. These preliminary analyses showed clear differences in health and health potential between social classes irrespective of whether class was measured at birth, at 16 or at 23 years of age. Social mobility within and between generations was related to height, but this did not explain the differences in height between social classes at age 23.

Here, these analyses are extended by focusing more closely on the health of specific groups of people who were either mobile or stable in terms of their social class. Analyses of social class differences in health at age 23 which controlled for social class in childhood are presented for a wider range of health indicators than published previously. We also investigate whether conclusions would be similar using housing tenure as an alternative indicator of socio-economic circumstances and social position during childhood and early adulthood. By broadening the range of health and socio-economic indicators used, we hope to obtain a clearer understanding of which conclusions might be more widely generalisable.

Subjects and methods
Sample and measures
The NCDS and most of the variables in these analyses have been described in detail in our previous paper and elsewhere (see Davie *et al.*, 1972; Fogelman, 1983; and Shepherd, 1985). NCDS is a longitudinal study of all people in Great Britain who were born in the week 3–9 March 1958. Following the original perinatal study (Butler and Bonham, 1963), the National Children's Bureau studied the cohort at ages 7, 11, 16 and 23. During the school years information

was obtained by means of parental interviews, medical examinations, school questionnaires, attainment tests and personal questionnaires. A substantial personal interview was conducted when the cohort was 23.

The present analyses draw on information about:

Socio-economic measures:

(a)   Social class at birth and 16, based on the father's occupation at the time of follow-up (individuals with no male head of household were excluded from the analyses);

(b)   Social class at 23, based on the subject's current or most recent occupation;

(c)   Housing tenure at 7, 16 and 23, classified as 'owner-occupier', local authority tenant', 'private rented tenant' or 'other' (information on housing tenure was not collected at birth);

Health measures:

(d)   Self-reported height at 23, summarised by the proportion who were 'short', defined here as falling below 1.676 metres for men and 1.524 metres for women – the lowest deciles for each sex.

(e)   'Malaise' inventory score, at 23 derived from a self-completed screening instrument on which scores of 7 or more have been suggested to indicate depression (see Rutter *et al.*, 1970; Rutter *et al.*, 1976);

(f)   Self-rated health at 23, described as either 'excellent', 'good', 'fair', or 'poor'; represented in the figures and tables as the proportion with the latter two responses;

(g)   Hospital admissions between the ages of 16 and 23 which involved an overnight stay on more than one occasion (reported by the subjects at 23); and

(h)   Psychiatric morbidity (but excluding mental handicap) between ages 16 and 23, derived from answers to questions in the 23-year interview on health problems which had required regular medical supervision, hospital admission, or specialist consultation.

Response patterns

A total of 12,537 people were successfully retraced and interviewed when they were 23. This represents 76 per cent of all those members of the study who were alive and still living in Britain. Analyses of response have been reassuring (see, for example, Shepherd, 1985). Those remaining in the study at age 23 tended to be more often from middle-class backgrounds, and to have grown up in smaller families and better housing circumstances. However, such contrasts with non-respondents are usually small. A more serious bias at age 23 is a substantial under-representation of those from ethnic minority backgrounds.

The data analysed here are drawn from several stages of the study. Only individuals with information on all relevant variables have been included and, as a result, there is a substantial reduction in the sample size. Response analyses demonstrate that subjects with information on relevant combinations of variables differ only trivially from the original cohort. For example, of the 16,969 individuals whose father's occupation at the time of their birth is known, 17.0 per cent were in Social Classes I or II, and 21.3 per cent were in Classes IV or V. Just over 8,000 subjects have complete social class data at birth, 16 and 23, of whom 16.9 per cent were in Classes I or II at birth and 21.0 per cent in Classes IV or V. Similarly, for those with data on housing tenure at ages 7, 16 and 23, 17.4 per cent were in Classes I or II and 20.6 per cent in Classes IV or V at birth.

Perhaps more surprisingly, there is little difference in response patterns according to whether the subjects' fathers were socially mobile. For example, of those whose fathers were in the same social class at the time of the subject's birth as when they were 16, 79.6 per cent have data on their own social class at 23. For those in a lower social class when the subject was 16 than at birth, 78.9 per cent have data at 23 as compared with 78.8 per cent for those who were in a higher social class.

Although such figures do not guarantee that the underlying relationships in which we are interested would not differ for those with missing data, they do suggest that this is unlikely.

Social mobility, stability and health
Social class at birth and at age 23
We have already shown the extent of mobility during childhood and subsequent intergenerational mobility (Power et al., 1986). The pattern to emerge which was of particular interest from the point of view of social mobility and health was the surprisingly high proportion of the sample who had stayed in the same social class at birth, 16 and 23. Of the 647 sons and 671 daughters of men in Social Classes I and II at the time of the child's birth, 336 (51.9 per cent) and 441 (65.7 per cent) were in Social Classes I and II at 16 and were in nonmanual occupations at 23. Nearly one-third (589) of the 1,902 sons of fathers in Social Class IIIM at birth were in Social Class IIIM at 16 and 23. Nearly one-third of the daughters of men in this class at their birth remained in the class until 16 and were subsequently found in Social Class IIIN.

The relationship of health and health potential to social mobility was also examined in this earlier analysis and clear differences were

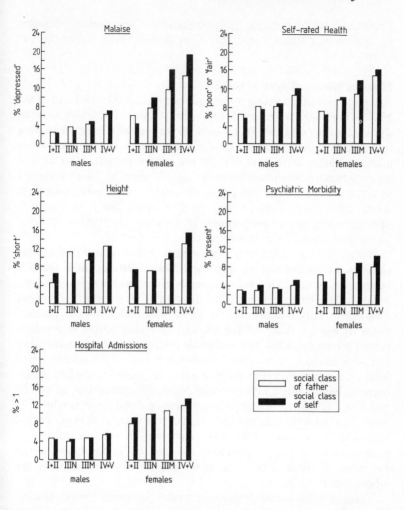

Figure 16.1 Differences in malaise, self-rated health, height, psychiatric morbidity and hospital admissions measured by own social class at age 23 and by father's occupation.

found, irrespective of whether social class was measured by father's occupation at the time of birth or by own social class at age 23. Those in lower, less skilled social classes reported worse health at 23 for most of the health indicators (see Figure 16.1). The differences observed for malaise, self-rated health and height appeared to be greater than those found for psychiatric morbidity and hospital admissions. Differences were greater and more consistent for women than men.

For most health measures, excluding height, they appeared stronger in relation to current social class than in relation to social class at birth.

Housing tenure at ages 7 and 23

Although parental housing tenure was not recorded at the birth of the NCDS member, from age 7 onwards it suggests marked stability during childhood (Table 16.1). Over 90 per cent of subjects who were in owner-occupied accommodation at age 7 were in owner-occupied accommodation at 16, and over 80 per cent of subjects who were in local authority accommodation at age 7 were in local authority accommodation at 16. Parents in privately rented accommodation when the cohort member was aged 7 were likely to move in approximately equal proportions into owner occupation or local authority tenure by the time their child was aged 16.

While, during childhood, the category 'other' comprised mainly subjects in institutions or accommodation tied to their parent's occupation, at age 23 it consisted mainly of respondents who were still living in their parental home. Classification by own tenure is therefore meaningful only when based on those who had left their parents' home by age 23. Also, for the majority of young people in privately rented accommodation this would be a transient situation and they can be expected to have moved subsequently into owner occupation or local authority tenure. For these reasons, our analyses of relationships between health and health potential and housing tenure at ages 7, 16 and 23 are restricted to comparisons between those subjects who at 23 were already owner-occupiers or local authority tenants (33 per cent of men and 55 per cent of women). However, in view of differences between socio-economic groups in the rates of leaving home and in marrying (Kiernan, 1986), this is not a representative sample of the whole cohort.

Turning now to differences in health between tenure groups, Figure 16.2 shows marked and consistent differences between owner-occupiers and local authority tenants for the five health measures used in our earlier work, with owner-occupiers having generally better health at 23. The only exception to this is psychiatric morbidity for men classified by housing tenure at age 7. Otherwise, differences appear to be similar to the social class differences shown in Figure 16.1. In general, housing tenure at age 23 is a better discriminator of health than housing in childhood, with the exception of height. As in Figure 16.1, the greatest differences are observed for malaise and self-rated health, and for female rather than male subjects. Although part of the differences between young men and young women may be related to the relative proportions of each sex in local authority and

Table 16.1 Housing tenure at ages 7, 16 and 23 by sex (number with complete data)

Tenure	Tenure at 16	Men					Women				
		O.O.	L.A.	P.R.	Other	Total	O.O.	L.A.	P.R.	Other	Total
				Tenure at 23					Tenure at 23		
O.O.	O.O.	361	69	253	922	1605	657	100	275	566	1598
	L.A.	19	8	8	35	70	29	23	4	25	81
	P.R.	5	3	6	18	32	10	5	10	9	34
	Other	3	2	2	6	13	12	1	4	2	19
	Total	388	82	269	983	1720	708	129	293	602	1732
L.A.	O.O.	81	21	32	131	265	125	28	28	64	245
	L.A.	257	235	132	695	1319	445	399	138	402	1384
	P.R.	9	0	3	7	19	8	10	3	5	26
	Other	10	7	2	5	24	9	4	3	8	24
	Total	357	263	169	838	1627	587	441	172	479	1679
P.R.	O.O.	37	12	16	72	137	61	12	26	34	133
	L.A.	42	30	12	68	152	48	37	20	52	157
	P.R.	27	10	10	77	124	49	20	15	32	116
	Other	3	4	2	22	31	14	2	4	12	32
	Total	109	56	40	239	444	172	71	65	130	438
Other	O.O.	11	1	4	12	28	10	3	6	8	27
	L.A.	2	5	1	9	17	5	13	2	7	27
	P.R.	4	1	0	5	10	6	0	1	2	9
	Other	8	7	4	20	39	12	11	5	9	37
	Total	25	14	9	46	94	37	27	14	26	100
Total	O.O.	490	103	305	1137	2035	853	143	335	672	2003
	L.A.	320	278	153	807	1558	527	472	164	486	1649
	P.R.	45	14	19	107	185	73	35	29	48	185
	Other	24	20	10	53	107	47	18	16	31	112
	Total	879	415	487	2104	3885	1500	668	544	1237	3949

Notes: O.O – Owner-occupied
L.A – Local authority tenure
P.R – Privately rented

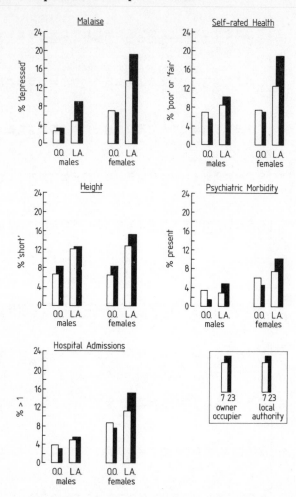

Figure 16.2   Differences in health between owner – occupiers and local authority tenants at age 23

owner-occupier housing at age 23, the similarity with observations by social class lends some credence to this pattern.

Similar patterns of differences in health are observed when subjects are classified by socio-economic status early in childhood and at age 23, but with generally more distinct differences by status at 23 than in childhood. We now explore what patterns are observed for subjects whose socio-economic status remained stable and for those who were upwardly or downwardly mobile.

In what follows, we use the term 'stable' to refer to those whose

Table 16.2   Health at age 23 of those with stable social class at birth, 16 and 23

| Health indicator | Social class at birth, 16 and 23 | | | | | |
| | Men | | | Women | | |
	I +II (n=288)	IIIM (n=595)	IV + V (n=115)	I + II (n=209)	IIIM/N (n=631)	IV + V (n=115)
Height (% 'short')	2.7	11.9	13.0	5.3	9.4	19.2
Self-rated health (% 'poor' or 'fair')	4.8	9.1	11.3	4.8	8.6	15.2
Hospital admissions (% > 1)	3.5	3.7	5.2	6.2	8.6	12.8
Malaise (% 'depressed')	2.2	3.7	9.6	3.4	9.8	25.0
Psychiatric morbidity (% present)	3.5	2.7	5.2	4.8	5.2	8.8

class or tenure was the same across various combinations of points in their childhood (birth and 16 for class, 7 and 16 for tenure) and at 23 – the exact combination depending on whether we are examining stability during childhood or intergenerationally. Similarly, 'mobility' is used when class or tenure differed on these occasions. It must be acknowledged that this overlooks any additional changes which may have taken place between these points, but it seems reasonable to assume that other changes would not be substantial enough to alter our conclusions.

The stable
Table 16.2 compares the health of those subjects in Social Classes I and II at birth, 16 and 23 with those in Social Classes IV and V. For men, those in Class IIIM at each age are also presented. Since labour market opportunities for young women are different, data are presented for female subjects whose fathers were in Class IIIM during the subject's childhood and who were themselves in Class IIIN. For each of the health indicators the patterns are as expected with stronger differences in malaise, self-rated health and height than in psychiatric morbidity and hospital admissions, and more marked differences for women than for men.

Similar analyses are presented in Table 16.3 for subjects whose socio-economic circumstances, measured in terms of housing tenure, were stable during childhood and early adulthood. These suggest

Table 16.3   Health at age 23 of those subjects with stable tenure at ages 7, 16 and 23

Health indicator	Men		Women	
	Owner-occupiers (n=361)	Local authority tenants (n=235)	Owner-occupiers (n=657)	Local authority tenants (n=399)
Height (% 'short')	6.4	12.9	5.5	18.0
Self-rated health (% 'poor or fair')	5.0	9.8	5.6	20.4
Hospital admissions (% > 1)	3.9	7.2	7.9	16.3
Malaise (% 'depressed')	2.2	9.8	5.5	21.6
Psychiatric morbidity (% present)	1.1	2.1	4.3	11.0

similar patterns of differences to those found when social class was used as the index of socio-economic status.

It should be noted from Tables 16.2 and 16.3 that, despite the fact that our tenure analyses are restricted to local authority tenants and owner-occupiers, the numbers in the stable groups are substantially greater than when Social Classes I and II are compared with Social Classes IV and V. Nevertheless, the differences between these two tenure groups are generally of similar magnitude to those between the extreme social classes.

The intergenerationally mobile

The above analyses indicate that broadly similar observations about socio-economic differences in health and health potential are apparent when analyses are restricted to those subjects whose socio-economic circumstances remained stable during their childhood and early adulthood as when differences are presented by characteristics at birth or at age 23 for the whole sample. It may be the case, nevertheless, that subjects whose socio-economic circumstances changed had different patterns and that these patterns contribute to the overall differences observed.

We consider first those whose own social class at age 23 was different to that of their fathers during their childhood. In order to

Table 16.4   Health at age 23 and intergenerational mobility from Social Class IIIM

| Health indicator | Mobility between social class in childhood* and age 23 | | | | | |
| | Men | | | Women | | |
	Upwards (n=194)	Stable (n=595)	Down-wards (n=231)	Upwards (n=210)	Stable (n=631)	Down-wards (n=264)
Height (% 'short')	5.2	11.9	12.3	10.0	9.4	14.8
Self-rated health (% 'poor' or 'fair')	4.1	9.1	13.4	5.2	8.6	16.3
Hospital admissions (% > 1)	5.2	3.7	7.8	11.9	8.6	12.9
Malaise (% 'depressed')	1.5	3.7	7.4	6.2	9.8	16.7
Psychiatric morbidity (% present)	3.6	2.7	6.5	3.8	5.2	10.6

*Includes those in Class IIIM at birth and age 16.

hold constant the effect of father's social class, we focus on those whose fathers were in Class IIIM when the subject was born, and were still in the same class when the subject was 16. We then look at the health differences observed according to the pattern of intergenerational mobility (Table 16.4).

For both young men and young women, those in a higher social class at 23 than during their childhood reported better health than those in a lower social class at 23 than during childhood. For comparison, those in Class IIIM (IIIN for women at 23) throughout their lives are shown again in Table 16.4, and it can be seen that usually, but not always, they fall between the upwardly and downwardly mobile. For young men, the largest differences are for malaise, self-rated health and height; for young women they are for malaise, self-rated health and psychiatric morbidity.

These data confirm that intergenerational mobility is associated with differences in the health of upwardly and downwardly mobile groups. For men, the magnitude of these differences is generally similar to those observed in Table 16.2 between subjects who remained stable to age 23. For women, the differences observed for height, hospital admissions and malaise are substantially wider for the stable than the mobile, but for psychiatric morbidity they are greater for the mobile.

In our analyses based on intergenerational changes in tenure, we

Table 16.5   Health at age 23 of those whose tenure changed between childhood and 23

Health indicator	Tenure mobility between childhood and age 23			
	Men		Women	
	Upward* (n=257)	Downward+ (n=69)	Upward* (n=447)	Downward+ (n=100)
Height (% 'short')	9.4	10.5	10.8	8.1
Self-rated health (% 'poor or fair')	4.7	10.1	7.6	15.0
Hospital (% > 1)	2.3	2.9	7.0	13.0
Malaise (% 'depressed')	3.9	5.8	7.7	15.0
Psychiatric morbidity (% present)	0.8	8.7	4.7	9.0

* From local authority housing at ages 7 and 16 to owner-occupier at 23.
+ Fom owner-occupier housing at ages 7 and 16 to local authority at 23.

define upward mobility in terms of movement from local authority tenure to owner occupation and downward mobility as movement from owner occupation to local authority tenure.

In Table 16.5, there is no obvious evidence that downwardly mobile subjects are shorter than upwardly mobile subjects. Equally there is little difference in the proportions of upwardly and downwardly mobile men who had had more than one hospital admission. However, for other health indicators there are clear differences to support the hypothesis that subjects who were upwardly mobile between 16 and 23 were healthier at age 23 than those who were downwardly mobile.

However, the patterns in Table 16.5 are slightly different from those in Table 16.4. With the exception of men with psychiatric morbidity, the health differences between the mobile groups in terms of housing tenure tend to be smaller than for those groups which were mobile in terms of social class.

The mobile during childhood

So far, we have concentrated on intergenerational mobility, but the health of those whose parents were mobile during the subject's childhood is also of interest. Again, in the analysis of differences between social classes we focus only on those whose fathers were in Social Class IIIM in 1958. Table 16.6 is further restricted to young

Table 16.6 *Health at age 23 and social mobility during childhood for those in Class IIIM at birth and at 23* only*

Health indicator	Mobility between birth and age 16					
	Men			Women		
	Upwards (n=101)	Stable (n=595)	Down-wards (n=147)	Upwards (n=157)	Stable (n=631)	Down-wards (n=133)
Height (% 'short')	3.0	11.9	13.6	6.4	9.4	7.5
Self-rated health (% 'poor' or 'fair')	6.0	9.1	8.8	12.1	8.6	9.7
Hospital admissions (% > 1)	5.0	3.7	5.4	12.1	8.6	12.8
Malaise (% 'depressed')	3.0	3.7	4.1	6.4	9.8	9.8
Psychiatric morbidity (% present)	1.0	2.7	3.4	4.5	5.2	4.5

*Class IIIN for women at age 23.

men in Social Class IIIM and young women in Social Class IIIN at 23. This table shows health differences at 23 according to whether the father was in a higher, the same or a lower class when the subject was 16 than at the time of the subject's birth. The middle columns for each sex represent those subjects who were in this class at birth, 16 and 23, as in Tables 16.2 and 16.4.

The numbers of subjects experiencing upward mobility during their childhood is understated here because we have attempted to control for class at age 23 by restricting this analysis to those who, at 23, were in the equivalent class to that of their fathers when they were born. As shown in our previous paper, this is the most common experience. Within this restricted group, the differences in health between those subjects whose fathers were upwardly mobile and those who were downwardly mobile are relatively small (Table 16.6). The single exception is the proportion of young men who were short, which was substantially greater for those whose fathers were down-wardly mobile. For each of the other health measures, suggestions of better health for those subjects whose parents were upwardly mobile, as compared with those whose parents were downwardly mobile, are weak.

In terms of housing tenure we have compared the health at age 23 of subjects whose parents moved to and from owner occupation from when the subject was 7 to when they were 16 (Table 16.7). The only

Table 16.7   Health at age 23 of those whose tenure changed during childhood

| Health indicator | Tenure mobility between ages 7 and 16 | | | |
| | Men | | Women | |
	Upwards* (n=430)	Downwards+ (n=115	Upwards* (n=405)	Downwards+ (n=134)
Height (% 'short')	11.2	11.4	8.2	15.8
Self-rated health (% 'poor or fair')	9.8	10.4	10.6	15.0
Hospital admissions (% > 1)	4.0	1.7	11.4	10.5
Malaise (% 'depressed')	2.8	3.5	7.7	14.4
Psychiatric morbidity (% present)	4.9	7.0	6.2	9.0

* Owner-occupiers at 16 but not at age 7.
+ Owner-occupiers at 7 but not at age 16.

suggestion that men benefited from upward mobility during childhood is in the difference in the proportions with psychiatric morbidity between 16 and 23, but these differences are small in comparison with those noted in Table 16.5. Table 16.7 does, however, suggest that women whose parents moved into owner occupation were indeed healthier than those whose parents moved out of owner occupation.

These analyses of health in early adulthood and parental mobility appear to conflict in many respects. In both Tables 16.6 and 16.7 there is weak evidence supporting the suggestion that subjects whose parents were upwardly mobile during childhood tended to be taller and healthier at 23 than those whose parents were downwardly mobile. However, the patterns are inconsistent for each sex and for individual health indicators. To illustrate, use of social class suggested that, in terms of height, men benefited from the upward mobility of their parents – but not women; the opposite was the case when tenure was used as the index of socio-economic status. For women, the patterns appear much weaker in relation to social class than to tenure, but for men, with the exception of height, they are equally weak for both measures.

The explanation for these differences may well lie in the select groups on which we have focussed in these analyses. For social class we have ignored here the height and health of subjects born in social classes other than IIIM, ie nearly half the population. Similarly for tenure our analyses are based on an unrepresentative sub-set of the population (those who had moved out of the parental home), though less so for women than for men.

Health at age 23 controlling for circumstances in childhood
The foregoing has demonstrated some relationships between social mobility and health in early adulthood. The question still remains of the extent to which these relationships explain the social gradient in health at age 23. In this section we attempt to answer this by standardising the relationship between social position at 23 and health at 23 for earlier social position. This has been shown previously for one health measure only – that is height.

As regards the other measures, standardisation for earlier circumstances results in some reduction in the gradient at age 23, but this is by no means always substantial. For instance, ratios of observed and expected 'depressed' men were 0.56 and 1.62 in Social Classes I and II combined, and IV and V respectively. This narrowed to 0.65 and 1.45 after taking account of father's social class at birth and age 16. Controlling for earlier social class had not therefore totally 'explained' the class differences in the proportions of men 'depressed'.

The extent to which this applied to both sexes and each of the health and socio-economic measures is demonstrated in Table 16.8, which provides summary indices of the crude and standardised ratios. The index used, the Index of Dissimilarity (ID), measures the proportion of all cases which would need to be redistributed among the classes or tenure groups in order to achieve equal rates for all groups (Preston *et al.*, 1981). It is calculated from the following formula:

$$\text{Index of Dissimilarity} = \Sigma_i \frac{IO_i - E_i}{\Sigma O_i + \Sigma E_i}$$

Where O_i and E_i are the numbers of cases observed and expected in each category and summation is over all categories used in the comparison.

A limitation of this index is the lack of any measurement of direction of inequality. The index can, for example, give the same answer when differences between socio-economic groups favour the better-off or poorer groups, or even when there is no systematic pattern to the differences. This limitation is not critical here since the gradients are generally clear, from better health in Classes I and II to poorer health in Classes IV and V and, similarly, from owner-occupiers to local authority tenants (see Figures 16.1 and 16.2).

It should also be appreciated that the index weights according to the size of the groups being compared. In the case of the social class

Table 16.8   Index of dissimilarity, by sex and health indicator at age 23: crude and standardised* for socio-economic circumstances during childhood

Health indicator	Tenure		Social class	
	Men	Women	Men	Women
Height (% 'short')				
crude	8.9%	14.7%	12.1%	14.8%
standardised	5.2%	9.5%	7.1%	10.8%
Self-reported health (% 'poor' or 'fair')				
crude	15.2%	23.9%	9.8%	12.7%
standardised	14.0%	19.2%	7.9%	10.4%
Hospital admissions (%>1)				
crude	18.9%	14.3%	5.9%	6.8%
standardised	18.5%	12.5%	3.9%	6.0%
Malaise (% 'depressed')				
crude	26.6%	27.1%	16.6%	17.3%
standardised	23.0%	21.0%	11.8%	14.6%
Psychiatric morbidity (% present)				
crude	39.9%	19.9%	8.1%	11.8%
standardised	43.6%	18.4%	7.5%	10.6%

* Standardisation is based on data obtained at birth and age 16 for Social Class and age 7 and 16 for tenure.

analysis, the largest groups are IIIM for men and IIIN for women. Since these are at the centre of the scale this property will tend to make the index relatively less sensitive to the values in the extreme groups. This limitation has to be taken into account when interpreting Table 16.8. The measure does have the advantage of using rates for all social classes and tenure groups, rather than, as is commonly practiced, just comparing the extremes.

The crude ID shown in Table 16.8, summarises the class and tenure differences shown in Figures 16.1 and 16.2 for the five indicators used throughout these analyses. The standardised ID is based upon the rates that would be expected from the distribution of, respectively, social class at birth and 16, and tenure at 7 and 16. The table therefore shows the effect of controlling for social position in childhood, and further, it provides an indication of the proportion of inequality in health at age 23, which can be 'explained' by social position earlier in childhood.

Standardisation almost always reduces the ID, the single exception being psychiatric morbidity in men in relation to tenure. However, the reduction is rarely substantial.

It does appear that social gradients in height, and to a lesser extent 'malaise', are partially explained by the relationship with earlier circumstances, but the gradients of the other three measures of health considered here are almost independent of any additional effects of social position during childhood.

Discussion

In this chapter we have built upon the preliminary ideas and results presented in our earlier paper (Power *et al.*, 1986). By using housing tenure as an index of socio-economic status we overcome, at least in part, limitations arising from earlier use of social class alone. Housing tenure is itself limited by the relatively small, and biased, fraction of the cohort who by age 23 had already formed their own household; and also by the likelihood that subjects in privately rented accommodation would have moved to owner occupation or local authority tenure within a few years of the 1981 interview. The biases introduced in the tenure analyses are, however, different from those in analyses based on social class. In particular, there is a tendency for those in the most disadvantaged circumstances to marry and to set up their own household earlier in life than those from advantaged backgrounds, and consequently to feature in these analyses. As an illustration, subjects brought up by lone mothers would, if they had left home by age 23, be included in the analyses of tenure, but not of social class.

On the other hand, young women leave home earlier than young men, and this may confound some of the sex differences observed in the tenure analyses with differences which might be associated with earlier marriage and household formation.

The analyses we have presented do, nevertheless, make clearer the extent to which selective social mobility, as described by Stern (1983), might influence relationships between socio-economic circumstances and health. Our analyses of health differences at age 23 supported hypotheses that subjects who had been upwardly mobile, in terms of social class or housing tenure, between ages 16 and 23 were on the whole healthier than those who had been downwardly mobile. This was most marked and consistent for malaise and self-rated health. This conclusion is not likely to be affected by differences in the social origins of the mobile, since class of origin was held constant by limiting the analysis to those born to fathers in Class IIIM. It remains possible, however, that different patterns could be found for those mobile from other social classes.

Evidence for a relationship between mobility of parents and socio-economic differences in the health of their children when they are young adults was less marked than the findings associated with intergenerational mobility. Again, there were inconsistencies: malaise among women, and to a lesser extent psychiatric morbidity, varied with mobility during childhood to a greater degree than other health indicators. The present analyses do not, however, rule out the possibility that differences in health may have been found if we had used other measures of health at 23, or health in childhood.

Overall, the evidence presented here, demonstrating the relationship between mobility and socio-economic differences in health at age 23, does not necessarily mean that mobility explains differences in health at 23. These differences must first be compared with those observed for subjects whose socio-economic circumstances remained relatively stable throughout childhood and early adulthood. This is a large group for whom health inequalities are not influenced by mobility. It is striking to note, therefore, that the gradients observed for this group were generally as large as, if not larger than, those between subjects who had been upwardly or downwardly mobile, inter- or intragenerationally.

For social mobility to be an important determinant of inequalities in health at 23, those who were mobile would need to be substantially different in terms of health at 23 from those who were stable, not just different from the group they were leaving but also different from the group they were joining. At the same time they would need to be numerous enough to influence the weighted averages. Although the upwardly mobile tend to be healthier than the downwardly mobile, the analyses we have performed thus far suggest that the differences between the incomers to the extreme groups and those who had always been in the extreme groups are not such as to determine the differences between the extreme groups, irrespective of the numbers who are mobile.

This is most clearly shown by our analyses which standardised gradients at age 23 for social circumstances during childhood. For most of the five health measures there was a reduction in the gradient, but there remained substantial differences in health at 23 which were not explained by the relationship with earlier social position.

Although the general direction of our findings is reasonably consistent, it is important to note that there are significant variations in detail according to which social measure or health measure was used, and between the sexes. Leon (1988), in a recent analysis of the social distribution of cancer, and Blaxter, in Chapter 10, have explained how indicators may represent different dimensions of socio-economic circumstances and health, respectively, and this is likely to be relevant to the measures used here. Consequently, some variation between the measures was to be expected. In particular, there was frequently a contrast between the patterns found in relation to height — a measure used in many studies as an indicator of general health in age groups up to early adulthood — and the other four health measures. In fact it is not surprising that a greater proportion of the differences in height between classes and tenure groups is explained by earlier circumstances. The other four health indicators can be taken to represent the more recent health experience of these young adults. Adult height, on the other hand, is likely to have been largely determined several years earlier, and thus be more influenced by earlier events and circumstances; genetic influences are also likely to have been greater (Foster *et al.*, 1983).

Social inequalities in height, and to a lesser extent malaise in early adulthood, appear from our analyses so far to be partially explained by social position in childhood. This is not so for hospital admissions, self-reported health or psychiatric morbidity. However, these are not yet firm conclusions. There are other aspects of childhood experience, such as family situation and size, which may influence the patterns we have found.

We have continued to use simple statistical approaches at this exploratory stage. However, it is already clear that, as soon as we complicate our 'model' further, and wish to quantify effects more precisely, more sophisticated multivariate approaches will be needed. In our further work we will build upon the tentative findings presented here and examine the mediating role of educational attainment between childhood circumstances, social position in adulthood and health, as well as the significance of health in childhood which must be expected to be a major influence on educational and occupational achievement and adult health.

Acknowledgements
This project on health and social mobility during the early years of life is funded by DHSS (Grant JS240/85/8). ESRC support for the NCDS User Support Group at City University is covered by Grant HO4250001. We are pleased to acknowledge both these sources.

References
Butler, N.R. and Bonham, D.G. (1963), *Perinatal Mortality*, Edinburgh: Livingston.

Carr-Hill, R.A. (1985), 'Health and income: a longitudinal study of four-hundred families', *Quarterly Journal of Social Affairs*, 1 (4), pp. 295–307.

Davie, R., Butler, N.R. and Goldstein, H. (1972), *From Birth to Seven*, London: Longman in association with National Children's Bureau.

Department of Health and Social Security (1980), *Inequalities in Health*, Report of a Research Working Group.

Fogelman, K. (ed.) (1983), *Growing up in Great Britain*, London: Macmillan.

Foster, J.M., Chinn, S. and Rona, R.J. (1983), 'The relation of the height of primary school children to population density', *International Journal of Epidemiology*, 2, pp. 199–204.

Illsley, R. (1986), 'Occupational class, selection and the production of inequalities in health', Quarterly Journal of Social Affairs. 2 (2), pp. 151–65.

Kiernan, K.E. (1986), *Transitions in Young Adulthood*, Proceedings of the British Society for Population Studies Conference on Population Research in Britain.

Leon, D.A. (1988), *The Social Distribution of Cancer. Longitudinal Study 1971–1975*, Series LS no. 3, London: HMSO.

OPCS (1986), *Occupational Mortality Decennial Supplement 1979–80 1982–83*, Series DS no. 6, HMSO.

Power, C., Fogelman, K. and Fox, A.J. (1986), 'Health and social mobility during the early years of life', *Quarterly Journal of Social Affairs*, 2 (4), pp. 397–413.

Preston, S.H., Haines, M.R. and Pamuk, E.R. (1981), 'Effects of industrialisation and urbanisation on mortality in developed countries' in *Solicited Papers*, 2, IUSSP 19th International Population Conference, Manila 1981, Liege.

Rutter M., Tizard, J. and Whitmore, K. (1970), Education, Health and Behaviour, London: Longman.

Rutter, M., Tizard, J., Yule, W. and Graham, P. (1976), 'Isle of Wight studies: 1964–1974'. *Psychological Medicine*, 6, pp. 313–32.

Shepherd, P. (1985), *The National Child Development Study: An introduction to the background to the study and the methods of data collection*, NCDS Working Paper no. 1, Social Statistics Research Unit, City University.

Stern, J. (1983), 'Social mobility and the interpretation of social class mortality differentials', *Journal of Social Policy*, 12 (1), pp. 27–49.

Wilkinson, R.G. (1986), 'Socio-economic differences in mortality: interpreting the data on their size and trends' in Wilkinson R.G. (ed.), Class and Health: Research and Longitudinal Data, London: Tavistock.

17 Steps towards explaining social differentials in morbidity: the case of West Germany
Johannes Siegrist

Introduction

Confronting the confusion about the issue of equity in health, we should first state what we are not talking about. Taking Mooney's distinctions of equity (Mooney, 1983) we obviously do not talk about equal health expenditures per capitum nor do we consider equal costs of health care under comparable health need. However, it seems that three dimensions of equity in health are of special importance in the area of morbidity and mortality differentials in developed industrialised countries:

1. equal health resources available for different socio-economic groups under conditions of comparable need for health care;
2. equal utilisation of health resources by different socio-economic groups under conditions of comparable need for health care;
3. equal exposure of different socio-economic groups to health hazards, and equal resistance.

Explaining social differentials in morbidity/mortality within a country means separating the effects of these three conditions as far as possible. As these conditions are located at different levels (institutional, societal, individual), it is difficult to compute respective information in a meaningful way.

This chapter concentrates on material of one industrialised western country: the Federal Republic of Germany (FRG). It first shows that few, if any, social differentials in morbidity/mortality are expected to result from unequal health resources available under conditions of comparable need for health care. This leaves the two other dimensions (utilisation, exposure and resistance) as the two major predicting areas. The second section focuses on current sociological knowledge on social differentials in utilisation behaviour in the FRG. Although conclusions may be preliminary, it seems that different utilisation patterns are not able to explain morbidity/mortality differentials in a substantial way, at least for the last 20 years.

In the third section, the main section of this chapter, we first deal with types of data and concept available in explaining different health hazards. We then present selected socio-epidemiologic results on differentials in morbidity (and partly mortality) from selected diseases. The chapter ends with a set of conclusions relating to conceptual and methodological weaknesses in the current state of knowledge as well as with suggestions for further scientific developments in the field.

Health resources in the Federal Republic of Germany

West Germany is a country with a long tradition of social security programmes. In the nineteenth century sickness funds for workers were already established, and social security programmes were expanded to include risks such as early retirement, unemployment and widowhood. Several legal reforms improved the situation for underprivileged socio-economic groups, first in 1911, and especially after the Second World War. Since the late 1950s more than 90 per cent of the population have been covered by public health insurance, and there is free access to a medical care system with one of the highest proportions of physicians available. Screenings for several cancers and preventive services during pregnancy and early childhood were introduced during the 1960s, after a period of nationwide build-up of rehabilitation programmes for the sick working population. Efforts were made by occupational medicine to minimise detrimental effects of toxic substances at work, and public preventive activities, including large vaccination programmes, were established. The numbers of physicians and nurses, hospital beds and private practices increased considerably and the socio-political movement during the late 1960s and early 1970s transformed social policy into a very expansive welfare state. Thus conditions in general seemed to be favourable to health for all by the year 2000, especially since economic prosperity persisted for about 30 years.

Indicators of wealth such as mean income, job availability and security, good housing conditions (including sanitary facilities and heating), potential for recreation, hobbies, travelling etc. suggest that this welfare system has positive effects on health and on life expectancy during adulthood.

Figures 17.1 and 17.2 give crude information on survival curves for males and females in 1871–80, 1949–50 and 1977–79 in West Germany. It can be seen that the last 30 years still had a remarkable effect on the survival of men under age 70 and of women in all age-groups. In addition, it can be seen that trends toward 'rectangular' shape are stronger in women than in men, and stronger in the late 1970s than earlier, whereas by the age of 85–90 only small effects are left for the development during the last 100 years (which supports the notion of biological determinants of life in old age – i.e. with a

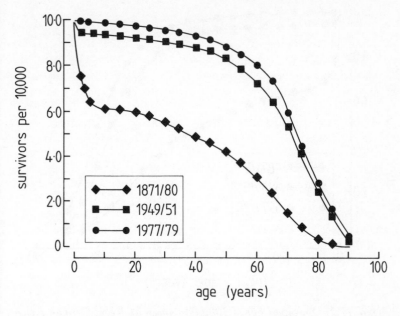

Figure 17.1 Survivors out of 100,000 men at age x: German Reich 1871–80, Federal territory 1949–51, Federal Republic of Germany 1977–79

Source: Schach, E., 1983.

maximum of between 85 and 100 years). Avoidable mortality thus essentially relates to premature death in middle adulthood as well as in advanced age up to 85 years.

Although a closer look at the West German health care system would require much more space, we think that the following information is essential for an evaluation of the present situation. In 1983, 93 per cent of the population were covered by public health insurance, about 5 per cent by private health insurance, and the remaining 2 per cent relied on welfare funds or on subsidiary support from the state. Virtually nobody is left without basic health insurance although the quantity and quality of services included vary considerably. There is no restriction as to age; old people are covered in a similar way. Working people who fall sick get their regular income during a consecutive period of 6 weeks. After that time a special sick fund operates which usually covers up to 70 per cent of regular income. The system of ambulant health care actually offers sufficient physicians in every rural and urban area in the country with a mean number of 440 inhabitants per physician. There is free choice of ambulant physicians, regardless of type of qualification or speciality

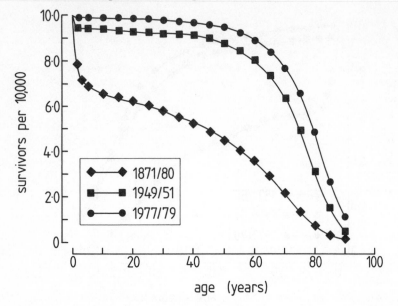

Figure 17.2   Survivors out of 100,000 women at age x: *German Reich 1871–80, Federal territory 1949–51, Federal Republic of Germany 1977–79.*

Source: Schach, E., 1983.

although waiting-time in some specialities (for example gynaecology, psychiatry, psychotherapy) is inevitable. Emergency services are now developed to a degree that every region has its own operating centre equipped with sufficient numbers of helicopters and emergency cars.

Hospitals provide even too many beds and their technical standard is becoming increasingly better. A few diagnostic (e.g. tomography) and therapeutic techniques (e.g. cardiac surgery, transplantation) are very scarce but the majority of medical expertise is available by and large. Special emphasis is given to extended rehabilitation services – for example after myocardial infarction and bypass surgery as well as for different patient groups with chronic degenerative diseases.

Critical aspects of the West German health care system include, among others, neglect of primary prevention – for example at the level of schools, occupational institutions, and ecology. They also include lack of coordination between the ambulant and the hospital sectors and disproportional income for a large number of physicians who support the oligopolistic structure of the health economy (drug industry and medical techniques).

Despite these critical aspects, the current level of medical care in the FRG seems reasonable and is available equitably to the large majority of the population. As a consequence it is unlikely that social differentials in morbidity/mortality can be attributed to unequal availability of health resources. Of course, since formal availability and real utilisation can be two different things, a more detailed approach to the study of health care utilisation is needed.

Utilisation of heath care and the question of social inequality

The question of under- versus over-utilisation of health services has been answered differently during the last two decades. In the 1960s, there was evidence of a pronounced social gradient in utilisation behaviour in several countries. This picture has now changed. Even in a country with large economic differentials in health care like the USA, medical sociologists observe a decline in the social gradient: members of lower socio-economic strata demonstrate similar rates of doctor-visits as do members of high socio-economic strata (Monteiro, 1973; Cockerham, 1986). Some studies report an inverse U-shaped relationship between social status and consultation of doctors, leaving middle-class members at the top (Angermeyer, 1982). Of course, assimilation of utilisation between socio-economic groups does not mean equal level of care. We have to take into consideration differences in the quality of care provided as well as a higher morbidity in the lower classes which would require disproportionate utilisation. Yet observed differences, even small ones, cannot be sufficiently explained by economic constraints. Rather socio-cultural, psychological and geographical conditions play a crucial role (see below).

Several studies of under-utilisation in West Germany are now available. Some of the significant findings are briefly summarised in this section.

Poor people (i.e. those with an income up to 60 per cent of mean income per capita) visit physicians less frequently than wealthier people. In those who visit a doctor, duration of treatment is longer than in wealthier people, indicating probably more severe health conditions. Poor people also prefer general practitioners and participate less in the specialised medical services (Brennecke, 1980).

Most striking differences are present in the field of prevention and screening programmes. Genetic counselling, for example, is used significantly more often by parents with higher educational degrees. Parents with an academic degree are six times over-represented in the user population as compared to their proportion in the general population; parents with only elementary school education are twice under-represented (Theile, 1977).

Number of contacts with a physician during pregnancy is signifi-

Table 17.1   Perinatal mortality and stillbirth by number of visits of physician during pregnancy (documentation includes 356 cases of perinatal mortality and 163 cases of stillbirth)

Number of visits:	0–6	7–9	10–12	13+	
– Perinatal mortality 0/00	35	12	6	7	P<0.001
– Stillbirth 0/00	14	6	3	4	P<0.001

Source: Collartz *et. al.*, 1983.

cantly related to social class and education of the mother (Collartz *et al.*, 1983): 32 per cent of lower-class mothers exhibit 0 to 6 visits, but only 9 per cent of middle- and upper middle-class mothers (p < 0.001). Of the latter, 77 per cent contact a physician during the first 3 months of pregnancy whereas 27 per cent of lower- class mothers delay into the second third and 5 per cent delay into the last third of pregnancy (p < 0.05).

A low rate of contact with physicians is critical because of its high statistical correlation with perinatal mortality and stillbirth, as illustrated in Table 17.1. In addition, perinatal mortality is higher if mothers' first contact takes place after 3 months of pregnancy. The same holds true for fatal outcomes. Results of this careful study indicate that the already existing risk of perinatal mortality among socio-economically or socio-culturally deprived mothers is critically increased by delayed utilisation of medical services during pregnancy.

Several other studies could be quoted which show higher utilisation, earlier visits and more preventive health and illness behaviour in higher educational and socio-economic groups. These studies, however, contain little additional information as they fail to offer explanations of this trend. Under given conditions of health insurance, economic explanations are of minor importance. Geographical location may account for some variance in the use of services; this has been demonstrated in the study on perinatal mortality. A large part of this variance may be explained by socio-cultural attitudes and behaviours related to broader socio-economic conditions. At least a couple of studies have tried to specify this proposition. In one such study it is argued that class-specific primary socialisation may generate different modes of body awareness and orientation towards the future. In middle- and upper-class families, skills and cognitive patterns related to deferred gratification and long-term planning favour preventive attitudes in the health field and symptom awareness, whereas coping techniques in blue-collar families are directed mainly toward actual problem solving, neglecting long-term prospective and preventive

Table 17.2 'Preventive attitude', socialised pattern of orientation and socio-economic class (N=165 men)

| | 'Involved in long-term individual concern' | | | |
| | Yes | | No | |
	Preventive	Non-preventive	Preventive	Non-preventive
–Upper and Middle class	24%	16%	41%	19%
–Lower class	9%	9%	35%	47%

CC = 0.28; p<0.01

Source: Kramer *et al.*, 1973.

concern (Kramer *et al.*, 1973). On the basis of structured interviews with 243 members of the middle and lower class, (study I N=78; study II N=165) it was shown that only 6 percent of lower-class members were identified as highly aware of symptoms and at the same time as involved in long-term individual concern. The percentage in the higher socio-economic group was four times as high. Similar trends were found with the variable 'preventive attitude' (see Table 17.2, Kramer *et al.*, 1973).

These results indicate a sort of cultural lag. Socio-cultural patterns of attitudes and behaviours resulting in under-utilisation of health services persist, although legal and economic constraints in the field of illness behaviour have disappeared.

So far we can summarise that the main burden of social inequality in this area is no longer under-utilisation of health services in situations of acute help-seeking, but lack of awareness of long-term concern about health. At present, the largest social differentials in the FRG arise from conditions such as absence of genetic counselling, low degree of prevention during pregnancy and early childhood, lack of medical knowledge, and inappropriate awareness of early symptoms. Although an unfavourable socio-economic background favours these attitudes, their immediate triggers are of a social–psychological nature (socialisation techniques, sub-cultural patterns, social perception) and are not necessarily related to insurance status, availability of health resources and the like.

It may well be that these deficiencies have a long-term impact on morbidity and mortality from chronic diseases. To our knowledge, no study has existed until now which could demonstrate such an effect. However, it is important to stress that it is probably the cumulative effect of insufficient preventive behaviour *and* unequal exposure to health hazards/unequal resistance which contributes to excess morbidity/mortality (see below).

For the present argument we may state that utilisation of health services, in the sense of acute help-seeking under need, is no longer different in the various social strata in the FRG and that only minor differences in health outcome are expected to result. One representative recent study even shows that patients over-utilise physicians in the latters' view; whereas patients judged about 30 per cent of their visits as 'urgent', or 'severe' only 18 per cent were judged in the same way by physicians (Schwartz *et al.*, 1984).

We turn back to the issue of preventive behaviour in the next section which deals with supposed main influences of social gradient on morbidity/mortality: different exposure and resistance.

Social differentials in exposure and resistance to health hazards
Data and concepts available
The assumption that exposure and resistance to health hazards can be equalised in different socio-economic groups clearly seems a Utopian one. However, excess mortality and morbidity between social classes have been minimised during the last decade and there are ways to reduce this excess further, at least to some degree. If characteristics of the social and natural environment as well as of the host (genetic, psychosocial) are important in determining excess vulnerability, scientific research in the area should provide clear knowledge of conditions, processes and outcomes of this vulnerability as a basis for health policy. This means that adequate theoretical models and empirical data should be made available.

Much of the nationwide and comparative research in the field until now is based on administrative data. These data are easily available from large groups and can be computed for longer time periods. Unfortunately they are not designed for scientific purposes and their quality therefore is severely limited. In the FRG, official morbidity and mortality data contribute very little to our questions, for the following reasons:

1. In official mortality statistics, even the crudest socio-economic indicators are lacking, thus leaving virtually no information on social differentials. In addition, as in other countries as well, data on mortality from specific causes are biased or inappropriate in several ways (multi-morbidity, diagnostic standards, classification problems, misreporting, etc.).
2. Morbidity data are available from sick-fund sources and rehabilitation agencies, but these data reflect utilisation and financial procedures in medical care offered rather than true prevalance or incidence. For example, every utilisation, regardless of whether

the same patient or different patients are considered, is recorded so that analyses based on individuals are almost unavailable.

3. Large data sets exist on differences between blue-collar and white-collar workers as these two large socio-economic groups are handled by two historically different rehabilitation agencies. However, the crude distinction between blue- and white-collar does not make sense in a sociological perspective and thus is of little use for the questions under consideration.

4. Subjective reports on health status from microcensus interviews are available but are of limited validity and reliability.

5. Despite high standards in scientific epidemiology in the period before the Second World War and national socialism in West Germany, the destruction of this discipline by national socialism has had a deep impact on the post- scientific development. Today there is still a very weak academic tradition of epidemiology in medicine and health policy in this country.

Equally critical problems arise from the academic disciplines themselves. Social epidemiology and medical sociology have until now tried hard to develop theoretically-grounded and methodologically-adequate measurements of social inequality. It has been stated repeatedly that the most telling weakness of traditional epidemiological research in the role of social factors in the etiology of disease is the oversimplification of social variables (McQueen *et al.*, 1982). Social variables are often treated as conceptually unitary or at best used as an index based on inadequate components. Differentials in morbidity and mortality from several chronic diseases have been documented by indicators such as level of education, income, occupational status, residential status, or subjective judgements of social positions. Data have been collected either on individual or on aggregate levels. Although results with simple indicators can be quite impressive, indicators themselves are not accurate measurements of real social life settings. Only very recently has sociology developed multidimensional concepts of social inequality which are now increasingly favoured, and which identify homogeneous socio-economic strata by means of causal models (Blau, 1977). In these models unidimensional hierarchy is no longer a useful approach to the study of inequality. Socio-structural configuration seems to cluster around sociologically meaningful concepts such as degree of control and autonomy (especially in the work-setting) (Kohn *et al.*, 1983) or degree of social resources under conditions of insecurity. Medical sociology and social epidemiology still suffer from a lack of multidimensional analysis of phenomena of social inequality and of related theoretically meaningful concepts. The same holds true for the issue of static versus dynamic concepts. There is a considerable lack of longitudinal cohort studies which would tell us more about the interaction between exposure to health hazards and resistance and coping processes over time. Researchers in the field are becoming increasingly aware of the need to study careers or time patterns of stressful experience rather than stable characteristics.

The following information is thus based on severe limitations. However, we try to highlight at least some of the approaches which might be appropriate in dealing with explanations of observed social differentials in morbidity and mortality. The next sub-section concentrates on administrative data on mortality in the FRG while the following sub-section focuses on socio-epidemiologic studies which search for causes of social differentials in disease, in which cardiovascular diseases serve as a prominent example.

Morbidity/mortality differentials in administrative data

Unlike the United Kingdom, nationwide official statistics in the health field, based upon a sociologically meaningful system of occupational, income or educational classification do not exist. Therefore we have to compute evidence from a variety of sources some of which are restricted to smaller samples. However, we think that good quality data can compensate to some extent for limited generalisability.

Two recent epidemiological studies exist, which show systematic relationships between educational and occupational status and mortality. Although restricted to two large cities they show an impressive gradient in age-adjusted mortality rate for socio-economic groups. Trends are most pronounced in the age categories 45–66 years. Unskilled workers show the highest, professionals the lowest rates. This holds true for total mortality – for mortality from liver cirrhosis (ratio between lowest and highest socio-economic group: 7.3:1 in the age-group 50–55); for mortality from ischaemic heart disease (ICD 410–414; ratio 2.5:1); and for mortality from lung cancer (ratio 5.2:1 in the respective age group) (Neumann *et al.*,1981).

Still, occupational data are very crude in this analysis, and several sources of bias are not controlled in an appropriate way.

The next step consists of analysing the impact of socio-economic differentials on mortality/morbidity at the level of more precise occupational characteristics. Best and most recent materials are available from a nationwide study on occupational characteristics of 22,689 male patients who first experienced and survived acute myocardial infarction (abbreviated AMI;ICD 410) between 35 and 64 years (Bolm-Audorff *et al.*, 1983). Data are analysed on the basis of the social security system for the years 1977 and 1978; they cover about 90 per cent of all enrolled male patients surviving AMI during

Table 17.3   *Blue-collar occupations significantly (P<.001) over-represented among male patients with AMI* (age 35 to 64) as
compared with the age-adjusted male working population in
West Germany (N=10,482)*

Occupational group	Observed	Expected	O/E ratio
Metal polishing, annealing and galvanising workers	209	64.7	3.23
Sawyers and woodworking machinists	225	80.0	2.81
Precision instrument makers	141	63.7	2.22
Unskilled workers, assembly-line workers	1,805	870.0	2.07
Miners	340	172.4	1.97
Furnacemen and rolling mill workers	193	105.3	1.83
Mechanics	588	481.7	1.22

Note:
* Acute myocardial infarction

Source: Bolm-Audorff *et al.*, 1983.

these two years. The basic occupational characteristics of these
patients were recorded according to the official West German occupational classification system. As the data are not organised by category,
computation for each of the 86 occupational categories of the official
classification system were made. Relative distributions of occupational
categories among the patient group, as well as among the control
group, were calculated, and differences between observed (AMI
group) and expected (control group) frequencies were tested by Chi-
square. The control group consisted of the total West German male
working population aged 35 to 64.

Results on occupational differentials in morbidity from AMI are
presented in Table 17.3 for blue-collar workers and in Table 17.4 for
white-collar workers. Over-represented blue-collar occupations
include metal workers, sawyers and woodworking machinists, precision instrument makers, unskilled workers, miners and furnacemen.
Over-represented white-collar occupations are technical assistants,
air-traffic controllers and pilots, porters and guards, sales managers
and bank and insurance brokers. The same results were found for the
age-adjusted sub-groups, indicating that these results are largely
independent of age.

Further exploration revealed that occupations with night-shift work
were significantly over-represented in the group of AMI patients (o-e
ratio=1.27), but no significant effect was found for piece-work
combined with shift-work if analysed independent of occupation
groups.

Table 17.4   White-collar occupations significantly (P<0.001) over-represented among male patients with AMI* (age 35 to 64) as compared with the age-adjusted male working population in West Germany (N=12,207)

Occupational group	Observed	Expected	O/E ratio
Technical assistants	354	111.2	3.18
Aircraft and ship pilots; air-traffic and ship controllers	120	69.9	1.72
Porters, guards	522	357.9	1.46
Sales managers, e.g., brokers, advertising agents	266	186.8	1.42
Bank and insurance brokers	491	359.4	1.37
Clericals	2,181	1,889.3	1.15

Note:
* Acute myocardial infarction

Source: Bolm-Audorff *et al.*, 1983.

Table 17.5   Occupations significantly (P<0.001) over-represented among female patients with AMI (age 35 to 64) as compared with the age-adjusted female working population in West Germany (N = 2,296)

Occupational group	Observed	Expected	O/E ratio
Workers in bakeries, confectioners	12	2.1	5.58
Unskilled workers, subsidiary workers	241	70.9	3.39
Merchants in service sector	22	7.8	2.82
Nurses and related health personnel	104	72.7	1.43

Source: Bolm-Audorff *et al.*, 1983.

Analogous data were collected for female patients with AMI in the same age/occupation categories (n=2296). Table 17.5 shows results which must be interpreted with caution due to the small numbers. However, for the two larger groups over-represented in the sample, job stress due to high workload (nurses) and/or job insecurity (unskilled workers) seems to be one possible factor contributing to higher incidence of AMI.

Although this system of occupational classifications still lacks sociologically meaningful specificity, data nevertheless give some evidence of occupational coronary risks. The combination of noise and psychomental work stress (for example, time urgency, low margin of control) may account for some variation in blue-collar coronary

Table 17.6 Mean age of retirement due to sickness or disability in new cases of blue-collar and white-collar annuity insurance in 1982 (selected diagnoses; males only)

	Blue-collar	White-collar
– Cancer of respiratory organs	52.8	54.9
– Diabetes mellitus	53.8	56.3
– Essential hypertension	57.8	59.6
– Ischaemic heart disease	55.7	57.1
– Cerebrovascular diseases	55.8	57.2
– Obstructive lung disease	56.5	57.6
– Duodenal and gastric ulcer	55.6	58.5
– Alcoholic liver cirrhosis	50.9	54.7
– Degenerative skeletal disease (Dorsopathia, spondylosis, etc.)	56.7	57.6

Source: Verband Deutscher Rentenversicherungsträger, 1983.

morbidity, and especially for the high incidence in metal workers, miners and woodwork machinists. Job insecurity, as reflected in a high incidence rate among unskilled workers may be of additional relevance (for further exploration see the next sub-section; see also Siegrist *et al.*, 1987). The over-representation of air-traffic controllers, sales managers, bank brokers, among others, may be partially related to psychomental workloads such as heavy responsibility, time urgency, interruptions and inconsistencies of demands, high concentration requirement and again, to some extent, to job insecurity. Thus these data give some further information on links between social inequality, occupational risks and disease outcome, especially in the cardiovascular field.

Another nationwide data source shows less favourable health conditions in blue-collar as compared to white-collar occupations, the criterion being early retirement due to sickness or to disability (Verband Deutscher Rentenversicherungstrager, 1983). In Table 17.6 mean age of premature retirement due to sickness or to disability is indicated for several disease conditions in new cases of blue-collar, as compared to white-collar, annuity insurance in 1982. In every disease category, blue-collar workers have a lower mean age of retirement than white-collar workers, indicating more severe impairment or at least more severe exposure to health hazards. This table contains information only for men; for women the case is less clear due to selective and more fragmentary occupational biographies.

Morbidity differentials in socio-epidemiological studies
It is difficult to assess the relative importance of different exposures

and resistance to health hazards in detail. Resistance, especially, is difficult to analyse, as genetic make-up appears to have a clear impact on the way individuals and even groups cope with health hazards. A still debatable issue in this regard is the etiology of mental disorders. For the FRG, a representative epidemiological study on rural adults has shown a moderate social class gradient in seven day prevalance of psychiatric disorders after controlling for health care utilisation (which, by the way, did not differ according to socio-economic status) (Fichtner *et al.*, 1985). However, in the lower classes, prevalence was higher in organic disease and alcohol-related disease but differences were small in depression and schizophrenia. The fact that the percentage of chronically ill people in a five-year follow-up was 40 per cent in the lowest class compared to 14 per cent in the upper class (Fichtner Weyerer, 1985) may give additional evidence to the drift or selection hypothesis of mental disorders, thus pointing to genetically (and environment-induced) impaired resistance, and to processes of social marginalisation operating in people who are already sick.

Yet, talking about resistance also includes psychosocial assets and coping mechanisms which have been related to the prevalance and incidence of a variety of diseases. Absence of socio-emotional support, of confidants and of close societal networks seems to aggravate health risks of environmental stressors (Siegrist *et al.*, 1986; Orth-Gomer *et al.*, 1983) as does the lack of psychological defence mechanisms such as stoicism and sense of coherence (Antonovsky, 1979), among others.

In this section, a sociological approach towards studying socio-environmental stressors in their relation to morbidity differentials is outlined, and selected results are shown. This approach is presented as an example of the kind of studies that are needed in order to overcome the insufficient state of the art.

The study briefly reported here investigates sociological and psychological predictors of premature cardiovascular risk and disease in middle-aged male populations. Three basic assumptions underlie this approach.

First, it is essential to define the quality of those experiences of social environment that cause emotional distress. We propose to restrict the term 'distress' to experiences of sustained physiological activation. Sustained activation occurs if an individual meets external demands without being able to control the demanding situation. Active coping under conditions of limited success and control has been shown to stimulate intense and long-lasting emotional reactions which, in turn, are associated with an activation of the autonomic nervous system and related neuro-hormonal responses (Ursin, 1984; Beamish *et al.*, 1985).

Second, external triggers of distressing experiences can be found in a variety of life circumstances, but those resulting from occupational life play a prominent role in explaining early cardiovascular disease in middle-aged populations. A recurrent daily workload characterised by time urgency, interruptions, responsibility or tensions at the work-site, and threats to occupational status, such as forced downward mobility or unemployment all reinforce long-lasting experiences of distress. Effects of these conditions on health can be worsened by the co-existence of chronic interpersonal difficulties and negative life events in private life.

Third, it is evident that different individuals may react in different ways to experiences of distress, and that the coping process is of crucial importance in determining possible health outcomes. Thus, it is the interaction between stressful external conditions and subjective appraisal and coping which determines the health impact of socio-emotional distress.

This third assumption can be specified more explicitly: in the context of occupational careers in middle adulthood, we have postu-lated that the presence of a specific style of coping with the demands of work increases emotional distress and sustained activation. This style of coping is expressed in a pattern of work-related attitudes that include overcommitment, perfectionism, competitiveness, vigorous efforts to meet goals and inability to withdraw from work obligations. It seems that this coping style reflects a high degree of need for control in challenging social situations. Individuals with this high degree of need for control may experience more sustained distress when exposed to adverse working conditions or even to threats to their occupational status than individuals with little need for control (Matschinger *et al.*, 1986).

This assumption has been tested in a prospective study on cardio-vascular risks in 416 male blue-collar workers aged 25–55 (mean 40.8±9.6) who were initially free from coronary events. These workers were observed over a period of three years in three panel waves (final sample N=310). The purpose of the study was to relate levels and changes in cardiovascular risk factors (especially blood pressure and blood lipids) and manifestation of new coronary events to several indicators of sustained distress.

Results presented in Figure 17.3 show the most relevant part of a linear structural model where effects of the latent factor 'vigour' (of the scale that measures need for control) on systolic blood pressure are expressed in terms of gamma-coefficients. The respective model takes into account some well known risk factors of high blood pressure (age, overweight, smoking). In Figure 17.3, estimates are shown for two distinct groups of blue-collar workers: a group of low-status unskilled workers with low occupational stability (n=75) and a group of skilled

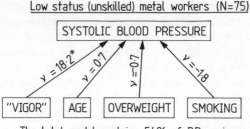

Low status (unskilled) metal workers (N=75)

SYSTOLIC BLOOD PRESSURE

γ = 18.2*   γ = 0.7   γ = 0.7   γ = -1.8

"VIGOR"   AGE   OVERWEIGHT   SMOKING

The total model explains 54% of BP variance

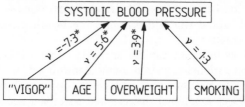

Higher status (skilled) metal workers (N=147)

SYSTOLIC BLOOD PRESSURE

γ = -7.3*   γ = 5.6*   γ = 3.9*   γ = 1.3

"VIGOR"   AGE   OVERWEIGHT   SMOKING

The total model explains 26% of BP variance
* p < 0.05

*Figure 17.3   Effects of 'vigour' on systolic blood pressure: linear struc-
tural models for healthy blue-collar workers*

Source: Matschinger et al., 1986.

workers with higher status and higher occupational stability (n=147).
In keeping with our assumption, a significant positive effect of vigour
on blood pressure was found in the sub-group suffering from chronic
unfavourable working conditions (upper part of Figure 17.3; gamma
coefficient = 18.2; p. <0.05), whereas no positive effect was observed
in the group of workers with higher status (lower part of Figure 17.3).
It is quite remarkable that the interaction model (stressful context
plus distress-inducing coping) was able to explain considerably more
of the observed variation in systolic blood pressure (54 per cent) than
the model based on coping style without the stressful context (26 per
cent) (Matschinger *et al.*, 1986; Siegrist, 1987).

Another important cardiovascular risk factor was level of blood
lipids, and especially low-density cholesterol (LDL). Unskilled
workers in the prospective study exhibited significantly higher mean
levels of LDL compared to skilled workers, after controlling for
weight, age and cigarette smoking. And again, presence of vigorous
coping attitudes at the workplace under restricted occupational
autonomy showed a direct effect on level of LDL, as demonstrated in
Figure 17.4. This effect, however, is restricted to a considerably large

Men with (mild) hypercholesterolemia (N = 90)

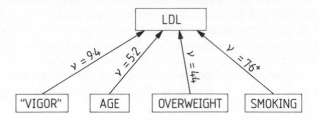

Men with hormocholesterolemia (N = 168)

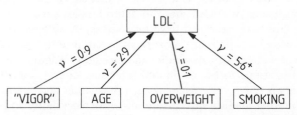

Figure 17.4   Effects of 'vigour' on low-density cholesterol (LDL) in hypercholesterolemic aid normocholesterolemic low-status blue-collar workers

Source: Matschinger *et al.*, 1986.

sub-group already at risk due to presence of mild hypercholesterolemia (upper part of the linear structural model presented in Figure 17.4; gamma-coefficient = 9.4; p <0.05).

Thus, a cumulative effect may be operating between somatic cardiovascular risks due to nutrition or genetic influence and psychosocial distress.

In another statistical approach with data from the same study, we have recently found that blood lipids are associated with indicators of severe occupational distress. By means of analysis of variance with repeated measurement, mean level of atherogenic LDL-HDL (ratio between low-density and high-density cholesterol) was highest in those sub-groups of blue-collar workers who suffered from both unfavourble external working conditions (occupational instability, excessive work demand) and subjective appraisal of workload. The finding covered a two-year period of observation, and the possible confounding effects of age, body weight and smoking were controlled. Again, the interaction effect was the most important statistical link between indicators of sustained distress and cardiovascular somatic risks (Siegrist *et al.*, 1988).

Examples like these demonstrate that refined sociological concepts and measurements are able to explain somatic risk conditions (such as high blood pressure, hypercholesterolemia) to a considerable degree although they are part of a multi-factorial approach. They may be useful in understanding causal effects of social stress on cardiovascular morbidity/mortality and thus in breaking down broader concepts such as socio-economic status (indicating social inequality) into more specific and relevant components. In the long run, refined knowledge of this kind enables us to address interventionist approaches specifically to sub-groups at high risk.

Conclusions

Present knowledge in the field of social inequality and health is far from conclusive. We need more in-depth studies which are able to separate effects of restricted health resources, of different utilisation behaviour and of different exposure and resistance to health hazards on disease vulnerability, morbidity and mortality. Administrative data are, and continue to be, of limited scientific interest, both because they contain only crude sociological information and because they usually present medical information of restricted validity and reliability. It is difficult to agree upon identical measurement techniques which would be a prerequisite of meaningful comparisons within and between countries. And it is difficult to find appropriate conceptual devices for the effects on health of those dimensions of social inequality which create excessive exposure to health hazards and which minimise resistance.

Sociology tries hard to define those conceptual devices in advanced industrial societies where traditional indicators of socio-economic status have lost significance and where the dominant role of occupational life is increasingly weakened. It seems that rapid social change prevents sociology from finding successful (more or less stable) conceptual devices. To my mind, it is this latter fact of rapid social change that gives new weight to the role of social and psychological coping skills in situations of social instability and uncertainty. As stated earlier in this paper, socio-structural configurations of social inequality seem to cluster around psychosocial resources under conditions of increased instability and insecurity. Threats to social (and especially occupational) status, which cannot be compensated for by alternative actions, become dangerous stressful stimuli for premature development of disease, as we have shown in the case of cardiovascular somatic risk factors. It is hoped that transdisciplinary research on these important topics can be intensified both within and between comparable countries. It is also hoped that available knowledge will have an impact on health policy, especially on primary and secondary prevention of chronic diseases.

References

Angermeyer, M. (1982), *Vergleichende Untersuchungen zum Schichtspezifischen Krankheitsverhalten*, unpublished report, Hannover.

Antonovsky, A. (1979), *Stress and Coping*, San Francisco: Jossey Bass.

Beamish, R.E., Singal, P.K. and Dhalla, N.S. (eds) (1985), *Stress and Heart Disease*, Boston, Dordrecht, Lancaster.

Blau, P.M. (1977), *Inequality and Heterogeneity*, New York.

Bolm-Audorff, U. and Siegrist, J. (1983), 'Occupational morbidity data in myocardial infarction', *Journal of Occupational Medicine*, 25,. pp. 367.

Brennecke, R. (1980), *Armut, Gesundheitsbeschwerden und Inanspruchnahme von Gesundheitsleistungen*, unpublished report, Frankfurt.

Cockerham, W.C. (1986), *Medical Sociology* 3rd edn., New Jersey: Englewood Cliffs.

Collartz, J., Hecker, H. and Oeter, K. (1983), *Perinatalstudie Niedersachsen und Bremen*, Munich, Vienna, Baltimore.

Fichtner, M.M. and Weyerer, S. (1985), *Die Oberbayerische Follow-Up Felduntersuchung*, unpublished report, Munich.

Kohn, M.L. and Schooler, C. (1983), *Work and Personality*, New Jersey: Norwood.

Kramer, A. and Siegrist, J. (1973), 'Soziale Schicht und Krankheitsverhalten' in Enke, H. and Pohlmeier, H. (eds), *Psycho-Soziale Rehabilitation*, Stuttgart, p. 119.

McQueen, D. and Siegrist, J. (1982), 'Social factors in the etiology of chronic disease: an overview', *Social Science and Medicine*, 16, p. 352.

Matschinger, H., Siegrist, J., Siegrist, K. and Dittmann, K.H. (1986), 'Type A as a coping career – Toward a conceptual and methodological redefinition' in Schmidt, T.H., Dembroski, T.M. and Blumchen, G. (eds), *Biological and Psychological Factors in Cardiovascular Disease*, Berlin, Heidelberg, New Heidelberg, New York, London, Paris, Tokyo, p. 104.

Mooney, G.H. (1983), 'Equity in health care: confronting the confusion', *Effective Health Care*, 1, p. 179.

Monteiro, L.A. (1973), 'Expense is no object . . . Income and physician visits reconsidered', *Journal of Health and Social Behaviour*, 14, p. 99.

Neumann, G. and Ledermann, A. (1981), 'Mortalitat und Sozialschict', *Bundesgesundheitsblatt*, 243, p. 173.

Orth-Gomer, K., Perski, A. and Theorell, T. (1983), 'Psychosocial factors and cardiovascular disease: a review of the current state of our knowledge' unpublished manuscript, Stockholm.

Schach, E. (1983), *Die Enthropie als Mass in der Bevölkerungsund Gesundheitsstatistik*, unpublished report, Annual Meeting of German Association of Medical Statistics.

Schwartz, F.W., Robra, P.P., Meye, M.R., Henke, K.D. and Behrends, C.S. (1984), *Medizinische Orientierungsdaten*, Köln.

Siegrist, J., Siegrist, K. and Weber, I. (1986), 'Sociological concepts in the etiology of chronic disease: the case of ischaemic heart disease', *Social Science and Medicine*, 22, p. 247.

Siegrist, J. (1988), 'Impaired quality of life as a risk factor in cardiovascular disease', *Journal of Chronic Diseases*, pp. 40, 571.

Siegrist, J., Matschinger, H., Cremer, P. and Seidel, D. (1987), 'Atherogenic risk in men suffering from occupational stress', Atherosclerosis, **69**, p. 211.

Theile, U. (1977), *Genetische Beratung*, Munich, Vienna, Baltimore.

Ursin, H. (1984), *Expectancy and activation: an attempt to systematise stress theory* unpublished manuscript.

Verband Deutscher Rentenversicherungsträger (ed.) (1983), *Statistik Rentenzugang 1982*, Frankfurt.

18 Way-of-life, stress, and differences in morbidity between occupational classes
Jeddi Hasan

Introduction

The 'materialist' explanation of social class differences in morbidity and mortality favoured by the *Black Report* (DHSS, 1980) emphasises the role of differences in specific socio-economic and physical features in the living conditions of the classes as causative factors. According to this view, the life circumstances of the lower classes employed in manual occupations are characterised by health risks associated, on one hand, with low income (quality of housing and food etc.), and on the other, with hazardous physical and social environments, especially at the workplace. These circumstances are also conducive to deleterious habits, such as smoking.

It is easy to see that a part of the morbidity differentials are, indeed, related to specific environmental influences (e.g. occupational accidents and diseases) or to behavioural differences between the classes (e.g. smoking). For a variety of presumably deleterious environmental features our knowledge of possible pathogenic influences and mechanisms is, however, poor or non-existent. We do not, for example, know how years of heavy physical labour affect health. This, and the remarkable similarities in the social class distribution of death and disease in most causes and diagnostic groups, has prompted a search for more general aetiological determinants of any one of many diseases which would affect the probability of falling ill and dying. The notion of a general susceptibility to disease has been invoked (Cassel, 1976), which would be modified (also) by psychosocial influences (stress), and play a part in producing the observed social class gradients in disease and death (Syme and Berkman, 1976).

The utility of published mortality data for the study of these questions is limited by the '. . . crude grouping together of diverse occupations into social classes, and by the failure to account for other risk factors' (Marmot *et al.*, 1984). Also, large categories of morbidity which are not reflected in mortality are left out of these studies. In the following, I shall try to contribute to the discussion with some results from a research programme designed to explore the life circumstances and morbidity differentials between occupational classes within a single industrial complex situated in one town.

The study population

A preliminary questionnaire designed to obtain background data was mailed in 1971 to all 4,570 employees of the four metal industry factories of Valmet Oy (a state-owned company) in Jyvaskyla, Central Finland. The factories include a wide variety of production branches and working environments, ranging from foundry and heavy engineering to precision engineering. Eighty-four per cent of the men and 90 per cent of the women replied. The study population was restricted to those who had been employed for at least 15 months before 1 February 1972, in order to include only persons with some experience of the work and of the working environments.

The employees were classified into four groups on the basis of their occupation, education, work task, and position in the organisation:

1. upper white-collar (managers),
2. lower white-collar (clerical),
3. skilled blue-collar, and
4. semi-skilled blue-collar workers.

There were no women in managerial positions nor in the skilled occupations.

The sample was selected systematically from those who returned the questionnaire and were willing to participate in a health examination. For the sampling, the employees (n=2653) were stratified into groups according to sex, age (three groups: born in 1946 or later; born between 1926 and 1945, and born in 1925 or earlier), and occupational class (four groups). The selection was made at equal intervals, separately from each stratum (stratified disproportional systematic sampling). Some persons selected for the sample subsequently refused or left their employment during the period of the health examination. They were replaced by those next in order on the list. 155 such changes – 17.2 per cent of the sample – were necessary. The size of the final sample was 902. Its characteristics and the sampling scheme have been described in detail (METELI, 1975; Parvi, 1977). The distribution of people into occupational classes is seen in Table 18.1.

The data

Information was obtained by questionnaire and interviews on the socio-economic characteristics, occupational history, working conditions, leisure-time activities, and health-related habits of the people in the sample. Data on pensions, absenteeism, and accidents were obtained from factory records. Ergonomic observations, as well as physiological and environmental measurements, were perfomed at the workposts of people in sub-samples (see METELI, 1977; Parvi, 1977; Manninen, 1977; Aunola *et al.*, 1978).

In the spring of 1973, the people in the sample participated in a health examination including questionnaires, interviews, clinical examinations by a physician and physiotherapist, and fitness tests. Electrocardigrams at rest and during exercise were recorded and blood pressure measured. Blood samples were taken for analyses.

Chronic illness was defined as an affirmative answer in a questionnaire to the question: 'Have you at present any permanent illness or impairment? The person was asked to name the illness(es), and during the clinical examination the physician tried to confirm it and to assess its chronicity, mainly by interview. The diagnosis of coronary heart disease (angina pectoris/infarction) was based on questionnaire answers, physician's interview, ECG-recordings, and hospital records (see Parvi, 1977; Aro, 1981).

The Stress Symptoms Score was the sum of the following 18 items in the questionnaire on symptoms experienced during the preceding year, rated according to frequency of occurrence from 0 to 3 (seldom or never-often or continuously): heartburn or acid troubles; loss of appetite; nausea or vomiting; abdominal pains; diarrhoea or irregular bowel function; difficulties in falling asleep or awakening at night; nightmares; headache; sexual unwillingness; dizziness; tachycardia or irregular heart beats; tremor of hands; excessive perspiration without physical exertion; dyspnoea without physical exertion; lack of energy or depression; fatigue or feebleness; anxiety or nervousness; irritability or fits of anger.

These symptoms were selected from various treatises on mental stress and its psychosomatic manifestations. The criteria for selection were somewhat arbitrary. Most symptoms are known or assumed to be common in people undergoing stressful life periods (see Aro, 1981).

Results
Way-of-life
I have selected some results from the surveys into Table 18.1. For almost all of the indices of socio-economic characteristics, working conditions, and health-related habits, there is a stepwise gradient from the highest to the lowest occupational class, such that the lower the class the more scarce are the available social and material resources, the more prevalent or intense are the known or presumed harmful or stressing features in the working conditions (and vice versa for the presumably favourable features), and the more common are the health-endangering habits (the opposite, again, being true for presumably health-promoting habits). The only exceptions from a regular gradient in this list are the higher prevalence of exhaustion after work in the upper than in the lower white-collar class, and the seemingly

Table 18.1 Indices of way-of-life by sex and occupational class[1]

| | Occupational class[2] | | | | | |
| | Men | | | | Women | |
	1	2	3	4	1	2
Socio-economic base						
Attended only primary school (%)	0	21	59	75	30	95
Median income (Fmk 1973)	1667	1113	885	785	707	639
Commodity ownership (index $\bar{x}$)[3]	3.5	2.9	2.2	1.4	2.4	2.3
Housing level (index $\bar{x}$)[4]	3.0	2.6	2.0	1.8	–	–
Ever unemployed at least 3 months (%)	8	13	22	32	9	19
Work						
Distance from home to work ($\bar{x}$, km)	2.1	2.7	3.2	5.2	2.8	3.0
Energy consumption ($\bar{x}$, kj/min)[5]	–	9.4	12.7	15.4	6.8	10.7
Physically strenuous work (%)	1	5	64	74	4	57
Lifetime physical strain ($\bar{x}$)[6]	1.3	1.9	2.8	3.0	1.3	2.4
Ergonomic drawbacks (index $\bar{x}$)[7]	–	0.7	3.8	4.2	1.2	3.9
Noise level above 74 dB (A) (%)[8]	0	9	70	78	2	54
Polluted breathing air (%)	9	33	63	67	13	58
Bruising & chafing objects (%)	0	1	11	16	1	9
Shiftwork (%)	1	9	34	37	4	30
Forced pace (%)	6	25	34	44	31	46
Pauses at will (%)	65	48	34	29	33	21
Monotony (%)	1	17	22	39	39	54
Interesting job (%)	87	63	46	28	36	24
Exhausted after work (%)	34	28	40	49	21	37
Habits						
Smoking regularly (%)	23	32	37	38	20	27
Intoxicated at least monthly (%)	8	16	25	24	3	2
Vigorous physical exercise (%)[9]	40	37	24	23	42	22
Active & creative hobbies (%)[10]	78	68	49	46	36	10
(n)	(103)	(155)	(187)	(167)	(142)	(151)

Notes:
[1]Data from questionnaire, except where indicated; standardised by age when necessary.
[2]Occupational class: 1=upper (managers), and 2=lower white collar; 3=skilled, and 4=semi-skilled blue collar.
[3]Based on ownership of dwelling, car, TV, telephone, motor-/sailboat, and summer cottage (range: 0–6).
[4]Based on area/person, and availability of hot water, bathroom and toilet, and sauna (range: 0–4).
[5]Measured as oxygen consumption during work in a sub-sample (n=234, no managers) (see Aunola *et al.*, 1978).
[6]Based on questionnaire item in a detailed recapitulation of occupational history (range: 1–4).
[7]Based on detailed structured observations and interviews at workplace in a subsample (n=660, no managers) (range: 0–9).
[8]Noise levels measured twice at the workposts of a sub-sample (n=320) (see Manninen, 1977).
[9]Based on detailed inventory of leisure-time physical activity, and average energy consumption in each type of activity. Only those activities for which the average coefficient of energy consumption exceeded 2000 kj/h are included (see Aro *et al.*, 1986).
[10]Based on detailed inventory and classification of leisure-time hobbies.

similar habits of heavy drinking in both blue-collar classes. Besides

Table 18.2   Age-standardised indices of well-being and morbidity by sex and occupational class[1]

	Occupational class[2]					
	Men				Women	
	1	2	3	4	1	2
Life dissatisfaction (index, z-scores)	−0.76	−0.31	0.15	0.38	−0.16	0.41
High Stress Symptoms Score (%)[3]	12	23	29	40	40	57
Self-appraised health 'poor' (%)	5	8	9	14	2	11
Chronically ill (%)	24	37	46	48	31	38
Systolic blood pressure ($\bar{x}$, mmHg)	135	141	141	142	134	139
Diastolic blood pressure ($\bar{x}$, mmHg)	77	77	76	76	76	76
Cholesterol ($\bar{x}$, mg/100 ml)	235	241	246	244	260	254
Triglycerides ($\bar{x}$, mg/100 ml)	129	143	141	142	93	107
Coronary heart disease (%)[4]	5	7	6	11	2	14
Chronic bronchitis (%)	3	3	8	10	1	3
Trunk flexion test ($\bar{x}$, times/30 sec.)	18	17	15	14	13	10
Chronic diseases of the musculoskeletal system (%)	7	8	17	18	8	21
Clinical findings in musculoskeletal system (index $\bar{x}$)[5]	1.0	1.3	2.0	2.3	1.3	2.6
Temporary disability (average sickness absence days per year)	4.2	7.5	14.4	16.0	7.0	18.0
Absenteeism due to accidents at workplace (%)	0	3	23	22	1	7
Disability pensions 1961–72 (annual average ‰[6]	4		9		3	14
(n)	(103)	(155)	(187)	(167)	(142)	(151)

Notes:
[1]Data from questionnaire and physician's examination, except where indicated.
[2]Occupational class: 1 = upper and 2 = lower white-collar 3 = skilled and 4 =semi-skilled blue-collar.
[3]Top third of index scores in the whole sample.
[4]Angina pectoris and infarction; based on questionnaire (Rose), physician's examination, ECG and hospital records.
[5]Score based on physiotherapist's systematic examination.
[6]From factory records; male white- and blue-collar classes combined.

educational attainment, the steepest gradients are found for many of the indices characterising conditions at work. With respect to some physical features of work and working environments one really does not see a gradient but rather a jump from one level to quite a different one when comparing the white- and blue-collar classes.

Well-being and morbidity

Some indices of well-being and morbidity are collected into Table 18.2. The indices show fairly consistent inverse gradients rising from the lowest figures for the upper white-collar to the highest ones for the lower blue-collar class. The gradients are steep for the indices of mental well-being and self-appraised health. They are fairly steep also for the prevalence of musculoskeletal disease and chronic bronchitis, suggesting a partly work-related aetiology. The characteristics of the working conditions are also reflected in the gradients of temporary disability and of disease due to occupational accidents. Chronic diseases of the musculoskeletal system were twice as common among the male and three times as common among the female blue-collar workers as in the respective white-collar groups. They were the most frequent cause of handicap at work. The gradients for morbidity in the cross-sectional sample are affected by the different rates at which people from the occupational classes (Table 18.2) had been prematurely pensioned off because of sickness: they become gentler.

Comment

The similarities in the distributions of socio-economic and occupational features presumably hazardous to mental and physical health in the ways-of-life of the occupational classes, on one hand, and the morbidity differences between the classes, on the other, are obvious. This raises questions about possible causal connections, which are difficult to answer on the basis of cross-sectional data. From what I noted in the Introduction, it follows naturally that we were especially interested in the fact that the distribution of abundant (presumed) stress symptoms (as well as the mean scores) between the occupational classes was also similar to those described above (Table 18.2). It seemed reasonable to assume that the multiple systematic differences between the occupational classes in exposure to various hazardous or strenuous features in their living and working conditions (Table 18.1) might be reflected as differences in experienced stress. If the stress –> susceptibility –> disease hypothesis contained some truth, this would contribute to the explanation of the occupational class differentials in morbidity.

The associations between indices of way-of-life and the Stress Symptoms Scores were moderate on an individual level (r =0.11–0.38). Multivariate analyses (MCA) indicated that different combinations of the indices explained from 5 to 30 per cent of the variation in the score in different groups. The explanatory power was greatest for some indices of working conditions (See Figures 18.1 – 18.3). We decided to study the associations between the presumed stress symptoms and morbidity by a follow-up of the sample described above.

The follow-up

The cohort examined in 1973 was invited to a similar health

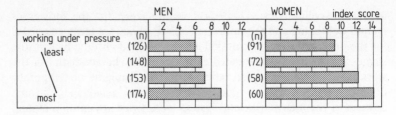

Figure 18.1   Stress symptoms according to piecework pressure or forced pace. Age-standardised means of index scores.

Source: Parvi, 1977.

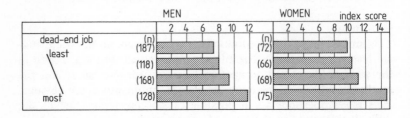

Figure 18.2   Stress symptoms according to work in uninteresting jobs with no prospects. Age-standardised means of index scores.

Source: Parvi, 1977.

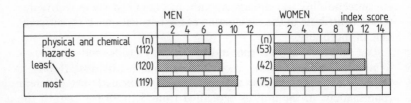

Figure 18.3   Stress symptoms in the blue-collar workers' groups according to adverse physical and chemical hazards. Age-standardised means of index scores.

Source: Parvi, 1977.

Table 18.3   *Age-standardised incidence rates (per 1,000 person-years)of chronic illness by sex and occupational class*

	Men				Women			
	White-collar		Blue-collar		White-collar		Blue-collar	
	Cases	Inci-dence	Cases	Inci-dence	Cases	Inci-dence	Cases	Inci-dence
Chronic illness	37	90.6	51	135.5	19	73.2	31	140.3
Myocardial infarction	3	6.7	10	8.7	1	1.3	–	–
Angina pectoris (Rose)	4	6.5	10	9.4	4	5.5	8	11.9
Chronic musculoskeletal disease (cumulative %)	5	4.5	12	11.5	6	3.0	16	6.5

examination in the spring of 1978. Of the original 902 persons, 154 were lost to the 5-year follow-up, 12 of whom had died. Some of the indices of morbidity in 1973 showed that the health of the living male blue-collar workers not participating in the follow-up may have been somewhat worse than that of the participants (see Aro, 1981). The male upper and lower white-collar groups, and skilled and semi-skilled blue-collar groups were combined for these analyses.

The 5-year incidence of new illnesses in those free of chronic disease at baseline by and large confirmed our previous findings as to the distribution of morbidity in the occupational classes (Table 18.3).

The incidence rates were higher in both blue-collar groups than in the respective white-collar ones; the relative risks for chronic illness in the male and female blue-collar groups were 1.5 and 1.9, respectively. Circulatory disease was the most commonly appearing new illness category in the male white-collar group (32 per cent), whereas an equal proportion of musculoskeletal diseases appeared among the male blue-collar workers. The latter were the most common new diseases in both female groups.

The association between the Stress Symptoms Score at baseline and incidence of chronic illness during the follow-up was strong in all groups except the white-collar females (Table 18.4).

Multiple logistic regression analyses showed that the Stress Symptoms Score remained a powerful predictor of chronic illness even after standardising for a range of variables in Table 18.1. This was also true for angina pectoris, particularly in the female groups, even when such presumed risk factors as relative weight, cholesterol, triglycerides, daily cigarette consumption, and physical activity were included in the model besides age and sex. However, the score appeared to have no or only negligible associations with the incidence of myocardial

Table 18.4   The association between three Stress Symptoms score levels and chronic illness assessed by the Mantel extension of the Mantel–Haenszel procedure

	b	X^2_1	
Men[1]	0.034	11.79	p<0.001
Women[1]	0.022	2.25	NS
White-collar[2]	0.037	10.39	p<0.001
Blue-collar	0.027	5.64	p<0.02
All[3]	0.029	12.60	p<0.001

Notes:
[1]Standardised by age and occupational class.
[2]Standardised by age and sex.
[3]Standardised by age, sex, and occupational class.
The assignment of the levels of the stress score has been made as follows:
0–4: (Low)=0; 5–10 (Moderate)=1; 11+ (High)=2

infarction and the change in systolic or diastolic blood pressure during the 5-year follow-up (Aro, 1984). Of the various chronic illnesses, the score was strongly associated with musculoskeletal diseases.

Discussion

The multidimensional social and occupational inequality that we have found in the characteristics of the occupational classes of this population, employed by the same industrial enterprise and living in the same geographic region, affords a glimpse into the conditions of the much more heterogeneous social classes in an industrial society, that have been described on a national level (for example, Reid, 1977; Townsend, 1979).

The physical and social inequalities in the living and working conditions of the occupational classes seem to be reflected in the distribution of morbidity between these classes. It would not seem unreasonable to infer that the latter results from the former. Can causal relationships be identified?

Prevailing medical thought considers that a large part of the diseases that constitute our indices of morbidity are of 'multiaetiological' origin. Accordingly, it would be futile to try to pinpoint a single cause for the higher prevalence of a given disease in the lower occupational classes. However, it could be possible, in principle, to prove that specific constellations of several causative factors are affecting the probability of the appearance of specific types of disease. Considering that almost all presumably health-endangering environmental characteristics in living and working conditions seem to accumulate in the lower occupational classes, such an aetiological background would result in the gradient of morbidity by occupational class which was observed for almost all types of disease. This type of aetiological background for the morbidity/mortality gradients by social class, the 'clustering of specific causes' has been considered (Marmot *et al.*, 1984).

The issue becomes more complex, however, if we accept the suggestion that not only can a variety of aetiological factors in different combinations elicit the development of a given disease ('multiaetiology'), but that a given aetiological constellation can also result in quite different disease outcomes in different individuals ('multipathogenecity': METELI, 1977; Parvi, 1977). A disease outcome would thus not only depend on the type of exposure causing it but also, very decisively, on the individual disposition of the exposed subject. We seem to deal with a situation where non-specific or multiple exposures elicit non-specific or multiple outcomes.

The regularities in the distributions of different features of life circumstances between the occupational classes and the correspondence of measures of these features within the classes suggest that they are interrelated in some consistent manner. Some principle seems to impose a regularity into the ensemble of characteristics of life in an occupational class along a general dimension of better/worse conditions. There is a strong impression that we are dealing with separate levels or systems of existence when comparing the occupational classes. The quantitative differences in separate features of the characteristics of the classes build up to qualitatively different entities when considered together. The values of separate variables gain meaning only by being considered in relation to all other variables, and within the context of the total conditions for each class, and the corresponding differences between the classes. There is not much point in trying to quantify the strength of association of single or even multiple indices of the life conditions of the classes with the indices of morbidity. The strong correspondence between the differences in the total characteristics of the living and working conditions of the classes, and the differences in total morbidity, do not appear as associations on the level of individuals, within the occupational classes.

We have tried this with multiple logistic regression models: strong associations between various characteristics of life circumstances and indices of morbidity disappear when occupational class is accounted for. Besides, there are formidable difficulties due to multicollinearity. For example, a scale describing hazardous physical and chemical influences from the work environment correlated with scales describing ergonomic drawbacks ($r = 0.91$), forced pace ($r = 0.57$), troublesome superiors ($r = 0.44$), and uninteresting tasks ($r = 0.54$).

This is not merely a technical difficulty: the clustering of characteristics on the level of individuals is a feature of real life.

I should like to suggest that what we are seeing here are relations within entities and differences between them. The (a) objective conditions, (b) subjective perceptions, (c) cognitions and (d) activities of the people in each occupational class constitute an entity, the properties of which are not reducible to the simple aggregate properties of its constituent parts. On the contrary, the parts acquire their properties from being parts of a given entity. This entity may be called the way-of-life of the occupational class. The differences in morbidity between the occupational classes are ultimately caused by the respective differences between the ways-of-life of these classes.

There is nothing mystical about the notion. It was forcefully put by Durkheim in his concept of a 'social fact' (Durkheim, 1950; see also Kosik, 1976 and Lieberson, 1985). To take a simple example: the fact that there are more cigarette smokers in a lower than a higher social class is not explained by any properties of the individuals in these classes as such. They acquire the property in question by being parts of the ways-of-life of the respective social classes. The risk of starting and continuing to smoke for an individual varies with the way-of-life of which he is a part. This can be studied empirically.

The ways-of-life of the social classes acquire characteristics from being parts of the larger system of the way-of-life of the whole society. Within the ways-of-life of the social classes, on the other hand, distinct sub-systems of the ways-of-life of (for example) occupational groups may be discerned, with characteristics acquired from being parts of the way-of-life of a social class. In modern industrial societies the ways-of-life of the social classes are divided into three interrelated main spheres: those associated with (i) work, (ii) the market and (iii) leisure (see Ottomeyer, 1977). Judging by our results, the white- and blue-collar ways-of-life would seem to differ most markedly in the sphere of work, including education.

The way-of-life is a dynamic structured system within which the interrelated parts and the whole are in continuous interaction with each other. In the evolution of the way-of-life the relations between its parts change perpetually; they are seldom either constant or linear. A change in one part of the system changes the whole, which acts on the other parts, and changes them and their interrelations. Causal associations are multidirectional and reciprocal. As a complex system, the way-of-life acquires, in addition, peculiar properties from its elementary parts being conscious purposeful actors. It follows that many important relations within the way-of-life cannot be characterised quantitatively but require symbolic representations with respect to the concept of meaning (significance).

We assumed that differences in the totalities of ways-of-life between the occupational classes are reflected as differences in the prevalence of the symptoms that form the Stress Symptoms Score. The score would represent a kind of synthesised expression of the intensities of environmental and personal stresses experienced by people. If there was some truth in the stress→susceptibility→disease hypothesis, the score would be a much stronger predictor of disease than any single feature in the living and working conditions of the people in the sample, and even stronger than many of these combined. The idea that differences in morbidity between the social classes might be partly caused by differences in experienced stress would thus be strengthened.

Our results seem, by and large, to lend some credence to these assumptions. The Stress Symptoms Score is clearly, albeit not very strongly, associated with many individual indices of way-of-life, and it is a strong predictor of future chronic illness. The score is also fairly strongly associated with smoking and alcohol consumption which supports the notion that at least some of the unhealthy habits more prevalent in the lower occupational classes may result from exposure to stressful environmental influences. The lack of association of these symptoms with the incidence of myocardial infarction and blood pressure change is somewhat confusing, as these have been considered as especially stress-related. The possible implications of this finding have been analysed elsewhere (Aro, 1981). Briefly, there is the possibility that the symptoms studied by us, whether or not they are symptoms of stress, lead to an increased use of health services and thereby increase the probability of becoming 'labelled' sick.

It must be noted, however, that if my argument about the ways-of-life of the occupational classes having the characteristics of entities is valid, then our analyses in the follow-up of the associations on an individual level between the Stress Symptoms Score and the various indices of morbidity are of limited value in explaining the differences between the classes. A more proper impression of the possible associations may be gained by looking at the distributions at the group level and noting their correspondence.

If the definition of the way-of-life as the totality of objective conditions, subjective perceptions, cognitions, and activities is accepted, it follows that the way-of-life may simultaneously be a cause and a consequence of the stress symptoms and morbidity. Disease is a deformation in the system.

One may, finally, ask in what kind of conceptual framework the causal links between way-of-life and morbidity may be understood. 'Stress' is a rather meagre and unidimensional concept burdened by vague over-use, and of little explanatory power. I have recently suggested that the study of the development and satisfaction of human needs might be helpful in this respect (Hasan, 1987). The suggestion includes the assumption that non-satisfied needs lead to physiological states, activities, and behaviours which increase the probability of disease and death. States of need may be said to increase 'general susceptibility' in more than a merely physiological sense. In the general case, socially determined needs are historically first formed and satisfied in the way-of-life of the highest social class of a socio-economically hierarchically organised society. From there they spread or are imposed downwards along the social hierarchy against a gradient of diminishing resources for their satisfaction. People in each lower class are therefore in a state of increasing (objective) relative deprivation (Townsend, 1979) in regard to those in the higher one(s). This gradient of increasing deprivation from the highest to the lowest class would then be a cause of the gradients in morbidity and mortality. In industrially highly developed societies the processes of development and satisfaction of needs are, of course, more complicated but the gradient of deprivation remains. The gradient of health is thus an inevitable feature of socio-economically stratified societies, although its steepness may vary between societies and historical periods. This conceptual construct seems to be helpful in attempts to understand, for example, British data on mortality experience by class. It might also serve as a base for a general theory of premature disease and death.

Acknowledgements

I have gleaned much of the data in Tables 18.2 –18.3 from the doctoral theses of Vesa Parvi (1977) and Seppo Aro (1981). Many people have worked in this research programme through the years, especially my associate, Professor Juhani Kirjonen.

References

Aro, S. (1981), 'Stress, morbidity, and health-related behaviour,' *Scandinavian Journal of Social Medicine*, Suppl. 25.

Aro, S. (1984), 'Occupational stress, health related behaviour, and blood pressure: a 5-year follow-up', *Prev Med* 13, pp. 333–48.

Aro, S., Räsänen, L. and Telama, R. (1986), 'Social class and changes in health-related habits in Finland in 1973–1983', *Scandinavian Journal of Social Medicine* 14, pp. 39–47.

Aunola, S., Nykyri, R. and Rusko, H. (1978), 'Strain of employees in the machine industry in Finland', *Ergonomics* 21, pp. 509–20

Cassel, J. (1976), 'The contribution of the social environment to host resistance'. *American Journal of Epidemiology*, 104, pp. 107–23.

DHSS, (1980), *Inequalities in Health*, Report of a research working group, London.

Durkheim, E. (1950 originally published in 1895), *The Rules of Sociological Method*, Glencoe: The Free Press.

Hasan, J. (1987), 'On the explanation of the differences in morbidity and mortality between the social classes – a conceptual framework for research', Abstract 107, XI

Scientific Meeting of the International Epidemiological Association 8–13. August, Helsinki, Finland.

Kosik, K. (1976), *Dialectics of the Concrete. A Study on Problems of Man and World*, Dordrecht: Kluwer.

Lieberson, S. (1985), *Making It Count*, University of California Press.

Manninen, O. (1977), *Environmental factors and employees' discomfort in three machine industry plants*, Finland: University of Tampere.

Marmot, M. G., Shipley, M. J., Rose, G. (1984), 'Inequalities in death – specific explanations of a general pattern?' *Lancet* i, pp. 1003–6.

METELI (Study Programme) (1975), *The Health Examination: Sampling, Methods, and Implementation (Terveystutkimus: otanta, mentelmät ja toteuttaminen. Jyväskylä).*

METELI (Study Programme) (1977), *Occupational Class, Working Conditions, and Morbidity Among Employees in the Engineering Industry (Ammattiasema, työolot ja sairastavuus metalliteollisuuden henkilöstöryhmissä. Jyvaskyla).*

Ottomeyer, K. (1977), *Ökonomische Zwänge und Menschliche Beziehungen*, Hamburg: Rowohlt.

Parvi, V. (1977), *Occupational Status, Working Conditions and Morbidity Among Employees in the Engineering Industry*, ser, A, 90, Acta Universitatis Tamperensis.

Reid, I. (1977), *Social Class Differences in Britain*, London: Open Books.

Syme, S. L., and Berkman, L. F. (1976), 'Social class, susceptibility and sickness', *American Journal of Epidemiology*, **104**, pp. 1–8.

Townsend, P. (1979), *Poverty in the United Kingdom*, Harmondsworth: Penguin Books.

19 Social inequalities in health: a complementary perspective
Aaron Antonovsky

Formulation of the question
We are all terminal cases. In this sense, there is no social inequality. The problems – moral, social and scientific – arise out of the observations that some, by no means a random sample, die before others, and/or, before death, suffer more often and/or more painfully from a wide variety of conditions to which the human organism is prone. This is overwhelmingly the way the problem is stated. The question asked shapes the search for etiological understanding.

But note that our workshops are not called 'Social Inequalities in Morbidity, Mortality and Inadequacies in Health Care'; nor are we alone in being euphemistic. *The Black Report* (Townsend and Davidson, 1982) preceded us. I have taken part in two UN–WHO expert groups, respectively referred to as 'The Meeting on Socio-Economic Determinants and Consequences of Mortality' and 'Mortality and Health Policy' – not longevity, not life expectancy.

Had we taken as our text Orwell's 'some are more equal than others', not 'some are less equal than others', our title would be more justified. Now, is all this semantics? The first of my two theses consists of a very urgent negative reply. I shall argue that, if we are to take our adopted title seriously, our deliberations and conclusions would be seriously affected. I do not wish to be misunderstood. Both the title we have taken and the one we have not, lead to errors of omission, not of commission. Or, to put it another way, we need both titles. (I could make the same point about the choice of 'inequalities' or 'equalities', but this will be left to the reader's imagination.)

One of the things we all share is that we like data as well as ideas. Let me, then, start with a few numbers. In 1982, the infant mortality rate per thousand live births in Israeli kibbutzim and moshavim was 5.4 (in over 6,000 live births), compared to the national rate among Jews of 11.6 (Israel Central Bureau of Statistics, 1985, 99). Kibbutz life expectancy at birth (1977) of males was 74.5 years (Leviatan and Cohen, 1985), compared to 72.7 in Japan (UN, 1982, p. 9), which ranked first in the world. Here is a sizeable population (115,000), engaged largely in hard physical labour, with machinery and chemicals, the males subject to military reserve duty till age 55, where smoking is widespread and diet is affluent – with a relatively remarkable health achievement. Or, to take a different statistic, which has been found to be a powerful predictor of survival of the elderly (Mossey and Shapiro, 1982), self-assessment of health. In 1982, 50.3 per cent of Americans 65 and over with a family income of $35,000 or more reported their health to be excellent or very good, compared to 28.9 per cent of those with an income of under $10,000 (US Center for Health Statistics, 1985, p. 108).

I cite these figures as a way of introducing my first thesis, namely: adoption of a salutogenic orientation is an essential step if we are to advance understanding of health inequalities and propose policies designed to increase equality in health. Ever since my first publication in this field almost two decades ago (Antonovsky, 1967), I have made a modest contribution to the pathogenic literature – i.e., to those studies aimed at demonstrating and explaining the causal relationship between location in the lower reaches of the social structure of a society and being sick, suffering and dying prematurely, as well as being disadvantaged in the use of health services. The dominant theme in this very considerable literature is that the health risk factors characterising the lives of the lower social classes are far greater than those found in the lives of the higher social classes. The former, far more than the latter, are exposed to pollution, hazardous work, overwork, damp housing, unemployment, psychosocial stressors, etc. When cultural–behavioural factors are cited, such as drugs, alcohol, smoking and poor diet, whether or not they are linked to the social structure, they too are seen as risk factors. *Lack* of exercise, *lack* of prenatal care, *lack* of access to health services – these are always what is emphasised. With regard to such psychosocial factors as alienation and powerlessness or social isolation, it is again the risk factor which is central. Of course data on the higher social classes are cited, but these are only given to point up the data on the lower social classes. Or, looking at another inequality, Waldron's (1976) paper, despite its title, is really about why men live shorter lives than women.

Again, I do not wish in the slightest to dispute the importance of a full identification and understanding of risk factors. My argument is, rather, that this pathogenic approach must be complemented by what I have proposed be called a salutogenic approach: identification and understanding of, first, protective factors, and, second, health-promoting factors. I have elsewhere (Antonovsky, 1984) analysed in detail the implications of this concept. Here I would consider it in terms of our present concern. Does it really make a difference if we think in terms of why some are *more* equal than others?

Implications of the salutogenic approach

The first reason, and perhaps the most underlying one, is in the realm of values and emotions. If we concentrate on the data of what in any given historical time *has been achieved*, such as the kibbutz data cited above, those of us still young enough in spirit to respond to unfairness in life without being Utopian will be aroused. If five out of a thousand kibbutz babies die in their first year, then there is no moral reason on earth to justify the fact that, among neighbouring Bedouin, 23 babies die. The psychological focusing on five, I propose, is more powerful in arousing emotion than when we think of 23. It alerts us to what can be achieved.

Second, the prevailing focus on risk factors expresses a philosophic assumption that, if only they could be got rid of, all would be well in the world. It is a contemporary version of a Rousseauean noble savage view of the world, one which maintains that the human organism is fundamentally healthy unless attacked by evil bugs, spirits or social conditions. The tragic view of the human condition is obliterated, with a few minor exceptions like congenital anomalies. (For very serious proponents of this view, see McKeown, 1979 and Fries and Crapo, 1981.) Unfortunately, there is very good evidence that the nature of human existence, both in terms of the inherent character of the organism and of the dynamics of physical and social environments, is such that risk factors will always be with us. A philosophical premise which sees perpetual health as almost just around the corner, if only we get rid of the current risk factors, is most shaky. It disregards AIDS and the Chernobyl explosion, and prevents exploitation of the concepts of adaptability (Dubos, 1959). It explains the preoccupation for the better part of two decades with life events research, as if it is high scoring which is decisive in producing illness.

Third, moving from the moral and philosophical levels to the level of research and action, a pathogenic approach generates hypotheses and programmes related to risk factors. It leads to concentration on the defects and dangers and inadequacies characterising the lives of those who are less equal, to wars on risk factors. In an era of poor sanitation, inadequate nutrition, terrible housing and the like, these were surely the burning issues. And for all too many, even in the industrialised world, they remain such. But in an era in which chronic diseases pose the dominant challenge, the search for understanding and controlling specific risk factors becomes relatively less important and less adequate for health promotion. It is this premise that led me (Antonovsky, 1972) to propose the concept of generalised resistance resources – i.e., a characteristic of any system, from the cellular to the societal levels, which is effective in combating a wide variety of threats (Antonovsky, 1979, p. 103), and hence in promoting health. In the past decade or so, the one type of resistance resource which has received a good deal of attention is social support, a concept which is only beginning to overcome theoretical and methodological inadequacy. At the same time, the exciting new field of psychoneuroimmunology (see Borysenko, 1984) has emerged. Unfortunately, the latter is largely alien to social scientists.

I am, then, proposing that a salutogenic orientation, a search for hypotheses about factors which not only inhibit disease but which promote health, is an essential tool in studying equalities in health. It would lead, in addition to studying why lower classes are sicker, to asking why the higher classes are healthier. The answers to the two questions are related, but different, and until we begin to ask the second question, we will be at a loss in fully tackling the issue of inequalities. Why do kibbutzim have such a low infant mortality rate? Why does Japan have such a low rate of cardiovascular disease mortality? Why are women healthier than men? Why do Mormons and Seventh Day Adventists have such superb health records? I suggest that it is not only because they are low on risk factors, but because they are also higher on protective or salutary factors. What these are is a question which has hardly begun to be asked.

Finally, I would suggest that our knowledge and understanding are inhibited when we limit our perspective and research efforts to establishing statistically significant differences on indicators of health and illness, or on risk factors, thereby ignoring the deviant case. Not all miners or poor people or elderly or Finns are sick or die prematurely, though the morbidity and mortality rates of these groups are higher than those of comparison groups. In fact, some of them are in splendid health and live long lives. Why? Thus, for example, the most striking datum for me in Lynge *et al.* (Chapter 8) is: 'The Finnish teachers only have a small excess mortality in comparison to male teachers in the other (Nordic) countries.' Why is this the case, when we know that overall, Finns have higher mortality rates? We generally do not study or even reflect on the deviant case, resting content with knowing that p is beyond the 0.01 level.

A tentative answer to the salutogenic question
I turn now to the presentation of my second thesis, which relates to a proposed answer to the salutogenic question. This will be done in two stages: a discussion of generalised resistance resources (GRRs), and second, consideration of the sense of coherence (SOC) concept. I propose that one crucial reason for some being more equal than others is that they have a stronger SOC: upper classes more than lower; Swedes more than Finns; whites more than blacks. (I confess that gender differences, both on health indicators and on the SOC, are too

complex to allow, at this stage, a simple comparison.)

For those of us who have worked on social class differences in health (or, rather, morbidity and mortality), and have not been content simply with descriptive epidemiology, class was always regarded as a zeroing-in variable. It was the 'What is it about social class?' that presented the real problem. But we always, from Booth to Black, focused on 'What is it about the poor?' Suppose we turn to 'What is it about the well-to-do that makes them healthier?' Many answers come to mind readily. First and foremost, they have more money, and money can buy goods and services that are good for the health. (I say this in full awareness of the dangers of an affluent diet.) Second, they probably have a healthier genetic endowment. Third, they have easier access to the best of health care available, and once in the medical care system, know their way around. Fourth, they are better educated and more literate, thus more able to exploit available health knowledge. Fifth, they have better police and fire protection. Less certainly, but plausibly, they may have more adequate social supports. Nor would it be irrelevant to speak of the health-enchancing consequences of prestige, deference and power in social relations.

In sum, I am proposing that the higher social classes have better health records than the lower social classes *both* because they are less subject to risk factors and because their lives are more often characterised by salutary factors. We know little about the latter because we have seldom designed our research in salutogenic terms. But a word must be said about the 'less subject to risk factors'. There is little doubt in my mind that this is by and large true. But the difference is not absolute. The direct class gradient on breast cancer and the seeming backward J-curve on coronary disease suggest that at least in some areas, matters are not so simple. Freedom to sleep under bridges or in the street, damp housing and not enough calories may be the 'prerogatives' solely of the poor, and occupational safety hazards and unemployment far more often confront manual workers than white-collar workers. But this is not to say that the well-to-do are not subject to living in polluted cities, psychosocial stressors at work, or the malnutrition of an affluent diet. They may be less so than others, but are not free of these risk factors. Moreover, the existential stressors of human existence are far from absent in anyone's life. The reader of this chapter is not likely to live in damp and cold housing or work in a physically dangerous place. But he or she surely knows what it is like to have an ageing parent with Alzheimer's disease, to live in an unhappy marriage, to have a Down's Syndrome child, to work in a driving competitive setting, and so on.

All of us, then, as human beings and as occupants of given locations in a social structure and culture, are subject to risk factors. Some, more than others, but none is free of them. Differential risk factor levels, particularly when combinations are taken into account (as they often are not, a point made by Blane, 1985, p. 438), make a major contribution to understanding inequalities in morbidity and mortality. But they do not bring us close enough to understanding the processes involved, not only because they lead us to forget about salutary factors, but also because, in this mode of thinking, we tend to forget that it is an *individual* human being who stays more or less healthy, who gets sick and who dies.

I do not wish to fall into the trap, as have so many of our colleagues who work in the field of what has come to be called behavioural medicine, of ignoring social epidemiology, of blaming the victim, of disregarding the structural–cultural sources of inequalities in health, and I will return to this issue. But the problem I would pose at this point is: how can we understand the fact that some individuals stay healthy or recover from illness, despite the high risk factor load inevitable in human existence, or the very high risk factor load confronted by some because of their positions in the social structure (or, sometimes, because of chance)?

To concretise what I mean, let me call your attention to one of the very few empirical studies I know which confronted this question (Werner and Smith, 1982). In 1955, Emmy Werner, an American developmental psychologist, initiated a 17-year study of all children born that year in the poorest of the Hawaiian Islands, Kauai. Werner's two earlier books had focused on the catalogue of distress, including physical illness, and its correlates. I cannot resist quoting from the introduction (p. 3) of the 1982 volume:

> Yet there were others, also *vulnerable* – exposed to poverty, biological risks, and family instability, and reared by parents with little education or serious mental health problems – who remained *invincible* and developed into competent and autonomous young adults . . . This report is an account of our search for the roots of their resilience, for the sources of their strength.

Posing the question in this way brings me back to the concept of GRRs. I can now state my tentative answer to the salutogenic question as follows. Those who are more equal than others are relatively successful in health matters in good part because they have managed to acquire a repertoire of GRRs which allows them to cope successfully with the risk factors in their lives. This is true, I suggest, on the group level (e.g., of social classes) and on the individual level (e.g., of those among the poor who do well in health terms).

Genetic and constitutional GRRs surely are relevant, but they are beyond my sphere of competence. In the course of my own work, as well as through familiarity with the literature, I was able to identify a number of phenomena which the data indicated served as GRRs. Thus, for example, in studying the adaptation of women in different ethnic groups, ranging from traditional to modern, to the variety of stressors in mid-life (Datan, Antonovsky and Maoz, 1981), our most fascinating finding was contrary to our alternative hypotheses. We had good reasons for expecting a direct relationship between the degree of modernity and adaptation (including physical health); we had equally good reasons for expecting an inverse relationship. But what we found was a J-curve: the most modern women (middle-class, Jewish, urban Israeli women born in central Europe) were best off; next best were the Israeli Arab village women. The worst off were those in cultural transition, those no longer traditional and not yet modern. Cultural stability, then, seemed to be a GRR.

The literature on social supports, despite all its theoretical and methodological problems, suggested that embeddedness in certain kinds of social networks served as a GRR. Brown's concept of a confidante (Brown and Harris, 1978) seemed relevant. One could go on (and I do so in detail in Antonovsky, 1979, Chapter 4). But I was left not only with the scientific demand for parsimony, but, more important, with the nagging sense that I had no culling rule to determine what was a GRR or, to put it another way, I did not understand *how* GRRs work in coping successfully with risk factors. The struggle with this problem led me, eventually, to the formulation of the sense of coherence concept, orginally presented in my 1979 book and carried much further in my new book (Antonovsky, 1987).

The sense of coherence

Perhaps the most precise stimulus to the development of the SOC concept came from reading Cassel's words (Cassel, 1977, 133). 'In human populations, increased susceptibility to disease should occur when, for a variety of reasons, individuals do not receive any evidence that their actions are leading to desirable and anticipated consequences.' It would take us too far afield to trace how, fascinated by systems theory and being salutogenically oriented, I found the concept of negative entropy useful, and came to a preliminary definition of a strong SOC as a way of looking at the world which allows one to make sense of the stimuli which constantly bombard one.

What the possession of GRRs does, what is common to them, is that they lead, over and over again, to a specifiable pattern of life experiences which I described as characterised by consistency, optimal balance of demands and available resources, and participation in decision-making in socially-valued activities. Those who repeatedly have such life experiences come to have a strong SOC. The SOC, as I now formally define it is (Antonovsky, 1987):

. . . a global orientation that expresses the extent to which one has a pervasive, enduring though dynamic feeling of confidence that (1) the stimuli deriving from one's internal and external environments in the course of living are structured, predictable and explicable; (2) the resources are available to one to meet the demands posed by these stimuli; and (3) these demands are challenges, worthy of investment and engagement.

The indicated three components of the SOC are called 'comprehensibility, manageability and meaningfulness'.*

For a preliminary sense of what I mean by the SOC, think of the British upper class in the pre- First World War era or, by contrast, of the Mexican poor living in a culture of poverty (which Lewis (1979) carefully distinguished from poverty *per se*). Or, to quote from Werner's (1982) study of the vulnerable but invincible youth, in which she identified 'a sense of coherence in their lives' (p. 154): 'There was structure and rules in the household, but space to explore in . . . an informal, multi-age network of kin, peers, and elders who shared similar values and beliefs, and from whom the resilient youth sought counsel and support . . . ' (p. 156).

Let me take a concrete example of how I think a person with a strong SOC, with a patterned expectation that the world can be made sense of, that resources can be mobilised, and that demands are challenges, may behave confronting a serious life stressor and, in behaving so, is more likely to maintain health than one with a weak SOC in the same stressor situation. A 40-year old steel worker is informed that his plant is to close and he is to lose his job. Endless negotiations to prevent the closing have proven fruitless. (Of course it would be more desirable were he living in a society in which plant closing was avoided or, if unavoidable, another job or paid retraining were immediately available. But this is all too often not the reality.) He speaks up at the union meeting, insisting that very careful track be kept of any attempt on the company's part to appropriate any or all of the severance pay, pension benefits or vacation and sick leave rights; he makes it clear that neither he nor his workmates, but rather incompetent management or general social conditions are to blame for the plant's failure; he examines the family budget, calculating what cuts can be made and how long savings might last; he discusses with his wife, who till now has preferred to stay home, whether she should look for a job and how the kids can pitch in; he re-examines whether this is not a good chance for a career shift and skill retraining; he does some of the things he'd wanted to do for a long time, without interfering with job hunting, now that some leisure time can be

*A feasible, reliable and seemingly valid 29-item scale to measure the SOC has been developed and appears in the Appendix of Antonovsky (1987).

anticipated; he contacts his uncle or an old army buddy for job leads; he rejoins the church choir and sings to let the pain ease; and he looks and looks not only for another job, but for one that might be more rewarding, for he is aware that he will be working for the next 25 years. I trust that in this example I have made it clear that having a strong SOC is not a passive adjustment to reality, but an active, creative way of coping in the real world.

There are no guarantees in life. But there are at least better chances for remaining healthy than if one begins to blame oneself, nag at the wife and kids, and drink heavily.

Conclusion

What I have done in this chapter is (1) present a different way of looking at the problem of social inequalities in health, which I call asking the salutogenic question; and (2) propose a parsimonious answer to this question, the sense of coherence. I have proposed that the SOC is a decisive variable in shaping the growth, reinforcement and maintenance of the human capital which determines the health fates of people. Two issues remain to be discussed briefly, before hinting at policy implications.

The SOC answer constitutes, at this stage, a hypothesis to be tested. It is, I believe, consistent with a great variety of data from both large-scale epidemiological and small-scale studies. The four preliminary studies which to date have been conducted, though not yet published, not only show that the instrument used to measure the SOC is reasonably good, but also support the hypothesis. Yet far more work must be done before I can be confident that I am on the right track of explaining why some are more equal than others. One suggestion is that the data prepared for this volume be examined with an eye toward testing the hypothesis, at least on the speculative level. In this respect, a piquant note; on the same day that I read Lynge's workshop paper (Lynge *et al.*), which reported that 'The Norwegian females are the most advantaged within the Nordic countries . . .', my newspaper carried a picture of the women in the new Norwegian Cabinet: 8 out of 18, including the Prime Minister. Might there not be a connection between the SOC of Norwegian women and the ambience of a society which gives women such political power? Of course, life expectancy is only one indicator of health. Full testing of the hypothesis would require better measures of health than our presently-available disease morbidity and mortality indicators.

Second, let us assume that the SOC hypothesis points in the right direction. We are then confronted with the question of the sources of a strong SOC. I have devoted a lengthy chapter to this question, in the context of a life cycle approach, in my new book (Antonovsky, 1987).

Above, I stated that it is individuals who become sicker and healthier. Here I would reiterate full awareness of the dangers of psychological reductionism. In proposing an individual dispositional orientation as a decisive factor in determining health status, I do not in the least wish to imply that such orientations can be abstracted from the social structures, historical contexts and cultures into which one is born and in which one grows up, works, relates to others, and lives out one's life. There is no contradiction between my own work and that of others on social class, and my present approach. The fact that one is born male in a professional family in Sweden, which has known no wars for many years, or born female to an unmarried adolescent mother in a Johannesburg African slum, with the respective relatively predictable life histories, is decisive in shaping the SOC.

Our series of Workshops, though conducted in scientific terms, was designed to suggest, to the extent possible, policy implications, in the hope that we would thereby be making a contribution to furthering health equalities. I submit that the approach I have presented in this paper is fully congruent with and may even underlie Illsley's (1986) thesis, which has generated considerable dispute. (For serious criticism of Illsley's thesis, see Pamuk, 1985.) In population and human terms, I understand Illsley to be saying, there has been a very considerable decrease in inequality in Britain in the last three decades, even if the data show unchanging differences between Classes I and V, for the simple reason that far many more human beings are now in the higher classes and far fewer in Class V. In my terms, what this means is that far fewer people are subject to the social conditions which vitiate the SOC, and far many more have been able to develop a strong SOC. It follows, then, that changing the population distribution in the class structure is a profound way to modify the SOC in the desirable direction. I am aware that this policy proposal is easily derivable without any thought of the SOC hypothesis. But what this hypothesis does is to explain *why* such a change will make a difference in the health of a population.

In similar fashion, one can formulate policies which are consciously designed to modify the strength of the SOC of those social groups which are disadvantaged. Reference can be made to many areas of life: trade union organisation, worker participation in management, the reorganisation of work life, the increasing participation of women in the labour force (though only under certain conditions which make paid work more meaningful than housework), recognition of the social value of the housewife role by the tax structure, and so on.

I would, however, end with one caveat. I have addressed myself to health as an outcome variable. But there are many cultural roads to a strong SOC. There are many concrete ways of living in which it can be expressed. There is a danger of identifying what is good for the health with what, in one's eyes, is good. But this is not at all necessarily the case. As I pointed out above, members of the pre- First World War British aristocracy, or Mormons, are very likely to be characterised by a strong SOC, and hence they should be relatively healthy. But this does not mean that one must be enamoured of the raj or of religion. The same is the case for a good member of 'the' party. The criteria for advocating a given social policy cannot be solely in terms of what is good for the health, but must also consider other values. Unfortunately, these do not always mesh smoothly.

References

Antonovsky, A. (1967), 'Social class, life expectancy and overall mortality', *Milbank Memorial Fund Quarterly*, **43** pp. 31–73.

Antonovsky, A. (1972), 'Breakdown: A needed fourth step in the conceptual armamentarium of modern medicine', *Social Science and Medicine*, **6**, pp. 537–44.

Antonovsky, A. (1979), *Health, Stress and Coping*, San Francisco: Jossey-Bass.

Antonovsky, A. (1984), 'The sense of coherence as a determinant of health' in J. D. Matarazzo *et al.* (eds), *Behavioral Health*, New York: Wiley, pp. 114–29.

Antonovsky, A. (1987), *Unravelling the Mystery of Health*, San Francisco: Jossey-Bass.

Blane, D. (1985), 'An assessment of the *Black Report's* explanation of health inequalities', *Sociology of Health and Illness*, **7** (3) pp. 423–45.

Borysenko, J. (1984), 'Stress, coping, and the immune system' in J. D. Matarazzo *et al.* (eds), *Behavioral Health*, New York: Wiley, pp. 248–60.

Brown, G. W. and Harris, T. (1978), *Social Origins of Depression*. London: Tavistock.

Cassel, J. (1977), 'The relation of the urban environment in health: toward a conceptual frame and a research strategy' in L. E. Hinkle Jr. and W. C. Loring (eds), *The Effect of the Man-Made Environment on Health and Behavior*, Atlanta: Center for Disease Control, Public Health Service.

Datan, N., Antonovsky, A. and Maoz, B. (1981), *A Time to Reap: The Middle Age of Women in Five Israeli Subcultures*, Baltimore: Johns Hopkins Press.

Dubos, R. (1959), *Mirage of Health*, New York: Doubleday.

Fries, J. F. and Crapo, L. M. (1981), *Vitality and Ageing*, San Francisco: Freeman.

Illsley, R. (1986), 'Occupational class, selection and the production of inequalities in health', *Quarterly Journal of Social Affairs*, **2**.2, 151–65.

Israel Central Bureau of Statistics (1985), *Statistical Abstract of Israel, 1984*, no. 35. Jerusalem: Central Bureau of Statistics.

Leviatan, U. and Cohen, J. (1985), 'Gender differences in life expectancy among Kibbutz members', *Social Science and Medicine*, **21** (5), pp. 545–52.

Lewis, O. (1979), 'The culture of poverty', *Anthropological Essays*, New York: Random.

McKeown, T. (1979), *The Role of Medicine* (revised edn), Princeton: Princeton University Press.

Mossey, J. M. and Shapiro, E. (1982), 'Self-rated health: a predictor of mortality among the elderly', *American Journal of Public Health*, **72** (8) pp. 800–8.

Pamuk, E. R. (1985), 'Social class inequality in mortality from 1921 to 1972 in England and Wales', *Population Studies*, **39** pp. 17–31.

Townsend, P. and Davidson, N. (eds) (1982), *Inequalities in Health: The Black Report*, Harmondsworth: Penguin.

United Nations (1982), *Levels and Trends of Mortality Since 1950*, New York: Department of International Economic and Social Affairs, 9, (ST/ESA/SER.A/74).

US National Center for Health Statistic (1985), *Current Estimates from the National*

Health Interview Survey, Series 10, no. 150, Washington: Public Health Service, 108.

Waldron, I. (1976), 'Why do women live longer than men?', *Journal of Human Stress*, **2** (1) pp. 2–13.

Werner E. E. and Smith R. S. (1982), *Vulnerable but Invincible: A Study of Resilient Children*, New York: McGraw-Hill.

Index